The GLMA Handbook on LGBT Health

The GLMA Handbook on LGBT Health

Volume 1: Societal Issues and
Health Promotion

Jason S. Schneider, MD,
Vincent M. B. Silenzio, MD, MPH, and
Laura Erickson-Schroth, MD, MA, Editors

Foreword by Hector Vargas, JD

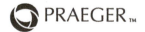 PRAEGER™

An Imprint of ABC-CLIO, LLC
Santa Barbara, California • Denver, Colorado

Library of Congress Cataloging-in-Publication Data

Names: Schneider, Jason S., editor. | Silenzio, Vincent M. B., editor. |
  Erickson-Schroth, Laura, editor.
Title: The GLMA handbook on LGBT health / Jason S. Schneider, Vincent M.B.
  Silenzio, and Laura Erickson-Schroth, editors ; foreword by Hector Vargas.
Other titles: Gay and Lesbian Medical Association handbook on LGBT health |
  Handbook on LGBT health
Description: Santa Barbara, California : ABC-CLIO, [2019] | Includes
  bibliographical references and index.
Identifiers: LCCN 2018043350 (print) | LCCN 2018044309 (ebook) | ISBN
  9780313395666 (eBook) | ISBN 9780313395659 (set : alk. paper) | ISBN
  9781440846847 (volume 1 : alk. paper) | ISBN 9781440846854 (volume 2 :
  alk. paper)
Subjects: | MESH: Sexual and Gender Minorities | Health Status | Health
  Services | Health Policy | United States
Classification: LCC RA564.9.H65 (ebook) | LCC RA564.9.H65 (print) | NLM WA
  300 AA1 | DDC 362.1086/64—dc23
LC record available at https://lccn.loc.gov/2018043350

ISBN: 978-0-313-39565-9 (set)
        978-1-4408-4684-7 (vol. 1)
        978-1-4408-4685-4 (vol. 2)
        978-0-313-39566-6 (ebook)

23 22 21 20 19   2 3 4 5

This book is also available as an eBook.

Praeger
An Imprint of ABC-CLIO, LLC

ABC-CLIO, LLC
147 Castilian Drive
Santa Barbara, California 93117
www.abc-clio.com

This book is printed on acid-free paper ∞

Manufactured in the United States of America

Contents

Foreword by Hector Vargas vii

Acknowledgments xi

CHAPTER 1
The Politics of LGBT Health *1*
Kellan E. Baker

CHAPTER 2
Interactions between Culture, Race, and Sexuality
in Health *39*
David J. Malebranche and LaRon E. Nelson

CHAPTER 3
Lesbian, Gay, Bisexual, and Transgender Public Health
and Epidemiology *61*
Randall Sell

CHAPTER 4
Transgender Medical Care in the United States:
A Historical Perspective *83*
*Madeline B. Deutsch, Marci L. Bowers, Asa Radix,
and Tamar C. Carmel*

CHAPTER 5
Exploring the Health Issues of LGBT Adolescents *133*
Travis A. Gayles and Robert Garofalo

CHAPTER 6
The Health of LGBT Elders *155*
W. Christopher Skidmore, Mark J. Simone, Manuel A.
Eskildsen, David O. Staats, and Jonathan S. Appelbaum

CHAPTER 7
Lesbian, Gay, Bisexual, and Transgender Parents *185*
Megan C. Lytle

CHAPTER 8
Preventive Health for Gay, Bisexual, and Queer Men *203*
Russell G. Buhr and Tri D. Do

CHAPTER 9
Sexual Health for Women *229*
Tonia Poteat, Dawn Harbatkin, and Alexis D. Light

CHAPTER 10
Sexual Health for Men *265*
Laura Erickson-Schroth, Richard E. Greene, and David Hankins

About the Editors and Contributors 295

Index 301

Foreword

When I joined GLMA: Health Professionals Advancing LGBTQ Equality as its executive director in 2010 (then known as the Gay and Lesbian Medical Association), the nation was on the cusp of very profound changes in how it would view and treat lesbian, gay, bisexual, and transgender (LGBT) people. "LGBT American" became part of the common dialogue. Same-sex couples would soon have the freedom to marry in every state, and the White House was lit in rainbow colors. We witnessed heightened awareness and understanding about transgender individuals and the pervasive challenges they face.

This revolution cascaded into all aspects of LGBTQ life, and LGBT health was no exception. Leading health care institutions and associations—including the National Academy of Medicine, Joint Commission, American Medical Association, and American Academy of Nursing, just to name a few—studied and adopted policies addressing the health and well-being of LGBT individuals. Health professional students of all disciplines demanded their schools provide more opportunities to learn about LGBT health. The federal government implemented initiatives ensuring LGBT inclusion in health and human services programs and funding opportunities, research and data collection, and nondiscrimination policies.

As I write this foreword today, however, we live in a dramatically changed political environment. So much of the progress we have experienced in LGBT equality and health has been stymied, and we are seeing formidable attempts to erode the gains we have made, particularly in areas such as nondiscrimination in health care access and coverage and inclusion of LGBT people in national health surveys. Like other civil rights movements, we are encountering an almost inevitable deceleration after a period of significant advances.

Through its nearly 40-year history, GLMA has endured many such peaks and valleys, but our role has remained constant: to engage the scientific expertise of our LGBTQ health professional members—physicians, nurses, advanced practice nurses, physician assistants, behavioral health specialists, dentists, and many others—in education and policy initiatives to improve the health and well-being of LGBTQ people. From the organization's roots focusing nationally on services and policy for people dying of AIDS to our present-day efforts to help organize mainstream health professional associations in support of policies promoting the health of LGBTQ people, GLMA has been at the forefront of efforts to advance LGBT equality and health equity nationwide.

It is with this history and spirit that GLMA and its members are proud to offer this resource, *The GLMA Handbook on LGBT Health*. Written by LGBT health care providers who provide care for LGBT patients and clients on a daily basis, the *Handbook* is purposefully crafted for members of the general public, including LGBT people, to bring the full scope of LGBT health concerns and prevention and treatment options into two volumes in plain, easy-to-grasp language. The *Handbook* also examines related public policy, political and resource/funding issues, and their impact on the health of LGBT people.

The *Handbook* covers a broad range of topics important to the health of LGBT people. Volume One begins with an essential grounding in LGBT health by delving into the public policy landscape and public health and research considerations for the LGBT community. You will also find chapters dedicated to preventive health and sexual health as well as to specific populations, including elders, families, youth, and transgender individuals. The intersections of race and sexuality and LGBT health worldwide are also explored. Volume One also probes a topic on the minds of all LGBT people, and that is fundamental to ensuring our health and well-being—finding health care providers who are welcoming of LGBT people. Volume Two looks at specific diseases, conditions, and interventions, including mental health concerns, eating disorders, substance use, cancer, sexually transmitted infections, intimate partner violence, and cardiovascular health.

The *Handbook*'s exploration of the interrelated connection between LGBT health and policy is imperative to understanding the issues of equality and dignity that the LGBT community continues to face. One cannot fully understand the policy importance of ensuring transgender people have access to basic human services, including bathrooms consistent with their gender identity, without understanding the serious physical and mental health implications of denying such access. Learning about the advances in HIV prevention and treatment is key to the efforts to reform laws that criminalize the transmission of HIV, many of which were adopted in the early days of the AIDS epidemic when so little was known about the virus. The sobering statistics on bisexual people and suicide point to the urgent need for client-centered services for this overlooked and extremely marginalized population within the LGBT community (Pompili, et al., 2014).

Equipped with this knowledge, LGBT people can be empowered in their interactions with health care providers, and everyone can be an advocate for LGBT health and equality. The *Handbook* shows that you do not need a medical, nursing, or other specialized degree to be an agent for change—just a willingness to learn and a commitment to put knowledge into action.

I would like to take this opportunity to express my deep appreciation to the editors—GLMA past president Jason Schneider, past board member Laura Erickson-Schroth, and member and former coeditor of the *Journal of the Gay and Lesbian Medical Association* Vincent Silenzio—for their tireless efforts on this publication. And my sincerest thank-you to the many GLMA members and supporters who volunteered to share their expertise as contributors to the *Handbook*. Your passion and dedication to your work is an inspiration to me and the entire LGBT health community.

I would also like to take a moment to honor the memory of Judy Bradford, a pioneer in LGBT health, whom we lost in 2017. She was the original author of this foreword. Judy's spirit permeates the chapters in the *Handbook*, and there is not one subject covered here that does not owe some gratitude to Judy's impressive body of work. Her optimism and vision as an LGBT health leader laid the groundwork for all that we have accomplished and will accomplish in the years ahead.

Like so many GLMA members through the years, Judy dedicated her professional life to improving the health and well-being of the LGBT community. She envisioned a world where the health needs of the LGBT community are fully integrated into policy discussions, training and education of health care professionals, research efforts, and, of course, in provider interactions with LGBT patients and clients.

The GLMA Handbook on LGBT Health is firmly behind this vision, offering central building blocks of information that lead us there. The *Handbook* is geared to action, so whether you are a part of the LGBTQ community or an ally, I hope you will join GLMA members and all supporters of LGBT health equity to do your part to support education, training, and policies to ensure that LGBT people receive the clinically and culturally competent care we need and deserve. Our health depends on it.

Hector Vargas, JD, Executive Director
GLMA: Health Professionals Advancing LGBTQ Equality

REFERENCE

Pompili, M., Lester, D., Forte, A., Seretti, M. E., Erbuto, D., Lamis, D. A., . . .
    Girardi, P. (2014). Bisexuality and suicide: A systematic review of the cur-
    rent literature. *Journal of Sexual Medicine*, *11*(8), 1903–1913. doi:10.1111
    /jsm.12581

Acknowledgments

The editors would like to particularly recognize the esteemed group of experts and scholars who gathered to complete this endeavor. Without the tireless dedication and patience of our contributors, the GLMA Handbook would not have come to fruition. Anna Artymowicz and Shea Nagle, both students at the University of Rochester School of Medicine and Dentistry, deserve special recognition for their heroic editorial assistance with several chapters. Finally, we owe significant thanks to Debbie Carvalko from ABC-CLIO for supporting this project throughout its extended timeline. Without her dedication and behind-the-scenes support, this publication would never have happened.

The chapters herein reflect the collective contributions of generations of health care professionals, scientists, public health researchers, advocates, and community members dedicated to the betterment of LGBTQ people everywhere. We stand on their shoulders.

For Judy

1

The Politics of LGBT Health

Kellan E. Baker

> Medicine is a social science, and politics is nothing else but medicine on a large scale. Medicine as a social science, as the science of human beings, has the obligation to point out problems and to attempt their theoretical solution; the politician, the practical anthropologist, must find the means for their actual solution.
>   —Dr. Rudolf Virchow (quoted in Friedlander, n.d.)

Policy is about visions, strategies, and decisions: it is a vehicle to turn knowledge into action and solutions. As the National Academy of Medicine asserts in each of its reports, "Knowing is not enough; we must apply. Willing is not enough; we must do." This transformation of ideas into activity is what gives policy its power to affect the characteristics and daily functioning of societies, communities, and individual people.

Policy operates at a number of different levels, from international treaties to protocols within a single organization. Important actors in American health policy include the federal executive branch of government, Congress, and the judiciary; state and territorial legislatures and gubernatorial administrations; tribal governments; municipal, county, and other local government systems; international entities such as the World Health Organization (WHO); and stakeholders such as hospitals, insurance companies, health care providers, advocates, and patients. This chapter focuses on health policy as it is developed and exercised by the federal govern-ment, particularly the U.S. Department of Health and Human Services (HHS), with regard to lesbian, gay, bisexual, and transgender (LGBT) populations.*

Because policy necessarily involves human agency, this chapter is also about the LGBT people and allies who have grappled with state power and its expression in policy—sometimes as subjects, frequently in resistance, and, increasingly, with the goal of harnessing policy's utility as a tool for creating change that benefits LGBT communities.

A SHORT HISTORY OF EARLY LGBT HEALTH ACTIVISM

Historically in the United States, policy was practiced upon LGBT people by a government that pathologized LGBT identities and criminal-ized LGBT lives. From the country's founding until 1961, same-sex sexual behavior was a felony in every state, and such prohibitions persisted in 14 states and Puerto Rico until the 2003 Supreme Court ruling in *Lawrence v. Texas* invalidated the anti-sodomy statutes that had long been used to per-secute sexual minorities. Beyond sexual behavior, as concepts of sexual orientation identity took clearer shape in the mid-20th century, homosex-uality was included as a "sociopathic personality disturbance" in the first *Diagnostic and Statistical Manual of Mental Disorders* (DSM) (American Psychiatric Association, 1952). For most of the last century, the federal government classified sexual minority people as national security risks and prohibited them from federal employment (Lewis, 1997).

Much of the hostility directed at lesbian, gay, and bisexual people has its roots in social sanctions against the transgression of established gender norms (Kimmel, 1996). These norms outline expected behavior for men and women in every aspect of their lives, from the toys they play with as children to the clothing they wear, the jobs they hold, and the intimate relationships they form with others—and they gave rise to laws such as prohibitions on marriage between two people of the same sex.

The consequences of rigid gender norms are also clear in the experi-ences of transgender people. Over the last 30 years, the term "transgender" has emerged as an umbrella term for people whose gender identity, which

---

* This chapter uses the term "LGBT" because of its widespread use in federal health policy. Other terms are also common, such as "lesbian, gay, bisexual, transgender, and queer" (LGBTQ) or "sexual and gender minorities" (SGM)—which encompasses LGBTQ people as well as groups such as intersex people and men who have sex with men but do not identify as gay or bisexual. The National Institutes of Health in par-ticular prefer the term "SGM."

is each person's deeply held internal identity as a man, a woman, or another gender, is different from the sex the person was assigned at birth (National Center for Transgender Equality, 2016b). Like lesbian, gay, and bisexual people, transgender people in the United States have long been subjected to discriminatory policies such as laws prohibiting "cross-dressing," forced institutionalization, and harmful "reparative" therapy that pathologizes gender variance and nonheterosexual sexual orientation (Meyerowitz, 2004). Many transgender people also need access to gender-affirming legal and medical procedures, meaning that transgender identities are heavily policed and dependent on aspects of policy such as state identity document laws and how health insurance companies interpret the diagnosis of gender dysphoria that remains in the DSM (National Center for Transgender Equality, 2016a).[1]

Whether through community organizing, political lobbying, or simply living their lives on their own terms, LGBT people have always found ways of resisting state-sanctioned mistreatment and policies that sought to exclude them from American society. In the 1960s and 1970s, these efforts became increasingly visible on the national policy scene. Activists such as Barbara Gittings and Frank Kameny, who filed the first civil rights claim based on sexual orientation in 1961 after he was expelled from federal employment for being gay, organized pickets to draw attention to discrimination against gay men and lesbians (Hunter, 2000). Crusaders such as Pauli Murray and Bayard Rustin were prominent in the movements for African American civil rights and women's liberation (Leighton, 2013), and activists such as the transgender rights pioneer Sylvia Rivera lived and organized at the intersections of race, gender, and LGBT rights (Sylvia Rivera Law Project, 2016).

A few years after the Compton's Cafeteria and Stonewall Riots that sparked the popular LGBT rights movement in the late 1960s, women's rights advocate Representative Bella Abzug and Representative Ed Koch introduced the Equality Act of 1974 (H.R. 14752), which was the first national legislative effort to prohibit discrimination on the basis of sexual orientation (Leclair, 2008). Though the bill did not pass, throughout the 1970s the goal of using the power of the political process to improve the circumstances of LGBT people's lives found numerous expressions in state- and local-level nondiscrimination campaigns, the founding of national advocacy organizations such as the National Gay Task Force (now the National LGBTQ Task Force) and the Human Rights Campaign Fund (now the Human Rights Campaign), and nationwide LGBT health organizing and advocacy (Myers, 2013).

An early milestone in LGBT health advocacy came in 1973, when activists secured the policy reversal that helped humanize sexual minorities in the popular imagination by removing homosexuality from the DSM

(Minton, 2002). In 1975, a wave of gay and lesbian affiliates of major health professional associations such as the American Nurses Association and the American Public Health Association began to appear, and the first national conference on gay health was convened in 1978 by the National Gay Health Coalition (NGHC), an entity that sought to bring together practitioners from various health-related disciplines working on sexual minority health issues (Mail & Lear, 2006). From this coalition came the National Gay Health Education Foundation, which was incorporated in 1980 and later operated as the National Lesbian and Gay Health Association until 1998. Another major sexual minority health professional organization, the American Association of Physicians for Human Rights, was founded in 1981 and became the Gay and Lesbian Medical Association in 1994. The organization is now known as GLMA: Health Professionals Advancing LGBT Equality.

In 1979, as part of the activities surrounding the first National March on Washington for Lesbian and Gay Rights, the NGHC organized the first formal dialogue between LGB health advocates and a sitting U.S. surgeon general (Mail & Lear, 2006). Policy proposals from this meeting included training for health care providers in the particular needs of sexual minority patients, research into specific health issues affecting sexual minority populations, and federal financial support for the community health clinics that had been founded in the 1970s in cities from Boston and Baltimore to Houston, Los Angeles, and San Francisco to provide LGBT culturally competent health care services. Clinics offering gender-affirming medical care for transgender people were also established in the 1960s and 1970s at the Johns Hopkins University and other major medical centers across the country, many with the support of transgender philanthropist Reed Erickson through the LGBT health-oriented Erickson Educational Foundation (Devor & Matte, 2007).

These early developments in LGBT health activism hint at the importance of health as a powerful tool for shaping and advancing a civil and human rights agenda. According to the World Health Organization, the enjoyment of the highest attainable standard of health is one of the fundamental rights of every human being (WHO, 1948). As Ronald Green argues, health is a primary good that is fundamentally and universally important to human well-being and capacity to enjoy other rights, such as the right to live, study, and work with safety and dignity and the right to form and protect a family (Green, 1976). Moreover, the power of health as a tool for human rights advocacy is distilled from the enormous body of evidence visible in the 20th century alone that human rights violations hurt people, make them sick, and often kill them. The lens of health thus has a unique ability to focus attention on the serious and far-reaching human consequences of a lack of respect for rights and dignity.

The rise of the HIV epidemic in the 1980s brought the connection between health and human rights for LGBT people into stark relief. Throughout the decade, as AIDS decimated LGBT communities and killed thousands of gay and bisexual men, the reaction from the federal government was silence (Shilts, 1987). Faced with official indifference, a coalition of activists founded the AIDS Coalition to Unleash Power, or ACT UP, in 1987. ACT UP quickly became associated with the Silence = Death Project, which declared, "Silence about the oppression and annihilation of gay people . . . must be broken as a matter of our survival" (Crimp & Rolston, 1990).

Throughout the remainder of the 1980s and into the 1990s, ACT UP employed a range of advocacy tactics to shatter that silence. These tactics included both "outsider" and "insider" activism: in addition to direct street action against relevant agencies within the U.S. Department of Health and Human Services (HHS), including the National Institutes of Health, the Food and Drug Administration, and the Centers for Disease Control and Prevention (CDC), some activists developed detailed knowledge of the workings of federal health policy and began to approach the issue of a national response to HIV from the perspective of policy advocacy (Crimp & Rolston, 1990).

POLICY PARADIGMS IN LGBT HEALTH

In order for social movements to advance via policy advocacy, advocates and policy makers must be able to employ a common language to define the terms and goals of the discussion. Peter Hall describes these shared cognitive frameworks as "policy paradigms." As he explains,

> Policymakers customarily work within a framework of ideas and standards that specifies not only the goals of policy and the kinds of instruments that can be used to attain them, but also the very nature of the problems they are meant to be addressing. . . . Policymaking in virtually all fields takes place within the context of a particular set of ideas that recognize some social interests as more legitimate than others and privilege some lines of policy over others. (Hall, 1993)

In other words, LGBT health policy advocacy is made possible by specific concepts that both facilitate the description of health issues affecting LGBT populations and provide the vocabulary necessary to engage with policy makers in casting these issues as legitimate objects of government concern.

Over the last 30 years, two major policy paradigms have formed the backdrop for LGBT health advocacy. The first, which arose in the 1980s, is characterized by a focus on health disparities. The second, which is related to disparities but which has played a significant role in U.S. health policy making only since roughly 2010, has been termed the "Health in All Policies" paradigm.

The Disparities Paradigm

The dominant paradigm within which federal LGBT health policy advocacy took shape in the 1980s was growing political attention to health disparities, meaning observable population-wide patterns in which the health of some groups of people lags behind that of other groups. In his analysis of government-oriented LGBT health advocacy, Steven Epstein describes the manifestation of the disparities policy paradigm in biomedical research as "inclusion-and-difference" (Epstein, 1996). In his account, the salient feature of this paradigm is the argument made to the National Institutes of Health (NIH) that federally supported biomedical research agendas should *include* specific population groups that experience disparities—such as LGBT populations—in order to describe the *differences* between these groups that warrant population-specific research.

In relation to policy, research is not an end in itself. As Vanessa Gamble and Deborah Stone note, social issues do not become matters of political concern just because research, even government-funded research, shows they exist. After research reveals problems, they write,

> Problems . . . must be converted into political issues by leaders (grassroots, community, political, religious, and intellectual). Then they must be defined in a way that government can do something about them with the kind of tools it has at hand (legislation, regulation, taxation, financing, public education). Only then does a problem begin to make its way through the political process as something to which government develops a specific policy response. (Gamble & Stone, 2006)

Thus, the means by which the disparities paradigm came to include LGBT populations are rooted in the history of the federal response to health disparities both in research at NIH and in policy across HHS. Beginning in the 1980s, the push to address health disparities via federal policy focused first on disparities related to race and ethnicity. Over the next 30 years, the disparities paradigm in federal health policy making gradually expanded to encompass other disparity factors as well, including sexual orientation and gender identity.

In 1979, the Department of Health, Education, and Welfare (DHEW)[2] released its first national public health agenda, *Healthy People: The Surgeon General's Report on Health Promotion and Disease Prevention*, which trumpeted the fact that the United States underwent an epidemiologic shift in the 20th century that saw dramatic drops in the incidence of infectious disease and substantial accompanying gains in life expectancy (U.S. Surgeon General, 1979). What the report mentioned only in passing, however, was that these gains were not evenly distributed across the U.S. population: specific population groups, particularly African Americans, experienced persistent disparities in disease incidence, health outcomes, and longevity.

It is important to note that not all health differences are disparities. The fields of medicine and public health have long recognized that human beings vary as widely in health as they do in every other attribute, and numerous factors give rise to health differences between people and, in the aggregate, among population groups. Margaret Whitehead offers the example of the role of human aging in the greater incidence of coronary heart disease in adults who are 70 years old versus those aged 20 (Whitehead, 1992); another example is the higher likelihood that HIV transmission occurs from an insertive to receptive sexual partner rather than vice versa (Jin et al., 2009). These differences are not health disparities. Rather, the concept of "disparities" invokes health differences that are unjustifiable, avoidable, and remediable by policy intervention.

As research documenting racial and ethnic health disparities mounted, political and public pressure for a government response grew (Gamble & Stone, 2006). In 1985, Secretary of Health and Human Services Margaret Heckler formally placed these disparities on the federal government's policy agenda by convening the Task Force on Black and Minority Health and, shortly thereafter, by establishing the Office of Minority Health within HHS (Heckler, 1985). By the time HHS published the second Healthy People report in 1990, reducing disparities had become one of the federal government's three overarching health goals (HHS, 1990). A wave of policy activity related to racial and ethnic disparities followed in the 1990s, including the establishment of the Office of Minority Health and Research at NIH, increased federally supported data collection around race and ethnicity, and the creation of specific federal programs dedicated to developing effective strategies for addressing racial and ethnic disparities (Gamble & Stone, 2006).

The early years of official federal recognition of racial and ethnic health disparities also saw increasing policy action around disparities affecting women. In 1985, HHS convened a Task Force on Women's Health Issues and charged it with looking at, in language mirroring the discussions around racial and ethnic disparities, "areas where the circumstances for women are unique, the noted condition is more prevalent, the interventions are different for women than for men, or the health risks are greater for women than for men" (HHS, 1985).

A central finding of the report was that breast cancer was the leading cause of death among women ages 35 to 54. In the 1970s, advocacy around breast cancer was still focused on dispelling the stigma attached to a disease that was considered "unspeakable" in polite company (Osuch et al., 2012). But by the 1980s, activists such as the black lesbian writer Audre Lorde had begun to rage against public censorship of the identity, image, and sexuality of women with breast cancer (Lorde, 1980), foreshadowing the fight against official erasure of the experiences of gay and bisexual men with AIDS. Throughout the 1980s, breast cancer advocates became increasingly vocal and visible and helped drive developments in a broader federal policy agenda around women's health, such as the establishment of the NIH Office of Research on Women's Health in 1990, the creation of the HHS Office of Women's Health in 1991, and provisions in the 1993 NIH Revitalization Act requiring all NIH-funded clinical research studies to include women and racial and ethnic minority groups.[3]

By the end of the 1990s, the relevance of the disparities paradigm for addressing LGBT health concerns through federally supported research and policy was clear. As Epstein describes, for instance, researchers investigating disparities among diverse populations of women—including lesbians—worked with HHS to generate the momentum that resulted in the 1999 Institute of Medicine report *Lesbian Health: Current Assessment and Directions for the Future* (Epstein, 1996; Institute of Medicine Committee on Lesbian Health Research Priorities, 1999). This report, which was funded by the NIH Office of Research on Women's Health with contributions from the Office of Women's Health at the Centers for Disease Control and Prevention, was the first major federally funded policy publication to specifically focus on any aspect of LGBT health aside from HIV/AIDS among men who have sex with men.

In 2000, the third iteration of the federal government's nationwide once-a-decade public health agenda, Healthy People 2010, called for the elimination of health disparities and included, for the first time, sexual orientation (though not gender identity) as a disparity factor (HHS, 2000). This important step came about after concerted advocacy by LGBT community organizations, which reacted strongly when almost all references to sexual orientation were deleted from an initial draft. Ultimately, sexual orientation was included as a factor in the data tables for 29 of the 467 objectives, though these data were ultimately unavailable for any objective because none of the federally supported surveys used to establish benchmarks and measure progress for the Healthy People plans reliably asked questions about sexual orientation (Epstein, 2007).

The inclusion of sexual orientation in Healthy People 2010 was followed by publications from several HHS divisions that reflected the growing status of sexual orientation and gender identity as "legitimate" disparity factors in federal health policy and research. In 2001, for instance, the Substance Abuse and Mental Health Services Administration developed the first federal publication that addressed the full spectrum of LGBT identities, and the Health Resources and Services Administration (HRSA) contributed funds toward the *Healthy People 2010 Companion Document for Lesbian, Gay, Bisexual, and Transgender Health*, which was a quasi-official accompanying volume for the federal Healthy People plan. Also in 2001, NIH released its first program announcement soliciting proposals for research specifically on "lesbian, gay, bisexual, transgendered [sic], and related populations" (NIH, 2001).

The most substantial evidence of the evolution of the federal disparities policy paradigm to include LGBT health was the *HHS Strategic Plan on Addressing Health Disparities Related to Sexual Orientation* (HHS, 2001). This plan, which was compiled by a committee composed of representatives from across the agency, first makes its case for both scientific and political legitimacy by laying out a roll call of documented disparities affecting LGBT populations, including HIV/AIDS among gay and bisexual men and breast cancer among lesbians and bisexual women, as well as issues such as mental health and substance use concerns, gaps in access to insurance and health care, and exposure to violence. It then recommends a range of interventions that adopts almost every existing marker of progress in the 20-year-old federal health disparities agenda, including development of a broad LGBT population-oriented research agenda at NIH, initiation of nationwide population-level data collection related to sexual orientation and gender identity, and establishment of a dedicated Office of LGBT Health at HHS to create and manage specific programs across the department to address LGBT disparities.

Unfortunately, this comprehensive federal plan to address LGBT health disparities was suppressed by the incoming George W. Bush administration and never publicly released. Under the Bush administration, federal LGBT health policy struggled through a period of faltering political commitment to addressing LGBT health disparities, rollbacks of sexual orientation and gender identity data collection, and purges of LGBT content from NIH research agendas (Scout, 2013). While political attention to some health disparities continued in various forms, it would be almost a decade before LGBT health issues visibly returned to the national policy scene.

The Health in All Policies Paradigm: Social Determinants and Health Equity

The appearance of health disparities on the U.S. federal policy agenda in the 1980s generated interest not only in documenting and quantifying these disparities but also in clarifying their underlying causes. From a scientific perspective, this interest was not new. Throughout the 19th and

20th centuries, debate raged about whether biology (i.e., genetics) or social, political, and economic environments weigh heavier on the scales of individual and population health.[4] For its part, the Reagan administration framed ill health and disparities among black Americans and other racial and ethnic minority groups almost exclusively as the result of poor individual "life-style choices" (Krieger & Bassett, 1986). This mantra of "personal responsibility" left little room for large-scale socioeconomic forces: in the 1985 report from the HHS Task Force on Minority Health, for instance, even the section on "social characteristics" of communities of color focuses on individual behaviors such as "acculturation" to white-dominated society, personal eating habits, and coping strategies for dealing with stress, while eliding any discussion of what the stressors themselves may be (Heckler, 1985). In fact, the word "racism" is almost completely absent from the report's eight volumes.

As a growing body of research demonstrated over the next 20 years, however, the answer is not so simple. While personal choices such as smoking, sexual behavior, and seeking appropriate medical care have significant effects on health, these choices are themselves strong functions of the social, economic, and political conditions that shape the range of options to which people have access throughout their lives (Krieger 1994, 1999, 2001; Whitehead, 1992). These conditions—collectively referred to as the social determinants of health—are dynamic manifestations of the systems that distribute resources, protection, and power across society, and they mediate exposure to physical and mental health hazards such as economic deprivation, discrimination, violence, unhealthy environments, and inadequate medical care (Wilkinson & Marmot, 2003; WHO Commission on Social Determinants of Health, 2008). As a consequence, health disparities reflect the literal human embodiment of inequality in the daily conditions in which people grow up, form families, work, age, and die (WHO, 2011). Consideration of the social determinants of health introduces a moral and ethical dimension, frequently termed "health equity," into discussions of disparities and illuminates that health disparities are not only avoidable and unjustifiable—they are unjust (Braveman et al., 2011).

The trajectory of the HIV/AIDS epidemic in the United States exemplifies the evolving understanding that broad social, political, and economic forces underlie disparities far more than biological factors or individual choices can be said to do. Before a national understanding of health disparities was well established, pundits and politicians in the early 1980s dismissed HIV as "gay-related immune deficiency" or "the gay plague" and implied that AIDS was punishment for insufficient personal responsibility among gay men for their own health (Clews, 2014). As HIV spread through the U.S. population, however, it became an infectious biomarker tracking the fault lines of what Paul Farmer calls "structural violence," meaning the inequity and discrimination that systematically marginalize people on the basis of factors such as sexual orientation, race, or gender and obstruct their ability to be healthy by depriving them of social and economic support, legal protections, and representation in political power structures (Farmer, 1999). In other words, health disparities such as differing rates of HIV illuminate the mechanisms by which societies decide whose lives matter.

HIV also demonstrates how social determinants bleed across identity boundaries and create particularly complex disparities for people who live at the intersections of multiple marginalized identities. Kimberlé Crenshaw coined the term "intersectionality" to describe how politically charged categories of difference such as race and sex intersect to produce discrimination and disparities greater than just the sum of racism and sexism (Crenshaw, 1989).[5] An intersectional perspective thus helps explain how racism and other social determinants affecting the distribution of power and privilege in society exacerbate disparities associated with sexual orientation and gender identity. More than 30 years of the HIV epidemic underscore the reality of the intersecting oppressions that give rise to health inequities: the only segment of the U.S. population in which documented new HIV infections continue to rise is among gay and bisexual men and other men who have sex with men, particularly young African Americans and Latinos (Centers for Disease Control and Prevention, 2015). Emerging evidence also indicates that black and Latina transgender women, who live at the intersections of racism, transphobia, and sexism, frequently experience severe unemployment, poverty, violence, and alienation from the health system, and may have the highest HIV prevalence of any population in the world (Baral et al., 2013; Poteat, 2015).

Because the roots of many social, political, and economic factors that give rise to health disparities lie outside the health system itself, addressing social determinants requires an integrated policy response from multiple sectors, including the economy, the environment, transportation, agriculture, immigration, and criminal justice. The term "Health in All Policies" has come into use to describe a policy paradigm that views optimizing the social determinants of health in order to promote well-being for all people as a fundamental building block of a thriving society and the shared responsibility of policy makers across all parts of government (Ståhl, Wismar, Ollila, Lahtinen, & Leppo, 2006). As the World Health Organization defines the term:

> Health in All Policies is an approach to public policies across sectors that systematically takes into account the health implications of decisions, seeks synergies, and avoids harmful health impacts in order to improve population health and health equity. Health in All Policies is founded on health-related rights and obligations and contributes to strengthening the accountability of policymakers for health impacts at all levels of policymaking. It improves

accountability of policymakers for health impacts at all levels of policymaking. It emphasizes the consequences of public policies on health systems,
determinants of health, and well-being. (WHO, 2013)

The Health in All Policies paradigm began to enter American health policy
around 2010 as it became clear that the magnitude of health disparities
had remained largely unchanged in the United States even after 30 years of
efforts to reduce them (Braveman et al., 2010; Satcher, 2010; CDC, 2011;
Institute of Medicine, 2013). This paradigm and its core principle of health
equity underscore the imperative for LGBT health policy advocates to
broadly fight for human rights and social justice, not simply to secure a
place for the LGBT population on a list of groups experiencing disparities
while leaving unchallenged the dynamics that fostered these disparities in
the first place. As Paula Braveman et al. write succinctly, "Health equity is
social justice in health" (Braveman et al., 2011).

The decennial Healthy People plans provide an example of the paradigm shift that has moved U.S. health policy from an ahistorical concept
of disparities as the result of individual choices and "lifestyle factors" to
more nuanced explorations of the role of systematic current and historical
inequities.

In 2000, Healthy People 2010 defined health disparities neutrally as
"differences that occur by gender, race or ethnicity, education or income,
disability, living in rural localities, or sexual orientation" (HHS, 2000).
While the text does foreshadow concepts of equity and health in all policies, it emphasizes that one of "the greatest opportunities for reducing
health disparities [is] empowering individuals to make informed health
care decisions" returning to the idea that poor choices by members of dis-
advantaged communities lie at the root of health disparities.

Ten years later, Healthy People 2020 defined a disparity very
differently—as:

> . . . a **particular kind** of health difference that is **closely linked with social,
> economic, and/or environmental disadvantage**. Health disparities
> adversely affect groups of people who have **systematically** experienced
> greater obstacles to health based on their racial or ethnic group; religion;
> socioeconomic status; gender; age; mental health; cognitive, sensory, or
> physical disability; sexual orientation or gender identity; geographic loca-
> tion; or other characteristics **historically linked to discrimination or
> exclusion** (emphasis added). (HHS, 2010)

This iteration of Healthy People is also the first to devote an entire topic
area to LGBT health, which places LGBT health disparities in the context
of the discrimination and oppression that LGBT people experience on the
basis of their sexual orientation and gender identity. Much remains to be
done to expose the role that societal prejudice and discriminatory public

policies have played in perpetuating these disparities and to shift the focus from chronicling disadvantages to fostering resilience. The equity lens of the LGBT health topic area in Healthy People 2020 is an important step toward health policies that move beyond offering minor fixes for discrete disparities to diagnosing and addressing the diseases of inequity and injustice in society at large.

AN OVERVIEW OF FEDERAL LGBT HEALTH POLICY BETWEEN 2009 AND 2016

The period between 2009 and 2016 was a particularly momentous time for federal policy related to LGBT health disparities and health equity. This section provides an overview of significant federal policy actions during this period that concern LGBT population health, including sexual orientation and gender identity data collection, the Affordable Care Act and other legislation, and policies and programs across the federal Department of Health and Human Services.

Data Collection about LGBT Population Health

Data are fundamental to health policy, especially with regard to health disparities. It is impossible to craft effective policies to promote health equity without evidence about the scope and impact of disparities. Key opportunities for gathering data about LGBT population health fall into at least four broad categories: research, survey data, administrative data, and medical records.

Research

Federally supported research was slow to take an interest in LGBT population health. A 2014 analysis showed that only one half of 1 percent of studies funded by NIH between 1989 and 2011 concern the LGBT population, and when studies focusing on HIV/AIDS and other sexual health concerns are excluded, the number drops to 0.1 percent of NIH-funded studies during these two decades (Coulter, Kenst, Bowen, & Scout, 2014).

In 2009, however, shortly after the beginning of the Obama administration, NIH requested that the Institute of Medicine (now the National Academy of Medicine) convene a study committee to comprehensively assess existing research in LGBT health and to document gaps and opportunities. The resulting report, *The Health of Lesbian, Gay, Bisexual, and Transgender People: Building a Foundation for Better Understanding*, invokes four conceptual frameworks—intersectionality, the life course, social ecology,

---

INSTITUTE OF MEDICINE REPORT RECOMMENDATIONS

1. NIH should implement a research agenda designed to advance knowledge and understanding of LGBT health.

2. Data on sexual orientation and gender identity should be collected in federally funded surveys administered by HHS and in other relevant federally funded surveys.

3. Data on sexual orientation and gender identity should be collected in electronic health records.

4. NIH should support the development and standardization of sexual orientation and gender identity measures.

5. NIH should support methodological research that relates to LGBT health.

6. A comprehensive research training approach should be created to strengthen LGBT health research at NIH.

7. NIH should encourage grant applicants to address explicitly the inclusion or exclusion of sexual and gender minorities in their samples.

---

and minority stress—to describe LGBT health disparities and offer recommendations for addressing them (Institute of Medicine Committee on LGBT Health Issues and Research Gaps and Opportunities, 2011).

In response to the report, NIH created an LGBT Research Coordinating Committee and later formally established a Sexual and Gender Minority Research Office (NIH Sexual and Gender Minority Research Coordinating Committee, 2015). The office's strategic plan outlines SGM health research priorities that include interactions between health risks and protective factors in groups such as older adults, youth, and communities of color; stigma and minority stress; resilience; depression and other mental health concerns; behavioral health and substance use; cancer; sexually transmitted infections; transgender health; and intersex conditions. In 2016, the Director of the National Institute for Minority Health and Health Disparities (NIMHD) cemented the application of the health disparities framework to SGM population health by formally designating the SGM population a health disparity population for research purposes (Pérez-Stable, 2016). This designation gives SGM population research a formal home within NIMHD and provides a rationale for NIH-funded disparities researchers to include a focus on SGM populations in their work.

Survey Data

According to estimates from the nationwide Gallup poll, in 2017 there were at least 10 million LGBT-identified people in the United States

---

SOME DATA ELEMENTS RELEVANT TO LGBT POPULATION HEALTH

- Gender expression
- Gender identity
- Gender pronoun
- Preferred name
- Relationship status
- Sex assigned at birth
- Sexual attraction
- Sexual behavior
- Sexual orientation identity
- Transgender status

(Gates, 2017). Despite the size of this population, data collection on sexual orientation and gender identity by the federal statistical agencies has historically been sparse. Throughout the 1990s and 2000s, only a handful of federally supported surveys asked questions about any aspect of LGBT identity or experience, and these efforts skewed heavily toward sexual behavior, and occasionally, personal identification as gay, lesbian, or bisexual, at the expense of more comprehensive and transgender-inclusive approaches (Sell, n.d.). With regard to same-sex relationships, even as states across the country began to extend legal relationship recognition such as civil unions, domestic partnerships, and eventually marriage to same-sex couples, the U.S. Census did not count same-sex couples until 2010 (Kreider, Bates, & Mayol-Garcia, 2017).

At the urging of LGBT health advocates who viewed data collection as a key priority, in 2011 the HHS Office of Minority Health released its first-ever "LGBT Data Progression Plan" to guide the addition of sexual orientation and gender identity questions to the agency's surveys (U.S. Office of Minority Health, 2011). The first step in this plan was the addition of a sexual orientation question to the agency's flagship health and demographic survey, the National Health Interview Survey (Division of Health Interview Statistics, 2014). CDC subsequently approved a sexual orientation and gender identity question module for states to use on their Behavioral Risk Factor Surveillance System questionnaires and added sexual orientation and sexual behavior questions to the core of the Youth Risk Behavior Survey (Baker & Hughes, 2016). Several other federal surveys, such as the National Survey of Drug Use and Health at HHS and the National Crime Victimization Survey at the Department of Justice, also began to include sexual orientation and gender identity measures during the Obama administration, and the Department of Labor began to test measures for use on the Current Population Survey.

In 2015, the Office of Management and Budget (OMB), the federal executive branch office that approves all agency data collection activities, convened the Federal Interagency Working Group on Improving Measurement of Sexual Orientation and Gender Identity to coordinate advances in collecting these data across the federal agencies. This working group, which was patterned after the OMB Interagency Working Group on Measuring Relationships in Federal Household Surveys that worked on the same-sex relationship questions on the 2010 Census, produced three reports summarizing existing practices and future recommendations for the use of sexual orientation and gender identity questions on federal surveys (Federal Interagency Working Group, 2016).

Changes to federal survey data collection on LGBT populations were an early indication that the Trump administration was not likely to continue the Obama administration's approach to LGBT health. In March 2017, for instance, the HHS Administration for Community Living announced that the National Survey of Older Americans Act Participants would be discontinuing the use of a question on sexual orientation (Centers for Medicare and Medicaid Services, n.d.; Morabia, 2017). In response to public outcry, the question was retained, but a previous proposal to expand the survey's approach to gender identity data was dropped. Around the same time, the administration also attracted criticism for deleting references to the proposed addition of sexual orientation and gender identity questions to the American Community Survey, the annual survey that took the place of the long-form Census questionnaire. Critics charged that the Census Bureau was responding to political pressure from the administration in rolling back this proposal, which had been formulated in response to federal agency interest in these data under the Obama administration (Wang, 2017).

Administrative Data

Administrative data are collected by programs, such as those funded by the federal government or state departments of health, to characterize the populations they serve. These data can also help monitor the effectiveness of nondiscrimination protections and cultural competency guidelines that include LGBT populations. Several administrative data systems at HHS, such as the Ryan White Program (Health Resources and Services Administration, 2014) and substance use prevention and treatment programs funded by the Substance Abuse and Mental Health Services Administration (Office of Applied Studies, 2010), collect some LGBT data. In 2016, the Health Resources and Services Administration added sexual orientation and gender identity data collection to the Uniform Data System, which all federally qualified health centers must use to report key demographic characteristics of the patient populations they serve (HRSA, 2016). The Trump administration, however, in 2017 reversed this trend by canceling the planned addition of sexual orientation and gender identity questions to the Annual Program Performance Report for Centers for Independent Living, an HHS-funded program that serves people with disabilities (Singh, Durso, & Tax, 2017).

Insurance claims are another important form of administrative data. In 2015, researchers in the Office of Minority Health at the Centers for Medicare and Medicaid Services (CMS) announced that they had successfully adapted an algorithm originally developed by the Veterans Administration to identify several thousand transgender people in Medicare claims data (Proctor, Haffer, Ewald, Hodge, & James, 2016). CMS used these data to explore the health and demographic profiles of transgender Medicare beneficiaries, which differ substantially from those of the cisgender Medicare population (Dragon, Guerino, Ewald, & Laffan, 2017). In particular, transgender Medicare beneficiaries are younger, more likely to be African American, and more likely to have a chronic condition such as depression, HIV, or chronic obstructive pulmonary disease.

Medical Records

Medical records are a major potential source for data on the health of LGBT populations. At the federal level, electronic health records (EHRs) were the focus of a major multistage initiative, the Incentive Program for the Meaningful Use of Electronic Health Records (known as "Meaningful Use"), which was launched under the HITECH Act in 2009 and overseen by CMS and the HHS Office of the National Coordinator for Health Information Technology (ONC). In 2015, CMS and ONC released final regulations governing Stage 3 of the Meaningful Use program that required all certified EHR systems to allow users to record, change, and access structured data on sexual orientation and gender identity (Office of the Secretary of HHS, 2015). The regulations note that this requirement will "help those within the patient's care team to have more information on the patient that can aid in identifying interventions and treatments most helpful to the particular patient," citing the example of a transgender man—a person who was assigned female at birth and identifies as male—who should be offered a cervical exam if he still retains a cervix (CMS, 2015). This aspect of the Meaningful Use program was continued under the Medicare Access and CHIP Reauthorization Act of 2015 (MACRA), which consolidated several physician incentive programs.

Legislative Approaches to LGBT Health

Many congressional efforts to address LGBT health disparities also historically centered on data collection. Then-representative Tammy Baldwin (D-WI), who was the first openly gay person to be elected to Congress, was a key champion of early efforts to push HHS to dedicate resources to sexual orientation and gender identity data collection. In 2009, Representative Baldwin introduced the Ending LGBT Health Disparities Act (ELHDA), an omnibus LGBT health bill that promoted LGBT research and data collection alongside priorities such as the routine incorporation of LGBT cultural competency in programs across HHS; the establishment of LGBT-inclusive nondiscrimination policies in federal health programs such as Medicaid, Medicare, the Federal Employees Health Benefits Program, and health services provided by the Veterans Administration; and the creation of an Office of LGBT Health within the HHS Office of Minority Health.

ELHDA was never enacted, but it represents a pivotal moment in congressional interest in combatting LGBT health disparities. Prior to ELHDA, no federal legislation had proposed to specifically address LGBT health disparities. Subsequently, however, legislation such as the Health Equity and Accountability Act (HEAA)—the comprehensive racial and ethnic minority health equity bill led by the Congressional Tri-Caucus[6]— began to consistently call for the routine collection of sexual orientation and gender identity data to help better understand and address LGBT health disparities. This evolution of the HEAA reflects growing awareness that populations experiencing health disparities are diverse and that racial, ethnic, and other disparities cannot be fully addressed in isolation from the disparities associated with stigmatized sexual orientation and gender identity.

In 2016, Congress passed the 21st Century Cures Act, which authorized billions of dollars in funding for NIH and included specific provisions directing NIH to undertake activities to improve the quality and quantity of research related to sexual and gender minority populations. Also in 2016, Senator Baldwin and Representative Raúl Grijalva (D-AZ) introduced the LGBT Data Inclusion Act, which is modeled on a 2010 House bill authored by Baldwin that would have expanded LGBT data collection at HHS. The 2016 legislation broadened its focus to all federal agencies and was reintroduced in both the House and the Senate in 2017.

The Affordable Care Act

Another major piece of legislation relevant to LGBT health is the Patient Protection and Affordable Care Act of 2010, commonly known as the

RESOURCES ON THE **ACA** AND **LGBT** POPULATIONS

Out2Enroll is a nationwide campaign that provides resources for LGBT people about their health insurance coverage options under the Affordable Care Act: www.out2enroll.org.

U.S. Department of Health and Human Services—*Transgender Health Care* (2016): www.healthcare.gov/transgender-health-care.

U.S. Department of Health and Human Services—*Outreach and Enrollment for LGBT Individuals: Promising Practices from the Field* (2015): https://aspe.hhs.gov/basic-report/outreach-and-enrollment-lgbt -individuals-promising-practices-field.

Center for American Progress—*Moving the Needle: The Impact of the Affordable Care Act on LGBT Communities* (2014): www.american progress.org/issues/lgbt/report/2014/11/17/101575/moving-the -needle/.

Kaiser Family Foundation—*Health and Access to Care and Coverage for Lesbian, Gay, Bisexual, and Transgender Individuals in the U.S.* (2014): http://kff.org/disparities-policy/issue-brief/health-and-access-to-care -and-coverage-for-lesbian-gay-bisexual-and-transgender-individuals -in-the-u-s/.

Substance Abuse and Mental Health Services Administration—Afford-able Care Act Enrollment Assistance for LGBT Communities: A Resource for Behavioral Health Providers (2014): http://store.samhsa. gov/product/Affordable-Care-Act-ACA-Enrollment-Assistance -for-LGBT-Communities/PEP14-LGBTACAENROLL.

Affordable Care Act (ACA). Though support for the law is a strongly partisan issue, the ACA is the single largest piece of federal legislation dealing with the American health system since the creation of Medicare and Medicaid in the 1960s—and, as then secretary of Health and Human Services Kathleen Sebelius asserted in 2011, "The Affordable Care Act may represent the strongest foundation we have ever created to begin closing LGBT health disparities" (Sebelius, 2011). Three major reasons that the ACA is important for advancing LGBT health are its support for data collection related to disparities, its reforms expanding the availability of insurance coverage, and its establishment of new nondiscrimination protections related to access to health coverage and care.

Disparities Data Collection in the ACA

Section 4302 of the ACA calls on all HHS-funded surveys and programs to collect data on several disparity factors, such as race, ethnicity, and disability.

It also grants HHS authority to collect "any other demographic data as deemed appropriate by the Secretary regarding health disparities." This opening for the secretary to initiate sexual orientation and gender identity data collection under the ACA was secured by LGBT health advocates who noticed that, while the House version of the health reform legislation included this open-ended phrase, the Senate version restricted data collection efforts under this provision to race, ethnicity, sex, disability status, and primary language. Because of the partisan controversy surrounding the law's passage, the two bills did not undergo the usual conference process where the House and Senate versions are compared and reconciled, and the Senate version largely became the final legislation. In response to advocate input, however, Senator Tom Harkin (D-IA) succeeded in changing the Senate language to reflect the flexibility of the House version, thus preserving a critical window for LGBT-inclusive implementation of this provision. The 2011 HHS LGBT Data Progression Plan referenced earlier was the agency's initial strategy for implementing ACA Section 4302 with regard to sexual orientation and gender identity data.

Availability of Insurance Coverage

When the Affordable Care Act was passed, almost 50 million Americans were uninsured, in addition to the large number of uninsured among the estimated 11 million undocumented immigrants living in the United States (U.S. Census Bureau., 2010; Wallace, Torres, Nobari, & Pourat, 2013). The ranks of the uninsured included many LGBT people: LGBT people are more likely than the general population to be uninsured (Gates, 2014), and immediately before many of the ACA's major insurance reforms took effect in 2013, one in three (34 percent) low- and middle-income LGBT people were uninsured (Durso, Baker, & Cray, 2013). One year later, this number had dropped to one in four (26 percent) uninsured, and in 2017 it had dropped to around one in five (22 percent) (Baker & Durso, 2017). Overall, there was a 35 percent decline in uninsurance among LGBT people with annual incomes less than $45,000 between 2013 and 2017.

The ACA facilitated access to health insurance coverage in two main ways—through an expansion of state Medicaid programs and through the establishment of new health insurance marketplaces. Together, these new options were intended to provide financial assistance to people with incomes up to 400 percent of the Federal Poverty Level (FPL): the ACA required Medicaid to cover those making up to 138 percent[7] of the FPL and made sliding-scale tax credits available through the IRS to assist those making between 139 and 400 percent of the FPL in paying the cost of their monthly premiums. In 2016, the FPL stood at $11,880 for an individual and $24,300 for a family of four.

The changes to the Medicaid program were intended to replace the pre-ACA system in which Medicaid coverage was only available to people who fit into a narrow group of predetermined eligibility categories, such as living with a disability, being pregnant, or having dependent children. Medicaid is jointly funded by the federal government and the states, and states were required to either use solely their own funds or obtain a federal waiver to cover childless adults who were not otherwise categorically eligible; before health reform, only five states offered full Medicaid coverage to this population (Kaiser Commission on Medicaid and the Uninsured, 2009). Because of these stringent eligibility requirements, people with HIV frequently could not get Medicaid coverage for HIV treatment until their health had deteriorated to the point where they became disabled by the disease progressing to AIDS (AIDS Action Council, 2004).

Further, Medicaid is a means-tested program, and states have historically had the leeway to set their own income eligibility standards. These standards are typically far below the poverty line. In 2010, the median Medicaid eligibility threshold for a working parent in a three-person household was 64 percent of the poverty level, or $11,718 per year, and eligibility thresholds in states such as Texas, Missouri, and Louisiana hovered around 25 percent of the poverty level, rendering a working parent with two children making more than $381 a month ineligible for coverage (Kaiser Commission on Medicaid and the Uninsured, 2011). The combination of narrow eligibility categories and highly restrictive income limits meant that many LGBT people were unable to access Medicaid coverage before the health reform law, even though LGBT people are significantly more likely than the general population be living in poverty (Baker, McGovern, Gruberg, & Cray, 2016).

When the Supreme Court ruled on the constitutionality of the ACA in June 2012, however, it decided that the federal government cannot compel the states to expand their Medicaid programs, effectively leaving the question of expansion to governors and state legislatures. By the beginning of the Trump administration in January 2017, 32 states and the District of Columbia had expanded their programs to cover all adults with incomes under 138 percent of the FPL (Kaiser Family Foundation, 2018).

In the states that did not expand Medicaid, the health reform law does not offer new options to help people with incomes under the poverty line, including poor LGBT people and their families, access coverage. There was no deadline for states to decide to move forward with the expansion, though states that delayed lost substantial amounts of federal funding: the federal government paid 100 percent of the costs of expansion between 2014 and 2016, and this percentage dropped slightly before settling at 90 percent in 2020 and beyond.

The other major coverage initiative under the Affordable Care Act was the creation of new health insurance marketplaces in every state. The marketplaces, which developed as a concept in conservative policy circles in the early 1990s, were intended to foster competition in insurance markets by allowing people to shop for private health insurance plans through a single streamlined interface that provides easy comparisons between different products (Butler, 1989). The ACA's marketplaces, which are modeled on the 2006 health reform effort overseen in Massachusetts by then governor Mitt Romney, provide income-based financial assistance in the form of tax credits that offset the cost of monthly premiums.

The intent of the ACA was that the states would run their own marketplaces, but the political environment around the reform effort led a majority of states to leave marketplace governance to HHS. As a result, in the 2017–2018 open enrollment period, only 12 states ran their own marketplaces; 11 states entered into a partnership with HHS, and 28 opted to use HealthCare.gov, which is the federally facilitated marketplace (Kaiser Family Foundation, 2018).

Access to Health Coverage and Care

Prior to the ACA, there were few federal laws providing oversight of insurance carrier activities, meaning that customers in most states had limited protections from high premiums, exclusions and limitations on coverage, and restricted access to health care providers. To address these concerns, the ACA prohibited practices such as medical underwriting to set premium rates, gender rating (the practice of charging women more than men for comparable coverage), exclusions based on preexisting conditions such HIV or cancer, the imposition of annual and lifetime limits on coverage, and the arbitrary withdrawal of coverage. The law also required all plans sold through any marketplace to be certified as qualified health plans (QHPs) under the oversight of a new federal Office for Consumer Information and Insurance Oversight. QHPs must meet a variety of requirements related to benefit design, marketing, and other aspects of coverage, including the ten categories of essential health benefits that all QHPs and all non-grandfathered plans in individual and small group markets in all states must cover. The regulations governing QHPs and the marketplaces explicitly prohibit discrimination on the basis of sexual orientation and gender identity. This means, for instance, that ACA-compliant plans could not refuse to insure same-sex couples together as a family even before the 2015 marriage equality ruling in *Obergefell v. Hodges* (CMS, 2014).

In addition to these broad reforms, the ACA established nationwide LGBT-inclusive nondiscrimination protections in health insurance and health care. Alongside the requirements that apply to QHPs and the marketplaces,

---

ESSENTIAL HEALTH BENEFITS UNDER THE ACA

1. Ambulatory patient services
2. Emergency services
3. Hospitalization
4. Maternity and newborn care
5. Mental health and substance use disorder services, including behavioral health treatment
6. Prescription drugs
7. Rehabilitative and habilitative services and devices
8. Laboratory services
9. Preventive and wellness services and chronic disease management
10. Pediatric services, including oral and vision care

ACA Section 1557 extends the protections of existing federal civil rights laws—including the Rehabilitation Act, which covers HIV status, and Title IX, which covers sex—to any entity or program receiving federal financial assistance or operated by HHS. Covered entities under Section 1557 include hospitals participating in Medicare or Medicaid; state health programs funded by federal grants; state Medicaid programs; federally qualified community health centers; HealthCare.gov and the state-run health insurance marketplaces; and all plans sold by health insurance carriers that participate in programs such as a health insurance marketplace, Medicare Part D or Medicare Advantage, and Medicaid managed care.

A regulation issued by the HHS Office for Civil Rights (OCR) in May 2016 expressly states that the sex nondiscrimination protections in Section 1557 protect LGBT, gender-nonconforming, nonbinary, and intersex people from discrimination in health insurance coverage and health care (HHS, 2016; Baker, 2016). In fall 2016, conservative legal groups challenged this regulation in court, and on December 31, 2016, a federal judge issued a nationwide injunction in *Franciscan Alliance, Inc. v. Burwell* prohibiting OCR from enforcing the provisions of the regulation that protect LGBT people, as well as provisions that were seen as expanding protections related to abortion access. As of 2018, the injunction remains in place while OCR revises the regulation (Keith, 2018). Regardless of the status of the regulation, however, the statute itself still prohibits discrimination on the basis of sex in health coverage and care, and numerous courts have clarified that discrimination on the basis of sexual orientation or gender identity is prohibited by federal sex nondiscrimination laws (U.S. Equal Employment Opportunity Commission, n.d.).

LGBT NONDISCRIMINATION IN THE ACA

- **Civil rights:** 42 U.S.C. § 18116 (ACA Section 1557) prohibits discrimination in any health program or activity, any part of which is receiving federal financial assistance, on the basis of race, color, national origin, age, disability, or sex.

- **Guaranteed issue:** 45 C.F.R. § 147.104(e) prohibits health insurance issuers in the individual, small group, and large group markets in any state from employing marketing practices or benefit designs that discriminate based on an individual's sexual orientation, gender identity, sex, race, color, national origin, disability, age, expected length of life, present or predicted disability, degree of medical dependency, quality of life, or other health conditions.

- **Essential health benefits:** 45 C.F.R. § 156.125(a) and (b) state that an issuer cannot claim to provide the essential health benefits as defined in Section 1302 of the Affordable Care Act if its benefit design, or the implementation of its benefit design, discriminates on the basis of an individual's sexual orientation, gender identity, sex, race, color, national origin, disability, age, expected length of life, present or predicted disability, degree of medical dependency, quality of life, or other health conditions.

- **Qualified health plans:** 45 C.F.R. § 156.200(e) states that a qualified health plan issuer must not discriminate on the basis of race, color, national origin, disability, age, sex, gender identity, or sexual orientation with respect to its qualified health plans.

- **Health insurance marketplaces:** 45 C.F.R. § 155.120(c) requires the health insurance marketplaces, including all their contractors, employees, and enrollment assisters such as navigators, to comply with all applicable nondiscrimination statutes and to not discriminate in any of their activities on the basis of race, color, national origin, disability, age, sex, gender identity, or sexual orientation.

Both the Section 1557 regulation and the ACA itself had a significant effect on the availability of health insurance coverage for transgender people in particular. Before the ACA, the majority of public and private coverage contained explicit exclusions denying transgender people coverage for a variety of services and treatments (Hong, 2002). As a result, transgender people frequently encountered denials of coverage for care that may be related to gender affirmation, such as hormone therapy and gender affirmation surgeries. They also faced denials for preventive screenings typically associated with only one sex, such as cervical Pap tests and mammograms, and sometimes for any care at all.

The 2016 OCR regulation on ACA Section 1557 clarified that transgender exclusions constitute prohibited sex discrimination in all public and private coverage subject to the ACA. Research indicates that the vast majority of plans in the federal insurance marketplace had already removed their transgender exclusions by the time of the injunction, and a subsequent study did not show that these changes were reversed following the court's action (Out2Enroll, 2017; Out2Enroll, 2018). States have also acted under the ACA and their own authority to prohibit transgender exclusions: between 2012 and 2017, insurance commissioners in 19 states and the District of Columbia issued bulletins prohibiting these exclusions in state-regulated plans (Baker, 2017). Fifteen states and D.C. similarly amended their Medicaid program rules during the same time period to affirm coverage for transition-related care.

Policies and Programs at the Federal Department of Health and Human Services

Though Congress and the White House dominate much of the news related to federal policy making, the federal executive branch agencies play a major role in policy making of all kinds. In particular, though Congress passes laws, much of the work of turning laws into functional everyday policy and practice is done by the agencies.

Under the Obama administration, HHS was particularly active in making policy related to LGBT health. The administration issued the first clear public signal of its interest in LGBT health in response to the experience of Janice Langbehn and her partner Lisa Pond: When Lisa suffered a brain aneurysm and collapsed during a family vacation to Florida in 2007, hospital staff told Janice that they were in an "anti-gay state" and barred her and the couple's three children from Lisa's bedside as she lay dying (Parker-Pope, 2009). The story began to be widely reported in the media a few years later, as a lawsuit filed by Langbehn made its way through the courts and the national movement around marriage equality for same-sex couples gathered momentum. In April 2010, President Obama issued a memorandum directing HHS to promulgate new nondiscrimination protections in family visitation for all hospitals participating in Medicare or Medicaid (Presidential Memorandum—Hospital Visitation, 2010). These protections established visitation rights for support people who do not fit narrow definitions of family, such as unmarried same- or different-sex partners, extended family members, and close friends (CMS, 2010).

The memorandum also directed the secretary of Health and Human Services to assess opportunities to address LGBT concerns through the agency's policies and programs. To fulfill this directive, then-secretary Sebelius convened the HHS LGBT Coordinating Committee composed of representatives from across the agency and initially cochaired by Assistant Secretary for Health Dr. Howard Koh, Assistant Secretary for Aging and

Administrator of the Administration on Community Living Kathy Green-lee, and Deputy General Counsel Ken Choe. Throughout the Obama administration, the committee worked with staff across the agency and with external stakeholders to initiate a wide range of policies and programs addressing LGBT health concerns. In addition to the advances in sexual orientation and gender identity data collection and research and the ACA-related nondiscrimination protections described earlier, between 2009 and 2016, the department completed the following notable achievements, among many others:

Staffing and Administration:

- Established the staff position of senior advisor for LGBT health within the Office of the Assistant Secretary for Health
- Updated the agency's equal employment opportunity policy to include sexual orientation and gender identity

Nondiscrimination Regulations:

- Promulgated a regulation requiring HHS grant recipients to abide by nondiscrimination requirements that include sexual orientation and gender identity
- Issued a policy stating that HHS employees are required to serve all people eligible for its programs, without regard to factors such as sexual orientation or gender identity

Reports and Strategies:

- Published a comprehensive report outlining the harms of sexual orientation and gender identity conversion therapy
- Addressed sexual orientation and gender identity disparities in high-profile reports and strategies such as the *National Healthcare Disparities Report, Women's Health USA*, the *Health Disparities and Inequalities Report*, and the *HHS Action Plan to Reduce Racial and Ethnic Health Disparities*
- Published numerous reports and briefs on health and human services issues affecting LGBT populations, particularly youth and elders
- Added new objectives to the Healthy People 2020 LGBT health topic area

Cultural Competency and Outreach:

- Incorporated sexual orientation and gender identity into the Culturally and Linguistically Appropriate Services (CLAS) Standards

- Promulgated a regulation requiring entities funded under the Runaway and Homeless Youth Act to be culturally competent in serving LGBTQ populations
- Conducted specific outreach to LGBT communities about affordable health insurance coverage options under the Affordable Care Act
- Convened listening sessions with the Indian Health Service on Native LGBT and Two Spirit issues
- Established a committee to promote LGBT cultural competency training modules

Research and Resources:

- Funded the establishment of the National Resource Center on LGBT Aging
- Established the Special Projects of National Significance "Enhancing Engagement and Retention in Quality HIV Care for Transgender Women of Color" Initiative
- Funded the establishment of the National LGBT Health Education Center to help community health centers serve LGBT patients

A fuller picture of the agency's LGBT health activities during the Obama administration, including the LGBT Coordinating Committee's annual reports outlining the previous year's priorities and laying out objectives for the next year between 2011 and 2016, can be found at www.hhs.gov/lgbt. Reflecting the policy paradigm of "health in all policies," it is important to note that many other federal executive branch agencies such as the Departments of Justice, Education, Labor, Agriculture, Homeland Security, Defense, and Housing and Urban Development, as well as the Veterans Administration and the Presidential Office of Personnel Management, also had active roles in policy making affecting LGBT health under the Obama administration and beyond.

LGBT FEDERAL HEALTH POLICY AFTER 2016

The election of President Trump in 2016 ushered in significant potential for changes in federal policy related to LGBT population health. As noted earlier, the administration gave early indications that it intended to roll back data collection on sexual orientation and gender identity on surveys such as the American Community Survey and the National Survey of Older Americans Act Participants. The administration also appointed a number of outspokenly anti-LGBT officials to senior staff positions, including Roger Severino as the director of the Office for Civil Rights at HHS

(National Public Radio, 2018). Director Severino, who formerly headed the DeVos Center for Religion and Civil Society at the Heritage Foundation, oversaw the launch of a new division within OCR in January 2018 to focus on enforcing federal laws that grant exemptions and protections to health care providers who claim a religious or moral objection to specific services (HHS, 2018). At the same time, OCR released a new proposed regulation that dramatically widened the scope of the agency's enforcement of religious exemption protections (HHS, 2018). These exemptions have often been associated with restrictions on abortion access, and critics of the new division noted that it may also hinder access to health care services commonly needed by LGBT people, such as care related to gender transition, fertility treatments for same-sex couples, and sexual health services such as HIV pre-exposure prophylaxis (Diamond, 2018).

On the legislative front, throughout 2017 the administration worked with the Republican congressional majority to enact legislation that would have amended substantial parts of the ACA. In late 2017, Congress passed Public Law No. 115-97, commonly known as the Tax Cuts and Jobs Act, which eliminated the ACA's individual insurance mandate. A 2017 analysis from the Congressional Budget Office (CBO) estimated that this change would be associated with 13 million people losing coverage by 2027 (CBO, 2017). Such an increase in uninsurance is a significant concern for the many LGBT people still struggling to access coverage: uninsurance across the entire LGBT population stood at 15 percent in 2017, compared to 7 percent among the general population aged 18 to 64 (Baker et al., 2017).

The Trump administration and Congress alone, however, do not determine the direction or impact of policy that affects LGBT health. Though this chapter has focused on federal LGBT health policy, many other government actors—including states, counties, Native American tribes, municipalities, and international entities—as well as private stakeholders play a significant role in designing policy and running programs that affect the health and well-being of LGBT communities. Regardless of the level at which it happens, policy making that seeks to understand and address LGBT disparities is critical to securing the health, safety, and well-being of LGBT people, families, and communities.

NOTES

1. In 2013, the diagnosis of gender dysphoria replaced Gender Identity Disorder (GID) in the DSM-5.

2. DHEW became the Department of Health and Human Services (HHS) in 1980.

3. The law technically leaves the definition of the term "minority" to the discretion of the director of NIH, but the statute and subsequent NIH guidance focus on

racial and ethnic minorities. NIH expanded this policy to include children in 1998, and in 2001 the policy with regard to women and racial and ethnic minorities was updated by the Minority Health and Health Disparities Research and Education Act (P.L. 106-525). This law also created the National Center for Minority Health and Health Disparities at NIH, required the Agency for Healthcare Research and Quality at HHS to conduct research on minority health and health disparities, and commissioned a report from the National Academy of Sciences regarding HHS-wide data collection on racial and ethnic minority health.

4. Nancy Krieger cites the example of the debate that began in the 1830s and 1840s about the poor health of black Americans: "Contrary schools of thought [asked]: is it because blacks are intrinsically inferior to whites?—the majority view, or because they are enslaved?" See Krieger, N. (2001). Theories for social epidemiology in the 21st century: an ecosocial perspective. *International Journal of Epidemiology, 30,* 668–677.

5. Crenshaw's work, which focuses on the example of the discrimination against black women that occurs at the intersections of race and sex, builds on more than a century of black feminist thought; see e.g., the speech by Sojourner Truth, "Ain't I a Woman?", delivered at a women's rights convention in 1851; Frances Beale's essay "Double Jeopardy: To Be Black and Female" (1969); and Angela Davis's *Women, Race, and Class* (1981).

6. The Tri-Caucus is comprised of the Congressional Black Caucus, the Congressional Hispanic Caucus, and the Congressional Asian Pacific American Caucus.

7. The law specified a threshold of 133 percent FPL, with a 5 percent income disregard, which makes the threshold functionally 138 percent of the FPL.

REFERENCES

21st Century Cures Act. (2016). Public Law 114-255.

Act to provide for reconciliation pursuant to titles II and V of the concurrent resolution on the budget for fiscal year 2018 ["Tax Cuts and Jobs Act"]. (2017). Public Law 115-97.

Administration for Children and Families. (2016). Runaway and homeless youth. *Federal Register, 81,* 93030–93064.

Agency for Healthcare Research and Quality. (2013). Priority populations. In *National healthcare disparities report.* Washington, DC: U.S. Department of Health and Human Services.

AIDS Action Council. (2004). Policy facts: Early Treatment for HIV Act. Retrieved from http://www.thebody.com/content/art33771.html

American Psychiatric Association. (1952). *Diagnostic and statistical manual of mental disorders.* Washington, DC: American Psychiatric Association.

Baker, K. E. (2016). LGBT protections in Affordable Care Act Section 1557. Retrieved from http://healthaffairs.org/blog/2016/06/06/lgbt-protections-in-affordable-care-act-section-1557

Baker, K. E. (2017). The future of transgender health coverage. *New England Journal of Medicine, 376*(19), 1801–1804.

Baker, K. E., & Durso, L. E. (2017). Why repealing the Affordable Care Act is bad medicine for LGBT communities. Retrieved from https://www.american progress.org/issues/lgbt/news/2017/03/22/428970/repealing-affordable -care-act-bad-medicine-lgbt-communities/

Baker, K. E., Durso, L. E., & Ridings, A. M. (2016). *How to collect data about LGBT communities.* Washington, DC: Center for American Progress.

Baker, K. E., & Hughes, M. (2016). *Sexual orientation and gender identity data collection in the behavioral risk factor surveillance system.* Washington, DC: Center for American Progress.

Baker, K. E., McGovern, A., Gruberg, S., & Cray, A. (2016). *The Medicaid program and LGBT communities: Overview and policy recommendations.* Washington, DC: Center for American Progress.

Baker, K. E., Singh, S., Mirza, S. A., & Durso, L. E. (2017) *The Senate health care bill would be devastating for LGBTQ people.* Washington, DC: Center for American Progress.

Baral, S. D., Poteat, T., Strömdahl, S., Wirtz, A. L., Guadamuz, T. E., & Beyrer, C. (2013). Worldwide burden of HIV in transgender women: A systematic review and meta-analysis. *Lancet, 13*(3), 214–222.

Braveman, P. A., Cubbin, C., Egerter, S., Williams, D. R., & Pamuk, E. (2010). Socio-economic disparities in health in the United States: What the patterns tell us. *American Journal of Public Health, 100*(Supplement 1), S186–196.

Braveman, P. A., Kumanyika, S., Fielding, J., LaVeist, T., Borrell, L. N., Manderschied, R., & Troutman, A. (2011). Health disparities and health equity: The issue is justice. *American Journal of Public Health, 101*(Supplement 1), S149–155.

Butler, S. M. (1989). *Assuring affordable health care for all Americans.* Washington, DC: The Heritage Foundation.

Centers for Disease Control and Prevention. (2011). CDC health disparities and inequalities report—United States, 2011. *Morbidity and Mortality Weekly Report, 60*(Supplement), 1–109.

Centers for Disease Control and Prevention. (2015). HIV among gay and bisexual men. Retrieved from http://www.cdc.gov/hiv/group/msm/

Centers for Medicare & Medicaid Services. (n.d.). National Survey of Older Americans Act Participants (NSOAAP): Years survey included sexual and gender minority (SGM)-related questions 2014–2016. Retrieved from https://www.cms.gov/About-CMS/Agency-Information/OMH/Downloads /SGM-Clearinghouse-NSOAAP.pdf

Centers for Medicare & Medicaid Services. (2010). Changes to the hospital and critical access hospital conditions of participation to ensure visitation rights for all patients. *Federal Register, 74,* 70831–70844.

Centers for Medicare & Medicaid Services. (2015). Medicare and Medicaid programs; Electronic Health Record Incentive Program—Stage 3 and modifications to meaningful use in 2015 through 2017. *Federal Register, 80,* 62761–62955.

Centers for Medicare & Medicaid Services, Center for Consumer Information and Insurance Oversight. (2014). Retrieved from https://www.cms.gov /CCIIO/Resources/Regulations-and-Guidance/Downloads/frequently -asked-questions-on-coverage-of-same-sex-spouses.pdf

Clews, C. (2014). HIV/AIDS: Why was AIDS called "the gay plague"? Retrieved from http://www.gayinthe80s.com/2014/04/1980s-hivaids-why-was-aids -called-the-gay-plague

Co-Chairs of the HHS LGBT Issues Coordinating Committee. (2016). LGBT health: Celebrating our progress and looking ahead. Retrieved from https://wayback.archive-it.org/8315/20170119102751/https://www.hhs .gov/blog/2016/06/09/lgbt-health-celebrating-our-progress-and-looking -ahead.html

Congressional Budget Office. (2017). Repealing the Individual Health Insurance Mandate: An updated estimate. Retrieved from https://www.cbo.gov /system/files/115th-congress-2017-2018/reports/53300-individualman date.pdf

Coulter, R. W., Kenst, K. S., Bowen, D. J., & Scout. (2014). Research funded by the National Institutes of Health on the health of lesbian, gay, bisexual, and transgender populations. *American Journal of Public Health, 104*(2), e105–112.

Crenshaw, K. (1989). Demarginalizing the intersection of race and sex: A black feminist critique of antidiscrimination doctrine, feminist theory and anti-racist politics. *University of Chicago Legal Forum*, 1, 139–167.

Crimp, D., & Rolston, A. (1990). *AIDS demographics.* Seattle: Bay Press.

DeSalvo, K. (2016). LGBT Health Awareness Week—Addressing LGBT health disparities across the board. Retrieved from https://wayback.archive-it.org /8315/20170119083141/https://www.hhs.gov/blog/2016/03/28/addressing -lgbt-health-disparities-across-the-board.html

Devor, A., & Matte, N. (2007). Building a better world for transpeople: Reed Erickson and the Erickson Educational Foundation. *International Journal of Transgenderism, 10*(1), 47–68.

Diamond, D. (2018). Trump administration dismantles LGBT-friendly policies. Retrieved from https://www.politico.com/story/2018/02/19/trump-lgbt -rights-discrimination-353774

Division of Health Interview Statistics. (2014). *A brief quality assessment of the NHIS sexual orientation data.* Centers for Disease Control and Prevention, National Center for Health Statistics. Hyattsville: U.S. Department of Health and Human Services.

Dragon, C. N., Guerino, P., Ewald, E., & Laffan, A. M. (2017). Transgender Medicare beneficiaries and chronic conditions: Exploring fee-for-service claims data. *LGBT Health, 4*(6), 404–411.

Durso, L. E., Baker, K. E., & Cray, A. S. (2013). *LGBT communities and the Affordable Care Act: Findings from a national survey.* Washington, DC: Center for American Progress.

Ending LGBT Health Disparities Act, H.R. 3001 (111th Congress, 2009).

Epstein, S. (1996). *Impure science: AIDS, activism, and the politics of knowledge.* Berkeley: University of California Press.

Epstein, S. (2007). Targeting the state: Risks, benefits, and strategic dilemmas of recent LGBT health advocacy. In I. H. Meyer & M. E. Northridge (Eds.), *The health of sexual minorities: Public health perspectives on lesbian, gay, bisexual, and transgender populations* (pp. 149–168). New York: Springer.

Farmer, P. (1999). *Infections and inequalities: The modern plagues.* Berkeley: University of California Press.

Federal Interagency Working Group on Improving Measurement of Sexual Orientation and Gender Identity in Federal Surveys. (2016, August). *Current measures of sexual orientation and gender identity in federal surveys.* Retrieved from https://s3.amazonaws.com/sitesusa/wp-content/uploads/sites/242/2014/04/WorkingGroupPaper1_CurrentMeasures_08-16.pdf

Federal Interagency Working Group on Improving Measurement of Sexual Orientation and Gender Identity in Federal Surveys. (2016, September). *Evaluations of sexual orientation and gender identity survey measures: What have we learned?* Retrieved from https://s3.amazonaws.com/sitesusa/wp-content/uploads/sites/242/2014/04/Evaluations_of_SOGI_Questions_20160923.pdf

Federal Interagency Working Group on Improving Measurement of Sexual Orientation and Gender Identity in Federal Surveys. (2016, October). *Toward a research agenda for measuring sexual orientation and gender identity in federal surveys: Findings, recommendations, and next steps.* Retrieved from https://s3.amazonaws.com/sitesusa/wp-content/uploads/sites/242/2014/04/SOGI_Research_Agenda_Final_Report_20161020.pdf

Franciscan Alliance, Inc. v. Burwell, no. 7:16-cv-00108-o (N.D. Tex. Dec. 31, 2016).

Friedlander, E. (n.d.). Rudolf Virchow on pathology education. Retrieved from http://www.pathguy.com/virchow.htm

Gamble, V. N., & Stone, D. (2006). U.S. policy on health inequities: the interplay of politics and research. *Journal of Health Politics, Policy, and Law, 31*(1), 93–126.

Gates, G. J. (2014). In U.S., LGBT more likely to be uninsured than non-LGBT. Gallup Well-Being. Retrieved from https://news.gallup.com/poll/175445/lgbt-likely-non-lgbt-uninsured.aspx

Gates, G. J. (2017). In U.S., More adults identifying as LGBT. Retrieved from http://news.gallup.com/poll/201731/lgbt-identification-rises.aspx

Gay and Lesbian Medical Association and LGBT Health Experts. (2001). *Healthy people 2010 companion document for lesbian, gay, bisexual, and transgender (LGBT) health.* San Francisco: Gay and Lesbian Medical Association.

Green, R. (1976). Healthcare and justice in contract theory perspective. In R. Veatch & R. Branson (Eds.), *Ethics and health policy* (pp. 111–126). Cambridge: Ballinger.

Hall, P. A. (1993). Policy paradigms, social learning, and the state: The case of economic policymaking in Britain. *Comparative Politics, 25*(3), 275–296.

Health Data Collection Improvement Act, H.R. 6109 (111th Congress, 2010).

Health Equity and Accountability Act, H.R. 3090 (111th Congress, 2009).

Health Resources and Services Administration. (2011a). SPNS Initiative: Enhancing engagement and retention in quality HIV care for transgender women of color, 2012–2017. Retrieved from http://hab.hrsa.gov/abouthab/special/transgenderwomen.html

Health Resources and Services Administration. (2011b). *Women's health USA.* Washington, DC: U.S. Department of Health and Human Services.

Health Resources and Services Administration. (2014). Transgender people. Retrieved from http://hab.hrsa.gov/abouthab/populations/transgenderfacts 2012.pdf

Health Resources and Services Administration. (2016). Proposed uniform data system changes for calendar year 2016. Retrieved from http://bphc.hrsa .gov/datareporting/pdf/pal201601.pdf

Heckler, M. M. (1985). *Report of the Secretary's Task Force on Black and Minority Health.* U.S. Department of Health and Human Services. Washington, DC: Government Printing Office.

Hong, K. E. (2002). Categorical exclusions: Exploring legal responses to health care discrimination against transsexuals. *Columbia Journal of Gender and Law, 11*(88).

Hunter, N. D. (2000). Sexuality and civil rights: Re-imagining anti-discrimination laws. *New York Law School Journal of Human Rights, 17,* 565–587.

Institute of Medicine. (2013). *U.S. health in international perspective: Shorter lives, poorer health.* Washington, DC: National Academies Press.

Institute of Medicine Committee on Lesbian, Gay, Bisexual, and Transgender Health Issues and Research Gaps and Opportunities. (2011). *The health of lesbian, gay, bisexual, and transgender people: Building a foundation for better understanding.* Washington, DC: National Academies Press.

Institute of Medicine Committee on Lesbian Health Research Priorities. (1999). *Lesbian health: Current assessment and directions for the future.* (A. L. Solarz, Ed.) Washington, DC: National Academies Press.

Jin, F., Crawford, J., Prestage, G. P., Zablotska, I., Imrie, J., Kippax, S. C., . . . Grulich, A. E. (2009). HIV risk reduction behaviours in gay men: Unprotected anal intercourse, risk reduction behaviours, and subsequent HIV infection in a cohort of homosexual men. *AIDS, 23*(2), 243–252.

Kaiser Commission on Medicaid and the Uninsured. (2009). *Where are states today? Medicaid and state-funded coverage eligibility levels for low-income adults.* Washington, DC: Kaiser Family Foundation.

Kaiser Commission on Medicaid and the Uninsured. (2011). *Holding steady, looking ahead: Annual findings of a 50-state survey of eligibility rules, enrollment and renewal procedures, and cost sharing practices in Medicaid and CHIP, 2010–2011.* Washington, DC: Kaiser Family Foundation.

Kaiser Family Foundation. (2018a). Current status of state Medicaid expansion decisions. Retrieved from http://kff.org/health-reform/slide/current-status -of-the-medicaid-expansion-decision

Kaiser Family Foundation. (2018b). State health insurance marketplace types, 2016. Retrieved from http://kff.org/health-reform/state-indicator/state -health-insurance-marketplace-types

Keith, K. (2018). ACA round-up: Section 1557 rule on horizon; CSR and Medicaid litigation updates; focus on employer mandate. Retrieved from https:// www.healthaffairs.org/do/10.1377/hblog20180219.671383/full

Kimmel, M. (1996). *Manhood in America: A cultural history.* New York: The Free Press.

Kreider, R., Bates, N., & Mayol-García, Y. (2017). *Improving measurement of same-sex couple households in Census Bureau surveys: Results from recent tests.* Retrieved from https://www.census.gov/content/dam/Census/library/working-papers/2017/demo/SEHSD-WP2017-28.pdf

Krieger, N. (1994). Epidemiology and the web of causation: has anyone seen the spider? *Social Science and Medicine, 39*(7), 887–903.

Krieger, N. (1999). Embodying inequality: a review of concepts, measures, and methods for studying health consequences of discrimination. *International Journal of Health Services, 29,* 295–352.

Krieger, N. (2001). Theories for social epidemiology in the 21st century: an ecosocial perspective. *International Journal of Epidemiology, 30,* 668–677.

Krieger, N., & Bassett, M. (1986). The health of black folk: Disease, class and ideology of science. *Monthly Review, 38*(3), 161–169.

Lawrence v. Texas, 539 U.S. 558, 123 S. Ct. 2472, 156 L. Ed. 2d 508 (2003).

Leclair, D. (2008). The road To ENDA: A brief timeline. Retrieved from http://www.ifge.org/?q=node/360

Leighton, J. E. (2013). *Freedom indivisible: Gays and lesbians in the African American civil rights movement.* (Doctoral dissertation). Retrieved from https://digitalcommons.unl.edu/cgi/viewcontent.cgi?article=1061&context=historydiss

Lewis, G. B. (1997). Lifting the ban on gays in the Civil Service: Federal policy toward gay and lesbian employees since the Cold War. *Public Administration Review, 57*(5), 387–395.

LGBT Data Inclusion Act, S. 3134 (114th Congress, 2016).

Lorde, A. (1980). *The cancer journals.* San Francisco: Aunt Lute Books.

Mail, P. D., & Lear, W. J. (2006). The role of public health in lesbian, gay, bisexual, and transgender health. In M. Shankle (Ed.), *The handbook of lesbian, gay, bisexual, and transgender public health: A practitioner's guide to service.* New York: The Haworth Press.

Medicare Access and CHIP Reauthorization Act. (2015). Public Law 114-10.

Meyerowitz, J. (2004). *How sex changed: A history of transsexuality in the United States.* Boston: Harvard University Press.

Minton, H. L. (2002). *Departing from deviance: A history of homosexual rights and emancipatory science in America.* Chicago: University of Chicago Press.

Morabia, A. (2017). American Journal of Public Health dossier on the erasure of the sexual orientation question from the National Survey of Older Americans Act participants. *American Journal of Public Health, 107*(8), 1203–1204.

Myers, J. (2013). *Historical dictionary of the lesbian and gay liberation movements.* New York: The Scarecrow Press.

National Center for Transgender Equality. (2016a). ID documents center. Retrieved from http://www.transequality.org/documents

National Center for Transgender Equality. (2016b). Transgender terminology. Retrieved from https://transequality.org/issues/resources/understanding-transgender-people-the-basics

National Federation of Independent Business v. Sebelius, 567 U.S. 519 (2012).

National Institutes of Health. (2001). Behavioral, social, mental health, and substance abuse research with diverse populations. Retrieved from http://grants.nih.gov/grants/guide/pa-files/PA-01-096.html

National Institutes of Health Sexual and Gender Minority Research Coordinating Committee. (2015). *NIH FY 2016–2020 strategic plan to advance research on the health and well-being of sexual and gender minorities.* Retrieved from https://dpcpsi.nih.gov/sgmro/reports

National Public Radio. (2018). Reporter says anti-abortion, anti-LGBTQ activists are shaping federal policy. Retrieved from https://www.npr.org/2018/01/25/580622864/reporter-says-anti-abortion-anti-lgbtq-activists-are-shaping-federal-policy

Neel, L. (2016). IHS hosts third public meeting to address LGBT2-S health issues. Retrieved from https://www.ihs.gov/newsroom/ihs-blog/may2016/ihs-hosts-third-public-meeting-to-address-lgbt2-s-health-issues

Obergefell v. Hodges, 576 U.S. ___ (2015).

Office of Applied Studies. (2010). Substance abuse treatment programs for gays and lesbians. Retrieved from http://media.samhsa.gov/data/spotlight/Spotlight004GayLesbians.pdf

Office of Planning, Research, and Evaluation. (2015). *LGBT populations: A snapshot of the knowledge base and research needs.* Retrieved from https://www.acf.hhs.gov/opre/resource/lgbt-populations-a-snapshot-of-the-knowledge-base-and-research-needs

Office of the Secretary of Health and Human Services. (2015). Edition health information technology (Health IT) certification criteria, 2015 edition base electronic health record (EHR) definition, and ONC health IT certification program modifications. *Federal Register, 80*, pp. 62601–62759.

Osuch, J. R., Silk, K., Price, C., Barlow, J., Miller, K., Hernick, A., & Fonfa, A. (2012). A historical perspective on breast cancer activism in the United States: From education and support to partnership in scientific research. *Journal of Women's Health, 21*(3), 355–362.

Out2Enroll. (2017). *Summary of findings: 2017 marketplace plan compliance with Section 1557.* Retrieved from https://out2enroll.org/out2enroll/wp-content/uploads/2015/10/Report-on-Trans-Exclusions-in-2017-Marketplace-Plans.pdf

Out2Enroll. (2018). *Summary of findings: 2018 marketplace plan compliance with Section 1557.* Retrieved from https://out2enroll.org/out2enroll/wp-content/uploads/2017/11/Overview-of-Trans-Exclusions-in-2018-Marketplace-Plans-1.pdf

Parker-Pope, T. (2009, May 18). Kept from a dying partner's bedside. *New York Times.*

Patient Protection and Affordable Care Act. (2010). Public Law 111-148.

Pérez-Stable, Eliseo J. (2016, October). *Sexual and gender minorities formally designated as a health disparity population for research purposes.* Retrieved from https://www.nimhd.nih.gov/about/directors-corner/message.html

Poteat, T. (2015). *Transgender people and HIV.* Geneva: World Health Organization.

Presidential Memorandum—Hospital Visitation. (2010). Retrieved from https://obamawhitehouse.archives.gov/the-press-office/presidential-memorandum-hospital-visitation

Proctor, K., Haffer, S. C., Ewald, E., Hodge, C., & James, C. V. (2016). Identifying the transgender population in the Medicare program. *Transgender Health, 1*(1), 250–265.

Satcher, D. (2010). Include a social determinants of health approach to reduce health inequities. *Public Health Report, 125*(Supplement 4), 6–7.

Scout. (2013). How far has LGBT health research progressed since Bush-era 'big chill'? Retrieved from http://www.huffingtonpost.com/scout-phd/how-far -have-we-come-in-l_b_4468902.html

Sebelius, K. (2011). Speech to the National Coalition for LGBT Health. Retrieved from https://wayback.archive-it.org/3924/20150211172934/http://www.hhs .gov/secretary/about/speeches/2011/sp20111017.html

Sell, R. (n.d.). Retrieved from http://www.lgbtdata.com

Shilts, R. (1987). *And the band played on.* New York: St. Martin's Press.

Singh, S., Durso L. E., & Tax, A. (2017). The Trump administration is rolling back data collection on LGBT older adults. Retrieved from https://www.american progress.org/issues/lgbt/news/2017/03/20/428623/trump-administration -rolling-back-data-collection-lgbt-older-adults

Ståhl, T., Wismar, M., Ollila, E., Lahtinen, E., & Leppo, K. (Eds.). (2006). *Health in all policies: Prospects and potentials.* Finland: Finnish Ministry of Social Affairs and Health.

Substance Abuse and Mental Health Services Administration. (2001). *A provider's introduction to substance abuse treatment for lesbian, gay, bisexual, and transgender individuals.* Washington, DC: U.S. Department of Health and Human Services.

Substance Abuse and Mental Health Services Administration. (2015a). *Ending conversion therapy: Supporting and affirming LGBTQ youth.* Retrieved from https://store.samhsa.gov/shin/content/SMA15-4928/SMA15-4928.pdf

Substance Abuse and Mental Health Services Administration. (2015b). LGBT training curricula for behavioral health and primary care practitioners. Retrieved from http://www.samhsa.gov/behavioral-health-equity/lgbt/curricula

Sylvia Rivera Law Project. (2016). Who was Sylvia Rivera? Retrieved from http:// srlp.org/about/who-was-sylvia-rivera

U.S. Census Bureau. (2010). Income, poverty, and health insurance coverage in the United States: 2010. Retrieved from https://www.census.gov/prod/2011 pubs/p60-239.pdf

U.S. Department of Health and Human Services (HHS). (1985). Report of the Public Health Service Task Force on Women's Health Issues. *Public Health Report, 100*(1), 73–106.

U.S. Department of Health and Human Services. (1990). *Healthy People 2000: National health promotion and disease prevention objectives.* Washington, DC: Government Printing Office.

U.S. Department of Health and Human Services. (2000). *Healthy people 2010.* Washington, DC: Government Printing Office.

U.S. Department of Health and Human Services. (2001). *Strategic plan on addressing health disparities related to sexual orientation.* On file with the author.

U.S. Department of Health and Human Services. (2010a). Healthy people 2020: Disparities. Retrieved from https://www.healthypeople.gov/2020/about /foundation-health-measures/Disparities

U.S. Department of Health and Human Services. (2010b). Lesbian, gay, bisexual, and transgender health. Retrieved from https://www.healthypeople.gov /2020/topics-objectives/topic/lesbian-gay-bisexual-and-transgender -health

U.S. Department of Health and Human Services. (2015). HHS partners with LGBT organizations to promote open enrollment activities during LGBT week of action. Retrieved from https://www.enewspf.com/latest-news /health-care-reform/hhs-partners-with-lgbt-organizations-to-promote -open-enrollment-activities-during-lgbt-week-of-action

U.S. Department of Health and Human Services. (2016a). Equal employment opportunity policy. Retrieved from https://www.hhs.gov/about/agencies /asa/eeo/policy/index.html

U.S. Department of Health and Human Services. (2016b). Health and Human Services Grants Regulation: 45 CFR Part 75. Retrieved from https://www.gpo .gov/fdsys/pkg/FR-2016-12-12/pdf/2016-29752.pdf

U.S. Department of Health and Human Services. (2016c). Nondiscrimination in health programs and activities: Final rule. *Federal Register, 81,* 31375–31473.

U.S. Department of Health and Human Services. (2016d). Poverty guidelines. Retrieved from https://aspe.hhs.gov/poverty-guidelines

U.S. Department of Health and Human Services. (2016e). Transgender health care. Retrieved from https://www.healthcare.gov/transgender-health-care

U.S. Department of Health & Human Services. (2018a). Conscience and religious freedom. Retrieved from https://www.hhs.gov/conscience

U.S. Department of Health & Human Services. (2018b). Protecting statutory conscience rights in health care; Delegations of authority. *Federal Register, 83,* pp. 3880–3931.

U.S. Department of Health and Human Services. (n.d.). Non-discrimination policy statement. Retrieved from http://web.archive.org/web/20111015061127 /http:/www.hhs.gov/asa/eeo/nondiscrimination/index.html

U.S. Department of Health and Human Services Departmental Appeals Board. (2014). NCD 140.3, Transsexual Surgery, Docket No. A-13-87, Decision No. 2576.

U.S. Department of Health and Human Services LGBT Issues Coordinating Committee. (2016). *Advancing LGBT health and well-being.* Retrieved from https://www.hhs.gov/programs/topic-sites/lgbt/reports/index.html

U.S. Equal Employment Opportunity Commission. (n.d.). Examples of court decisions supporting coverage of LGBT-related discrimination under title VII. Retrieved from https://www.eeoc.gov/eeoc/newsroom/wysk/lgbt_examples _decisions.cfm

U.S. Office of Minority Health. (2011a). *Action plan to reduce racial and ethnic health disparities.* Washington, DC: U.S. Department of Health and Human Services.

U.S. Office of Minority Health. (2011b). Improving data collection for the LGBT community. Retrieved from http://minorityhealth.hhs.gov/omh/browse .aspx?lvl=3&lvlid=57

U.S. Office of Minority Health. (2013). National standards for culturally and linguistically appropriate services in health and health care: A blueprint for advancing and sustaining CLAS policy and practice. Retrieved from

https://www.thinkculturalhealth.hhs.gov/pdfs/EnhancedCLASStandards
Blueprint.pdf

U.S. Surgeon General. (1979). *Healthy People: The surgeon general's report on health promotion and disease prevention.* Washington, DC: U.S. Department of Health, Education, and Welfare.

United States v. Windsor, 570 U.S. ___ (2013).

Wallace, S. P., Torres, J. M., Nobari, T. Z., & Pourat, N. (2013). *Undocumented and uninsured: Barriers to affordable care for immigrant populations.* Washington, DC: The Commonwealth Fund.

Wang, H. L. (2017). Census Bureau caught in political mess over LGBT data. *National Public Radio.* Retrieved from https://www.npr.org/2017/07/18/536484467/census-bureau-found-no-need-for-lgbt-data-despite-4-agencies-requesting-it

The White House. (2010). *National HIV/AIDS strategy for the United States.*

Whitehead, M. (1992). The concepts and principles of equity and health. *International Journal of Health Services, 22*(3), 429–445.

Wilkinson, R., & Marmot, M. (Eds.). (2003). *Social determinants of health: The solid facts.* Denmark: World Health Organization.

World Health Organization. (1948). Constitution of the World Health Organization. Geneva.

World Health Organization. (2011). Rio political declaration on social determinants of health. *World Conference on Social Determinants of Health.* Rio de Janeiro. Retrieved from https://www.who.int/sdhconference/declaration/en/

World Health Organization. (2013). *Health in All Policies (HiAP) framework for country action.* Geneva.

World Health Organization Commission on Social Determinants of Health. (2008). *Closing the gap in a generation: health equity through action on the social determinants of health.* Geneva.

2

Interactions between Culture, Race, and Sexuality in Health

David J. Malebranche and LaRon E. Nelson

> I really hope no white person ever has cause to write about me because they never understand Black love is Black wealth and they'll probably talk about my hard childhood and never understand that all the while I was quite happy.
>
> —Nikki Giovanni

In the past 40 years, we have seen remarkable cultural and political advances in lesbian, bisexual, gay, and transgendered (LGBT) health issues. In the early 1980s, the LGBT community mobilized on political, cultural, and health-related levels to address the HIV/AIDS epidemic. As time has moved on and further barriers in LGBT political rights and HIV prevention/treatment continue to be broken, the time has come to conceptualize LGBT health in terms that transcend HIV-centered models of pathology and illness and the hopeless repetition of the need to overcome "barriers" to illness and disease. Health initiatives that address specific LGBT-related concerns should be rooted in an acknowledgment of the fundamental social and structural issues underlying health outcomes while we also emphasize factors that encourage health and wellness. A key aspect of this acknowledgment is that LGBT health is not a universal concept without consideration of larger contexts of race, ethnicity, and culture that undeniably shape sexual orientation and expression as well as health experiences and outcomes. This chapter highlights how fundamental realities of race, ethnicity, and culture fluidly intersect with sexual desire, expression, and gender identity to impact the health of LGBT people in the United States.

CONCEPTUALIZING LGBT HEALTH: THE ROLE OF RACE AND CULTURE

Indeed, the current focus on LGBT health emerged most recently out of a context of extraordinary mobilization of efforts to survive a deadly HIV epidemic but also other health disparities, including adverse mental health, suicide, and hate crimes (Herek, 1989, 2009). This has resulted in many calling for federal, regional, and state-level initiatives targeting LGBT health (Mayer et al., 2001, 2008; Northridge, 2001; Epstein, 2003; Fikar and Keith, 2004), with some success in the development and sustainment of centers of LGBT health (Mayer et al., 2008). Survey research has supported the academic call for these initiatives, larger public support, and the need for increased LGBT sensitivity training, sexual history taking and cultural competency initiatives for medical personnel (Wilkerson, Rybicki, Barber, & Smolenski, 2011). Recent national surveys indicate that marriage equality, antigay discrimination, and HIV/AIDS are top priorities for LGBT populations in general (Battle & Crum, 2007). In order for any national list of LGBT health priorities to be wholly comprehensive and inclusive, however, it will have to address other variables that influence health among LGBT people who experience additional marginalization based on race/ethnicity, culture, and class, which are often overlooked in broader LGBT health discussions.

Historically, discussions of the intersection of race, ethnicity, and culture with LGBT health have narrowly focused on reports of higher rates of individual-level HIV-related risk behaviors among "people of color," often without consideration of larger social and structural contexts (MacWilliams-Brooks, 2008). This is particularly evident when discussing current racial disparities among Black men who have sex with men (MSM) and the HIV epidemic (Millett, Peterson, Wolitski, & Stall, 2006) but also is applicable to studies describing general sexual risk behavior, smoking, suicidal ideation, and poor mental health (Mimiaga et al., 2010). For instance, it is often speculated that higher rates of unprotected anal sex and multiple sexual partners among black MSM compared with other MSM contribute to the HIV racial disparity, but these assumptions are not supported in the research literature (Millett, Flores, Peterson, & Bakeman, 2007; Millett et al., 2006). Moreover, gay/bisexual men exhibit a higher prevalence of eating disorders compared to their heterosexual counterparts (Feldman & Meyer, 2007), and high rates of smoking, binge drinking, early pregnancy, and depression are often found among LGBT samples (Cochran, Mays, Alegria, Ortega, & Takeuchi, 2007; Herrick, Matthews, & Garofalo, 2010; Washington, 2002). Additionally, a small study of Native American two-spirited persons noted a higher prevalence of childhood sexual abuse and trauma, more psychological symptoms, use of mental health facilities, and alcohol/drug use than their heterosexual counterparts (Balsam, Molina, Beadnell, Simoni, & Walters, 2004). Studies like these are often presented in such a way as to implicate race and cultural behavior as the likely explanation for current health disparities. Unfortunately, this is often typical of the evidence base that medical and public health officials rely on, in part, to inform the ways in which we understand patients (McNair and Hegarty, 2010; Schulman et al., 1999). Clinician consumers of research must exercise caution against too easily accepting research interpretations of why these disparities persist, particularly when evidence exists for larger medical institutional and interpersonal dynamics impacting healthcare (Schulman et al., 1999). Furthermore, some have suggested that race is a purely social construction and there is very little clinically relevant genetic variation between people who have been categorized into different groups based on the color of their skin (Graves, 2011; Jorde & Wooding, 2004; Mountain & Risch, 2004; Parra, Kittles, & Shriver, 2004).

While many studies highlight overall LGBT behavioral outcomes with little consideration of diversity in race, ethnicity, and culture, there are some studies that incorporate analysis of this variety but often only highlight negative mental and physical health outcomes. For example, in an earlier study of African American and Latina women, minority sexual orientation (nonheterosexual) was associated with increased sexual risk behavior and less utilization or preventive health care services (Mays, Yancey, Cochran, Weber, & Fielding, 2002). In another study with Asian Pacific Islander (API)/Guam young adolescents, same-sex orientation was associated with higher risk of suicide attempts than their heterosexual counterparts (Pinhey & Millman, 2004). HIV-positive Black gay/bisexual men are more likely to have unprotected sex than their white counterparts, but not their Black heterosexual counterparts (Siegel, Schrimshaw, & Karus, 2004), and among a predominantly lower-income sample of Black HIV-positive women, those who were nonheterosexually identified were more likely to have unprotected sex, report income from sex work, and feel that community services neglected their needs than their heterosexual counterparts (Teti et al., 2008). In racially diverse LGBT samples of substance users (Senreich, 2010) and HIV-positive (Schuster et al., 2005) individuals, white participants reported less satisfaction and connection with community services as well as higher rates of perceived discrimination than their Black and Latino counterparts. Finally, among 106 participants from a Web-based survey, internalized racism and heterosexism were significant predictors of low self-esteem, but only internalized heterosexism was a predictor of psychological distress (Szymanski & Gupta, 2009).

What can we learn from these studies? First, there are different approaches to conduct research among LGBT populations that incorporate race, ethnicity, and culture, including intraracial comparisons based on sexual orientation or behavior or interracial comparisons among larger LGBT populations. Second, there is a relative overabundance of research that examines the health of LGBT people from within a disease-specific pathological focus. What is needed now are research efforts that move beyond the traditional focus on LGBT health problems toward the factors and racial/cultural assets that promote and preserve health.

Religion/Spirituality and LGBT Health

One aspect of race, ethnicity, and culture in LGBT life that often gets overlooked is the role of religion and spirituality. It is important to note the distinction between the two, as religion describes a set of principles, usually centrally organized and regulated by a person or group, both by which its members understand a spiritual reality and its connection to their experiences of the physical world, whereas spirituality describes an understanding and relationship to a spiritual reality that is exercised with autonomy and without external regulation (Foster, Arnold, Rebchook, & Kegeles, 2011; Rodriguez & Ouellette, 2000). While many discussions of LGBT communities and health center on negative narratives regarding homosexuality perpetuated by religious institutions (Lewis, 2003; Stokes & Peterson, 1998; Woodyard, Peterson, & Stokes, 2000), the larger acknowledgment of the importance of religion and spirituality as fostering resiliency is much less visible.

While the pejorative stance of many, albeit not all, religious institutions against homosexuality is well documented in the media and academic research, the focus has typically been on how societal and institutional sexual prejudice negatively influences the mental health, and perhaps the sexual behavioral patterns, of LGBT individuals (Stokes & Peterson, 1998; Chaney & Patrick, 2011). Moreover, research often highlights a higher level of "homophobia" among Black and Latino communities compared with white communities (Woodyard et al., 2000; Stokes & Peterson, 1998), despite evidence that these relationships may be mediated by other social variables such as education and religiosity (Lewis, 2003). Another angle of this dynamic that is often ignored, however, is how larger societal religious and faith beliefs play out in medical settings and may impact medical experiences as well. Among a sample of nursing students in the Midwest, relatively low levels of "homophobia" were observed, and high religiosity was associated with higher levels of homophobia, while knowledge of LGBT folks was associated with lower levels of homophobia (Dinkel, Patzel, McGuire, Rolfs, & Purcell, 2007). The authors, surprised with the lower homophobia scores among the sample, concluded that perhaps it reflected attitudes of neutrality or subtle heterosexism that could adversely impact their treatment of LGBT patients. A similar study noted that race (African American) and religious affiliation (Protestant) were both significantly associated with higher levels of homophobia and worse attitudes among MSW students (Logie, Bridge, & Bridge, 2007). Findings like these have led to cultural competency curricula for health professions education and training programs that incorporate diversity training in topics such as religion and sexual orientation in addition to traditional variable of race, culture, and gender (Lim et al., 2010; Banton, 2011).

On an individual level, religion and spirituality plays a key role in the overall health of LGBT persons' lives as well and not simply related to sexual prejudice experienced at religious institutions and organizations. Among 498 LGBT participants (24 percent Hispanic, 9 percent African American) at a New England Pride event, "spirituality" was defined largely in relational terms (God and self), and "religion" was defined in terms of communal worship and negative influences in the lives of peoples and communities (Halkitis et al., 2009). The authors also found that spiritual identities were more pronounced than religious identities among participants in the sample. Seventy-five percent of participants were raised in what they described as "religious" households, but only 25 percent held their current religious affiliations with the denominations in which they were raised. Their findings are not surprising and speak to the fluid nature of how religious upbringing intersects with sexual identification along the life journey, as well as how a more individualized sense of spirituality emerges among LGBT persons as a positive and resilient coping mechanism in their lives. In a study of 92 ethnically diverse (mostly African American) young male-to-female transgender women, Dowshen et al. (2011) found that participation in formal religious practices, even more so than one's spirituality, was associated with lower HIV-risk-related sexual behaviors. This notion of religion and spirituality being incorporated as a positive coping mechanism with life stressors has also been described among Black MSM, having implications not only for future sexual health initiatives but also for general health programs (Lubensky, Bradford, & Bland, 2008).

The literature on LGBT health and religion/spirituality is not limited to Christians and Protestants either (Hooghe, Dejaeghere, Claes, & Quintelier, 2010). Focus groups with Muslim men and women in Belgium, responsible persons for a large mosque, and four Muslim LGBT individuals revealed themes describing homosexuality as a "forbidden behavior"; however, participants also noted the importance of family and overall culture in religious beliefs and faith, not simply reflective of the religious institutions that one attends. Consequently, the notion of being open or "out" about being LGBT for many Muslim men and women is as much a familial issue as a personal one and also has implications for their status and health in larger communities and social institutions. For many in this qualitative study, individual rights as LGBT persons intersected with dense familial traditions of honor and one's duty to the larger community, making the notion of "coming out" a much more complex process with familial/community implications that go beyond traditional Eurocentric Western notions of this being solely an individual journey. This sense of a cultural clash of intersecting religious and sexual identities, particularly when considering Muslim LGBT persons, has been echoed in other studies as a type of "queer intersectionality" in which characteristics and tenets of Islam faith appear to threaten core European values (Rahman, 2010).

In examining Santeria, a system of beliefs reflecting an intersection of African Yoruba traditions with Roman Catholic and Native American indigenous customs, similar issues emerge. Practicing Santeria in the United States for LGBT persons may involve sexual minorities emphasizing the traditional "homophobic" teachings of the faith, and some have suggested that women and gays resist these discriminatory practices, just as African slaves embraced Santeria to combat the racism, slavery, rape, and violence perpetrated against them during the Diaspora (Vidal-Ortiz, 2005). Dealing with homophobia in Santeria cannot be neatly dissected from issues of sexism and racism that are also present. In other words, further examination is needed to address how white practitioners of the religion demand that homosexuals be entitled the opportunities to become *babalawos* (high priests or chiefs of the faith) yet do not demand that practitioners other than women work in the kitchen or equality in the racial hierarchies of these institutions. Oppression is oppression along several social lines and categories, and one cannot discuss LGBT rights or "sexual minorities," as the case may be, without also discussing the gender and racial inequities that exist simultaneously.

Reconceptualizing how religion intersects with race/culture and sexuality among LGBT communities also has important implications for clinical encounters. While many studies have described the negative influence of religion on the lives of LGBT individuals and their experiences in healthcare facilities, particularly Black gay men (Woodyard et al., 2000; Stokes & Peterson, 1998; Malebranche, Peterson, Fullilove, & Stackhouse, 2004), others have noted the importance of religion and/or spirituality as an indicator of resiliency or coping in various racial/ethnic communities

(Pitt, 2010; Rodriguez & Ouellette, 2000). In other words, all LGBT people do not share common stories of trauma from religious upbringings; nor do they all reject church or religious services. For many, religion and spirituality may be the cornerstone of how they conceptualize their self-identities or how they navigate maintaining their mental and physical health. Moreover, when religion is discussed among LGBT communities, we often only focus on Christianity, when a myriad religions/faiths are subscribed to by same-gender-loving people. When clinicians, public health officials and other agencies do not ask about aspects of religion/spirituality in the lives of LGBT persons, they may be missing important opportunities to develop health-promoting plans that best match the lived experiences and cultural assets of their patients.

Intersectionality: A Promising Paradigm for True LGBT Health

The most appropriate way to look at how race, culture, and ethnicity inform sexuality incorporates what we call an "intersectional" framework. Intersectionality emerged as a concept in the late 1970s and developed through early work of Kimberlé Crenshaw (Crenshaw, 1989, 1991), postulating that social identities (e.g., gender, race, and class) do not exist in separate compartments for individuals but rather in a fluid, intersecting manner. The early work from Crenshaw emerged from Black feminist theory and addressed how multiple social identities converged among women of color such that they were simultaneously subjected to multiple oppressions in the context of larger societal sexism, violence, and other forms of discrimination. However, this framework works well beyond a feminist critique and can be applied to how race, culture, and ethnicity intersect with and inform sexual desire, behavior, and expression.

In her seminal work, Kimberlé Crenshaw argues that gender, race, and class all play a role in the lives of women of color and their lived experiences through issues of public policy, immigration laws, and specific gender role expectations, among others (Crenshaw, 1989). She notes:

> The fact that minority women suffer from the effects of multiple subordination, coupled with institutional expectations based on inappropriate non-intersectional contexts, shapes and ultimately limits the opportunities for meaningful intervention on their behalf.

Intersectionality has become a core concept in women's studies since the 1970s and 1980s and has also extended out to include discussions of health policy issues and the lived experiences of lesbian women. Intersectional theory has also been applied to the issue of women's reproductive rights, sexuality, and abortion (Price, 2010), where the "pro-choice" movement in the United States may not resonate with many poor working-class women or women of color due to how race/class privileges and disadvantages contextualize political issues for women. Issues like abortion, reproductive rights, and the pro-choice movement cannot simply be seen through the lens of women's rights but should also consider how the social context and position of women factor into how they prioritize or engage in these political issues.

Recent work has incorporated social identity and sexuality as part of the intersectional matrix for women, pointing out the benefits of intersectionality approaches in research and interventions, particularly in the lives of black and Latina women (Schuster et al., 2005; Asencio & Battle, 2010). Moreover, the medicalization of sexuality, reproductive health, and HIV/AIDS has not only ignored lesbians in favor of highlighting the issues of solely gay men but also moves us away from a discussion of larger social factors that impact lesbian women's lives from a nonpathological perspective (Bowleg, Craig, & Burkholder, 2004; Teti et al., 2008). Social identities (e.g., Black, lesbian, and woman) are intersectional, and the subjective interpretation of researchers should acknowledge this intersectionality when doing work with Black lesbian populations in the future (Bowleg, 2008). To illustrate this point, among a sample of 92 Black lesbian women, internal factors (e.g., self-esteem, racial identification, and sexual identification) were more predictive of an active coping style to stress than external factors (e.g., social support and perceived availability of LGBT resources) (Bowleg et al., 2004). Finally, empirical work discussing the role of intersectionality in the "coming out" process (Bowleg, 2008) found that ranking sexual identity over racial identity positively predicted being "out and actively talking about" one's sexuality among a sample of 95 Black lesbian and bisexual women. However, it was also noted that: (1) decisions to "come out" were not individualistic decisions but involved considerations that included the influence of larger social, familial, and community contexts; and (2) the coming-out process emerged through the intersection of racial, gender, and sexual identities, not through keeping them separate.

While there have been few studies that directly utilize the concept of intersectionality with gay men, many researchers have addressed the concept indirectly, though often from a disease-specific or pathologic lens. From a theoretical perspective, some have called for an intersectional approach when addressing gay men's health and sexuality (Jaffe, 2009). And while the HIV epidemic mobilized the overall gay community and what is viewed by many to be gay civil rights, an unintended consequence was neglecting a research focus on LGBT communities that addressed larger issues from a nonmedicalized, nonpathological perspective. As a result, most of the intersectional research with gay men is within the context of HIV or other adverse health disparities. Public health literature comes close to bringing intersectionality to the forefront with LGBT populations when using the term "syndemics" to describe intersecting adverse health outcomes that inform each other, such as HIV, sexually transmitted infections (STIs), mental health, and substance abuse (Egan et al., 2011; Mayer et al., 2001, 2008). However, these considerations are still within a larger downstream medical framework of disease and illness and don't begin to capture the richness of how intersecting social identities influence some of the more resilient and affirming lived experiences of racially and ethnically diverse LGBT people.

Most studies about Black gay men tend to focus on explaining the HIV racial disparity among these men (Millett et al., 2007, 2006), with many highlighting the so-called "down-low phenomenon" that consciously or inadvertently pathologizes intersections of race, masculinity, and sexuality in an attempt to explain high HIV rates among Black women (Barnshaw & Letukas, 2010). However, Black gay men who possess more positive (i.e., integrated self-identification as being both Black and gay) reported higher levels of self-esteem, HIV prevention self-efficacy, stronger social support networks, greater levels of life satisfaction, and lower levels of male gender role and psychological distress than their counterparts who reported less positive (less integrated) Black and gay identity development (Crawford, Allison, Zamboni, & Soto, 2002). These findings suggest that it is not one social identity (i.e., racial versus sexual) that may predominate at all times but rather a fluid integration of these identities and backgrounds that sustain health. This sentiment has been echoed by other social scientists and public health advocates, emphasizing how Black LGBT individuals are uniquely positioned with feet firmly entrenched in both the civil and gay rights movements simultaneously (Battle & Crum, 2007; Battle, Bennett, & Shaw, 2004). If we do not consider the intersection of how race, culture, and ethnicity influences the sexual lives of LGBT individuals and communities, not only will individual health variables suffer but also larger communities, how our children our raised, and how we function in society (Cahill, Battle, & Meyer, 2003).

There are few studies that address this intersectionality approach among diverse populations of LGBT people, primarily focusing on HIV and other social/health stigmas, oppression, and the influence of religiosity. A qualitative study of 44 LGB individuals' experiences with hate-related crimes found that low-income LGB folks "of color" had more violent hate crimes perpetuated against them, but white, middle-class LGB interpreted their experiences as "more severe" (Meyer, 2010). The authors concluded that the social context of LGB folks is important in considering how they interpret and experience hate crime experiences. While this is an important conclusion to make, it falls short of truly addressing intersectionality for a couple of reasons. First, it is difficult to make comparisons regarding the lived experiences of LGB folks of diverse races and ethnicities who reside in different class distinctions—contrasting the experiences of middle-class LGB folks of all races/ethnicities would have provided for a more balanced analysis, as studying interclass differences among different racial groups may lead to solely race-based conclusions that do not consider the role of class at all. Second, one cannot look at Black, Latino, API, or Native American LGB persons and disentangle the experiences with racial and ethnic discrimination, immigration, and class from hate crimes based on sexual prejudice. Perhaps previous experiences with racism and other forms of discrimination prepare one for sexual prejudice hate crime experiences so that they don't seem as severe, or they do not leave as much of an impression.

Beyond sexual prejudice hate crimes, there has also been work looking at additional deficit model approaches to how intersectional identities may impact health. In addressing the HIV racial disparity among Black MSM, applying an intersectionality perspective acknowledges that racialized stigma may play a large role in their lives and that sexuality experiences vary by race (Haile, 2009). These experiences, in turn, provide context for feelings of self-esteem and self-efficacy, which can negatively influence sexual decision making and condom-use practices. Additionally, others have suggested that HIV stigma adds an additional level of intersectionality that further compounds trauma and stigma along economic, racial, and sexual lines (McTigue, 2010). Literature among Mexican American gay men has noted how issues of "machismo" (Diaz, Ayala, Bein, & Marin, 2001) intersects with social class, geography, and immigration (Thing, 2010) to assist in sexual identity formation. A LGBT People of Color Microaggressions Scale has been developed to address intersecting avenues of social oppression, noting that men scored higher than women and API scored higher than both African Americans and Hispanics (Balsam et al., 2011). A common theme through much of this work is not only a tendency to focus on how these intersecting racial and sexual identities are simply sources of trauma in the lives of diverse LGBT persons, but it often emerges from an overarching focus on sexual identity formation and "coming out" and how race, culture, and ethnicity seem to serve as "barriers" to this process. This bias can be problematic and is often seen in public health and social literature, as the authors and researchers are primarily white LGBT individuals whose primary social identification revolves around sexual identities, and it is through that lens that they view LGBT experiences of other racial and ethnic groups. For LGB individuals who are already racial/ethnic and gender minorities, distinct sexual identification may not be as important in social contexts as for white LGB people.

Interestingly, education and religion yield a few notable explorations of intersectionality among diverse LGBT people. Interviews with seven Black gay men attending predominantly white institutions (PWI) of higher learning found that the issue of how to "come out" regarding their sexual orientation played a role in their choice of school for college (Strayhorn, Blakewood, & DeVita, 2008). The authors discussed the issue of being a racial minority at the college competing with being the sexual minority at a predominantly black institution and how the men navigated and weighed the pros and cons of those environments in their personal lives. Similarly, an intersectionality analysis of a mixed-race (mother white, father Black) young man named "Tyson," who had attended racially mixed schools growing up, revealed how he had to navigate complex racial and class divisions among his peers as he developed his own personal identity along the way (Harper, Wardell, & McGuire, 2011). Tyson had to address fluid class identities as he changed schools due to his parents' changes in income over time, as well as to integrate his masculine, sexual, and spiritual identities in young adulthood. The authors conclude that embracing and addressing the complex intersecting identities among students in higher educational settings may be challenging (particularly the larger the institution), but policy and classroom modifications can begin to address the complexity of reconciling these sometimes competing identities by having students exposed to the concept of intersectionality and how it may impact their everyday lives.

Finally, the role of religion as an intersecting identity has come into focus in the lives of racially and ethnically diverse LGBT. As stated previously, the traditional narrative of how religion and spirituality operate in the lives of LGBT individuals usually describes the negative influence of homophobic and heterosexist rhetoric from the pulpit of Protestant churches (Malebranche et al., 2004; Stokes & Peterson, 1998; Woodyard et al., 2000). A content analysis of T. D. Jakes and his Potter's House interviews and sermons described a "Black Mega Church" and its disconnect with the black LGBT community (Chaney & Patrick, 2011). The study highlighted how transcripts of these interviews and sermons were vague and ambiguous when discussing LGBT inclusivity and same sex marriage in church, yet the Church claimed "tolerance" of same-sex behavior in larger media stories. However, there have been calls for a more overriding appreciation of the individual-level intersection of religion and spirituality in the context of qualitative and quantitative research with LGBT populations (Yip, 2008). Yip argues that the multiple social identities that one embraces and prioritizes are crucially important when considering how religious beliefs and traditions influence the lived experience of being homosexual. He uses his own personal example as a Chinese Malaysian, Muslim, self-identified "gay" man to emphasize how these intersecting aspects of his identity have helped facilitate his ability to do research on religion and spirituality among diverse LGBT populations. Yet Yip clearly states that his sexual orientation is not one of a "gay lifestyler" (where sexual identity assumes "master status" in all social contexts), but rather, his ethnicity is equal to, if not more salient than, his sexuality in everyday life. As with class and race, ethnicity (which often umbrellas religious formative contexts) may be viewed by nonwhite LGBT persons as a primary social identification over sexuality in everyday life.

MOVING BEYOND HIV AND SEXUAL HEALTH: CONSIDERATIONS OF RACE AND CULTURE

The goal of this chapter is not to describe the entire breadth of literature and work done on the intersection of race, culture, and sexuality but instead to highlight this often-overlooked issue when discussing larger LGBT health initiatives. Given the paucity of research on LGBT health initiatives overall, and the even fewer studies that acknowledge equal importance to the influence of the social contexts of race and culture on these initiatives, we would suggest several avenues for future directions. These suggestions are meant to be specific in intent but broad and conceptual overall in recognition that experiences and definitions of LGBT health may vary according to gender, race, culture, religion, geography, and myriad other variables.

1. Change how we conceptualize the relationship of race and culture with sexuality

The bias in current literature on LGBT health must first be acknowledged, then the wording changed to be more specific and appreciative of racial and cultural diversity instead of utilizing the generic term "of color" after "LGBT" to describe nonwhite persons. While this is a convenient term in terms of length and may assist in reducing reader confusion, it can also be dismissive and reductionist of the unique features of individual races and cultures that intersect with sexual expression. Moreover, we cannot view various social identities as always "competing" or conceptualizing race and culture as merely barriers or impediments to the "coming out" process or to a standard European definition of what it means to be LGBT. We must appreciate that sexual expression and identification is not necessarily pathologic if it comes in a different form than the mainstream "gay" version that has been socially constructed since the Stonewall era. What it means to be LGBT from within the context of various races and cultural backgrounds can mean different things at different times and highlights the drawbacks of viewing an individual from a dominant sexual identity context first without recognizing that culture, religion, and race are variables that exert an influence on an individual's formative experiences long before they are sexually aware enough to shape their own personal sexual identity politics. Once someone becomes sexually aware, the variables of race, culture, religion, and sexuality become more fluid and intersecting, but to ask how religion fits into the lives of LGB folks may be the wrong approach—we should be asking ourselves how our continuing evolving sexual awareness and identification emerges from a foundation of racial, cultural, class, religious, gender, and ethnic upbringings.

2. Promote a health research and intervention agenda that incorporates a true intersectional approach

While "intersectionality" has been a term incorporated when considering women's health issues and for more theoretical considerations of people's lived experiences, it is truly a framework deserving of attention when considering the larger context of promoting LGBT health and wellness. Historically we have viewed the civil rights movement and the gay rights movement as separate entities, while some have seen them as representing two sides of a similar coin of standing up to oppression, discrimination, and fostering social justice. While the parallel that discrimination is discrimination can be drawn between the racial and sexual civil rights movements, we must acknowledge that these are two very different and very distinct social movements. And, as such, racial and culturally diverse LGBT folks have to straddle the fence between both these important and intersecting social identities. LGBT health is a noble cause, and, yes, there are health disparities between LGBT folks and their heterosexual counterparts, but there are also many deep-rooted social, political, and health disparities that exist between racial and ethnic minorities and their white counterparts that are the consequence of years of entrenched institutional policies and preferences. These racial and cultural disparities do not simply go away if we decide to focus on LGBT health; nor are they disparities that can be placed lower on the hierarchy of health concerns. Health initiatives that emphasize LGBT issues must realize that these issues do not exist in silos and are not neatly compartmentalizable or separable from race and culture-specific health concerns. For racial and ethnic minorities who are also LGBT, both these disparities are pertinent to their livelihoods, and one should not stress one health agenda in favor of the other. LGBT health is much more than just sexual health, HIV and STI, and LGBT health, for racially and culturally diverse individuals, must consider conditions that are pertinent to all our intersecting social identities. We need research, both qualitative and quantitative, that promotes equal consideration of race and cultural variance with diversity in sexual orientation.

3. Adopt a resiliency approach to LGBT health among diverse populations

Historically, intersectionality emerged from a context of addressing the overlapping avenues of social oppression and discrimination (i.e., gender, class, and race) that impact the lives of women of color (Crenshaw, 1989; 1991). Moreover, this intersectionality has been couched in a predominantly biomedical framework that has emphasized diversity in race, culture, and sexuality from a pathological lens focused on HIV and STI. Over time, however, intersectionality as a concept has expanded to include other social considerations and variables such as sexuality, masculinity, and religion/ spirituality. As such, we must embrace a definition of intersectionality that begins to look at how these overlapping identities (particularly race, culture, class, and sexuality) have resilient qualities that enhance our health and meaningful existence, not just as overlapping identities that automatically equate to oppression and simply predict static outcomes of HIV, childhood sexual abuse, poor mental health, or alcohol/substance abuse outcomes. Moreover, instead of conceptualizing intersectionality as a cumulative or additive merging of these identities, we must examine how these identities have intrinsic benefits and drawbacks that may vary, work synergistically, or cancel each other out depending on the time, space, and location in which an individual is situated. For example, in larger society and general everyday life, how do the race and gender privilege identities of being white and male in the United States intersect with the stigma faced by being gay? The benefits of race and gender privilege may trump the stigma of being homosexual in a same-sex-affirming environment or space but may not in other heteronormative contexts. Similarly, a Latina lesbian from a working-class family may face adversity based on her gender, class, and culture in larger, white-male-dominated circles but may find solace and peace in a Hispanic community that affirms her cultural, religious, and ethnic identities at the expense of being "open" regarding her same-gender desire and identification. It is important to note the complexity of how these identities intersect, how they may or may not balance each other out, and ultimately how they are related to health when using an intersectional framework. The decisional balance of how intersecting identities work or do not work in different settings is key to understanding the context for health-related behaviors among LGBT individuals. There may not be a space where all of the identities that an individual comprises are either affirmed or stigmatized equally; in fact, the majority of spaces occupied by LGBT people in society will likely involve deciding which social identity is the priority for that moment in time. For better or for worse, the fluidity of how these identities are experienced, how they are prioritized, and which ones solicit affirmation versus stigma in varied settings is a reality that we cannot ignore. Accepting this will put us on track to embracing a more holistic definition of what LGBT health truly means in our diverse community.

4. Engage medical communities to redefine LGBT health as an intersectional approach to "cultural competency"

The phrase "cultural competency" has often been used to describe medical approaches to patient communication and care that heavily consider diversity in ethnic/cultural differences. Unfortunately, these approaches often do not include sexual diversity as a component of this competency. Similarly, calls for "LGBT" health initiatives have not been inclusive of the full racial/ethnic and cultural diversity within LGBT communities. We would call for a merging of these two approaches to health care, and if we are truly to embrace a holistic definition of providing "culturally competent" care to patients, this will include addressing how all aspects of cultural diversity influence health among patients, from racial/ethnic variation to diversity in sexual orientation and expression. Intersectional approaches to LGBT health should not be confined to theoretical considerations in textbooks and public health journals but should be applied in the clinical settings where many health discussions and treatment decisions are made. In this redefining of cultural competency, diversity in race/ethnicity, sexual orientation, gender identity, religion, and other personal characteristics should not be viewed as barriers to care from a traditional deficit-model perspective often held by medical communities. Instead, this diversity and complexity in the intersection of many social identities should be viewed from an assets approach, in which clinicians can capitalize on the diversity among LGBT patients so as to best serve all their health care needs, not just those centered on sexual health.

CONCLUSION

The intersection of race and culture with sexuality is an important concept that cannot be understated when discussing LGBT health. Instead of a strict pathological lens that associates nonwhite and non-European manifestations of same-sex behavior with HIV, alcohol abuse, or other adverse health disparities, we must embrace diversity in race and culture as the fertile foundation from which sexual expression grows and develops. Nikki Giovanni recognized that race/ethnicity and cultural differences are often seen as negative attributes when in fact, these differences are merely just variations of what is "normal" for many LGBT people. You cannot neatly extract the blackness from a Black MSM; nor can you carve out Islamic faith, beliefs, or practices from a Muslim lesbian when addressing their individual health concerns. LGBT individuals exist as complex persons—not just static entities within a master framework of sexual identification labels and culture, but fluid intersections of other racial, cultural, spiritual, and social identities that exist together to make them the whole of who they are.

REFERENCES

Asencio, M., & Battle, J. (2010). Introduction: Special issue on black and Latina sexuality and identities. *Black Women, Gender & Families, 4*(1), 1–7.

Balsam, K. F., Huang, B., Fieland, K. C., Simoni, J. M., & Walters, K. L. (2004). Culture, trauma, and wellness: A comparison of heterosexual and lesbian, gay, bisexual, and two-spirit Native Americans. *Cultural Diversity and Ethnic Minority Psychology 10*(3), 287–301. doi:10.1037/1099-9809.10.3.287

Balsam, K. F., Molina, Y., Beadnell, B., Simoni, J., & Walters, K. (2011). Measuring multiple minority stress: The LGBT people of color microaggressions scale. *Cultural Diversity and Ethnic Minority Psychology, 17*(2), 163–174. doi:10.1037/a0023244

Banton, M. (2011). Religion, faith, and intersectionality. *Ethnic and Racial Studies, 34*(7), 1248–1253. doi:10.1080/01419870.2011.582727

Barnshaw, J., & Letukas, L. (2010). The low down on the down low: Origins, risk identification and intervention. *Health Sociology Review, 19*(4), 478–490.

Battle, J., Bennett, N., & Shaw, T. C. (2004). From the closet to a place at the table: Past, present, and future assessments of social science research on black lesbian, gay, bisexual, and transgender populations. *African American Research Perspectives, 10*(1), 9–26.

Battle, J., & Crum, M. (2007). Black LGB health and well-being. In I. H. Meyer & M. E. Northridge (Eds.), *The health of sexual minorities* (pp. 320–352). Boston, MA: Springer.

Bowleg, L. (2008). When black + lesbian + woman ≠ black lesbian woman: The methodological challenges of qualitative and quantitative intersectionality research. *Sex Roles, 59*(5), 312–325. doi:10.1007/s11199-008-9400-z

Bowleg, L., Craig, M. L., & Burkholder, G. (2004). Rising and surviving: A conceptual model of active coping among black lesbians. *Cultural Diversity and Ethnic Minority Psychology, 10*(3), 229–240. doi:10.1037/1099-9809.10.3.229

Cahill, S., Battle, J., & Meyer, D. (2003). Partnering, parenting, and policy: family issues affecting Black lesbian, gay, bisexual, and transgender (LGBT) people. *Race and Society, 6*(2), 85–98. doi:10.1016/j.racsoc.2004.11.002

Chaney, C., & Patrick, L. (2011). The invisibility of LGBT individuals in black mega churches: Political and social implications. *Journal of African American Studies, 15*(2), 199–217. doi:10.1007/s12111-010-9153-y

Cochran, S. D., Mays, V. M., Alegria, M., Ortega, A. N., & Takeuchi, D. (2007). Mental health and substance use disorders among Latino and Asian American lesbian, gay, and bisexual adults. *Journal of Consulting and Clinical Psychology, 75*(5), 785–794. doi:10.1037/0022-006X.75.5.785

Crawford, I., Allison, K. W., Zamboni, B. D., & Soto, T. (2002). The influence of dual-identity development on the psychosocial functioning of African-American gay and bisexual men. *Journal of Sex Research, 39*(3), 179–189. doi:10.1080/00224490209552140

Crenshaw, K. (1989). Demarginalizing the intersection of race and sex: A black feminist critique of antidiscrimination doctrine, feminist theory and anti-racist politics. *The University of Chicago Legal Forum, 1*, 139–168.

Crenshaw, K. (1991). Mapping the margins: Intersectionality, identity politics, and violence against women of color. *Stanford Law Review, 43*(6), 1241–1299.

Diaz, R. M., Ayala, G., Bein, E., Henne, J., & Marin, B. V. (2001). The impact of homophobia, poverty, and racism on the mental health of gay and bisexual Latino men: Findings from 3 US cities. *American Journal of Public Health, 91*(6), 927–932.

Dinkel, S., Patzel, B., McGuire, M. J., Rolfs, E., & Purcell, K. (2007). Measures of homophobia among nursing students and faculty: A midwestern perspective. *International Journal of Nursing Education Scholarship, 4*(1). doi:10.2202/1548-923X.1491

Dowshen, N., Forke, C. M., Johnson, A. K., Kuhns, L. M., Rubin, D., & Garofalo, R. (2011). Religiosity as a protective factor against HIV risk among transgender women. *Journal of Adolescent Health, 4*(48), 410–414.

Egan, J., Frye, V., Kurtz, S., Latkin, C., Chen, M., Tobin, K., . . . Koblin, B. (2011). Migration, neighborhoods, and networks: Approaches to understanding how urban environmental conditions affect syndemic adverse health outcomes among gay, bisexual and other men who have sex with men. *AIDS and Behavior, 15*(0), 35–50. doi:10.1007/s10461-011-9902-5

Epstein, S. (2003). Sexualizing governance and medicalizing identities: The emergence of "state-centered" LGBT health politics in the United States. *Sexualities, 6*(2), 131–171. doi:10.1177/1363460703006002001

Feldman, M. B., & Meyer, I. H. (2007). Eating disorders in diverse lesbian, gay, and bisexual populations. *International Journal of Eating Disorders, 40*(3), 218–226. doi:10.1002/eat.20360

Fikar, C. R., & Keith, L. (2004). Information needs of gay, lesbian, bisexual, and transgendered health care professionals: Results of an Internet survey. *Journal of the Medical Library Association, 92*(1), 56–65.

Foster, M. L., Arnold, E., Rebchook, G., & Kegeles, S. M. (2011). It's my inner strength: Spirituality, religion and HIV in the lives of young African American men who have sex with men. *Culture, Health & Sexuality, 13*(9), 1103–1117.

Graves, J. L. (2011). Evolutionary versus racial medicine: Why it matters. In S. Krimsky & K. Sloan (Eds.), *Race and the genetic revolution: Science, myth, and culture* (pp. 142–170). New York: Columbia University Press.

Haile, F.-R. G. (2009). *Social stigma and HIV/AIDS in black MSM, health behavior and health education* (Doctoral dissertation, University of Michigan). Retrieved from https://deepblue.lib.umich.edu/handle/2027.42/64692

Halkitis, P., Mattis, J., Sahadath, J., Massie, D., Ladyzhenskaya, L., Pitrelli, K., . . . Cowie, S.-A. (2009). The meanings and manifestations of religion and spirituality among lesbian, gay, bisexual, and transgender adults. *Journal of Adult Development, 16*(4), 250–262. doi:10.1007/s10804-009-9071-1

Harper, S. R., Wardell, C. C., & McGuire, K. M. (2011). Man of multiple identities: Complex individuality and identity intersectionality among college men. In J. A. Laker & T. Davis (Eds.), *Masculinities in higher education: Theoretical and practical considerations* (pp. 81–96). New York: Routledge.

Herek, G. M. (1989). Hate crimes against lesbians and gay men: Issues for research and policy. *American Psychologist, 44*(6), 948–955.

Herek, G. M. (2009). Hate crimes and stigma-related experiences among sexual minority adults in the United States. *Journal of Interpersonal Violence, 24*(1), 54–74. doi:10.1177/0886260508316477

Herrick, A. L., Matthews, A. K., & Garofalo, R. (2010). Health risk behaviors in an urban sample of young women who have sex with women. *Journal of Lesbian Studies, 14*(1), 80–92. doi:10.1080/10894160903060440

Hooghe, M., Dejaeghere, Y., Claes, E., & Quintelier, E. (2010). "Yes, but suppose everyone turned gay?": The structure of attitudes toward gay and lesbian rights among Islamic youth in Belgium. *Journal of LGBT Youth, 7*(1), 49–71. doi:10.1080/19361650903507916

Jaffe, J. M. (2009). *Borderland bodies: Queering intersectional health activisms.* (Bachelor's thesis). Middletown, CT: Wesleyan University.

Jorde, L. B., & Wooding, S. P. (2004). Generic variation, classification, and race. *Nature Genetics, 36*(11), S28–S33. doi:10.1034/ng1435

Lewis, G. B. (2003). Black-white differences in attitudes toward homosexuality and gay rights. *Public Opinion Quarterly, 67*(1), 59–78.

Lim, R. F., Koike, A. K., Gellerman, D. M., Seritan, A. L., Servis, M. E., & Lu, F. G. (2010). *A four-year model curriculum on culture, gender, LGBT, religion, and spirituality for general psychiatry residency training programs in the United States.* Sacramento, CA: University of California, Davis School of Medicine. Retrieved from https://www.academia.edu/765843/A_Four -Year_Model_Curriculum_on_Culture_Gender_LGBT_Religion_and _Spirituality_for_General_Psychiatry_Residency_Training_Programs_in _the_United_States?auto=download

Logie, C., Bridge, T. J., & Bridge, P. D. (2007). Evaluating the phobias, attitudes, and cultural competence of master of social work students toward the LGBT populations. *Journal of Homosexuality, 53*(4), 201–221. doi:10.1080/ 00918360802103472

Lubensky, M. E., Bradford, T., and Bland, W. (2008, August). *Black Brothers Esteem's spiritual health initiative: Focusing on spiritual health to further HIV prevention and strengthen holistic health among African-American MSM (men who have sex with men).* Paper presented at the XVII International AIDS Conference, Mexico City, Mexico.

MacWilliams-Brooks, A. A. (2008). *Imagined bridges: Welfare rights collaboration among women of color and the LGBT community in Minnesota.* (Honors project) Macalester College. Retrieved from https://digitalcommons. macalester.edu/poli_honors/13/

Malebranche, D. J., Peterson, J. L., Fullilove, R. E., & Stackhouse, R. W. (2004). Race and sexual identity: Perceptions about medical culture and health-care among Black men who have sex with men. *Journal of the National Medical Association, 96*(1), 97–107.

Mayer, K., Appelbaum, J., Rogers, T., Lo, W., Bradford, J., & Boswell, S. (2001). The evolution of the Fenway Community Health model. *American Journal of Public Health, 91*(6), 892–894. doi:10.2105/ajph.91.6.892

Mayer, K. H., Bradford, J. B., Makadon, H. J., Stall, R., Goldhammer, H., & Landers, S. (2008). Sexual and gender minority health: What we know and what needs to be done. *American Journal of Public Health, 98*(6), 989–995. doi:10.2105/ajph.2007.127811

Mays, V. M., Yancey, A. K., Cochran, S. D., Weber, M., & Fielding, J. E. (2002). Heterogeneity of health disparities among African American, Hispanic, and Asian American women: Unrecognized influences of sexual orientation. *American Journal of Public Health, 92*(4), 632–639. doi:10.2105/ajph.92.4.632

McNair, R. P., & Hegarty, K. (2010). Guidelines for the primary care of lesbian, gay, and bisexual people: A systematic review. *Annals of Family Medicine, 8,* 533–541. doi:10.1370/afm.1173

McTigue, P. (2010). The challenge of HIV—Social stigma or disability? *Web Journal of Current Legal Issues.* Retrieved from http://webjcli.ncl.ac.uk/2010 /issue5/mctigue5.html

Meyer, D. (2010). Evaluating the severity of hate-motivated violence: Intersectional differences among LGBT hate crime victims. *Sociology 44*(5), 980–995. doi:10.1177/0038038510375737

Millett, G. A., Flores, S. A., Peterson, J. L., & Bakeman, R. (2007). Explaining disparities in HIV infection among black and white men who have sex with men: a meta-analysis of HIV risk behaviors. *AIDS, 21*(15), 2083–2091. doi:10.1097/QAD.0b013e3282e9a64b00002030-200710010-00011

Millett, G. A., Peterson, J. L., Wolitski, R. J., & Stall, R. (2006). Greater risk for HIV infection of black men who have sex with men: A critical literature review. *American Journal of Public Health, 96*(6), 1007–1019. doi:10.2105/ Ajph.2005.066720

Mimiaga, M. J., Reisner, S. L., Fontaine, Y. M., Bland, S. E., Driscoll, M. A., Isenberg, D., . . . Mayer, K. H. (2010). Walking the line: Stimulant use during sex and HIV risk behavior among Black urban MSM. *Drug and Alcohol Dependence 110*(1–2), 30–37. doi:10.1016/j.drugalcdep.2010.01.017

Mountain, J. L., & Risch, N. (2004). Assessing genetic contributions to phenotypic differences among "racial" and "ethnic" groups. *Nature Genetics, 36*(11), S48–S53. doi:10.1038/ng1456

Northridge, M. E. (2001). Editor's note: Advancing lesbian, gay, bisexual, and transgender health. *American Journal of Public Health, 91*(6), 855–856.

Parra, E. J., Kittles, R. A., & Shriver, M. D. (2004). Implications between skin color and genetic ancestry for biomedical research. *Nature Genetics, 36*(11), S54–S60. doi:10.1038/ng1440

Pinhey, T. K., and Millman, S. R. (2004). Asian/Pacific Islander adolescent sexual orientation and suicide risk in Guam. *American Journal of Public Health, 94* (7), 1204–1206. doi:10.2105/ajph.94.7.1204

Pitt, R. N. (2010). "Killing the messenger": Religious black gay men's neutralization of anti-gay religious messages. *Journal for the Scientific Study of Religion, 49*(1), 56–72.

Price, K. (2010). It's not just about abortion: Incorporating intersectionality in research about women of color and reproduction. *Women's Health Issues 21*(3, Supplement), S55–S57. doi:10.1016/j.whi.2011.02.003

Rahman, M. (2010). Queer as intersectionality: Theorizing gay Muslim identities. *Sociology 44*(5), 944–961. doi:10.1177/0038038510375733

Rodriguez, E. M., & Ouellette, S. A. (2000). Gay and lesbian Christians: Homo-sexual and religious identity integration in the members and participants of a gay-positive church. *Journal for the Scientific Study of Religion, 39*(3), 333–347. doi:10.1111/0021-8294.00028

Sanchez, J. P., Meacher, P., & Beil, R. (2005). Cigarette smoking and lesbian and bisexual women in the Bronx. *Journal of Community Health, 30*(1), 23–37. doi:10.1007/s10900-004-6093-2

Schulman, K. A., Berlin, J. A., Harless, W., Kerner, J. F., Sistrunk, S., Gersh, B. J., . . . Escarce, J. J. (1999). The effect of race and sex on physicians' recommendations for cardiac catheterization. *New England Journal of Medicine, 340*(8), 618–626.

Schuster, M. A., Collins, R., Cunningham, W. E., Morton, S. C., Zierler, S., Wong, M., . . . Kanouse, D. E. (2005). Perceived discrimination in clinical care in a nationally representative sample of HIV-infected adults receiving health care. *Journal of General Internal Medicine 20*(9), 807–813. doi:10.1111/j.1525-1497.2005.05049.x

Senreich, E. (2010). Differences in outcomes, completion rates, and perceptions of treatment between white, black, and Hispanic LGBT clients in substance abuse programs. *Journal of Gay & Lesbian Mental Health, 14*(3), 176–200. doi: 10.1080/19359701003784675

Siegel, K., Schrimshaw, E. W., & Karus, D. (2004). Racial disparities in sexual risk behaviors and drug use among older gay/bisexual and heterosexual men living with HIV/AIDS. *Journal of the National Medical Association, 96*(2), 215–223.

Stokes, J. P., & Peterson, J. L. (1998). Homophobia, self-esteem, and risk for HIV among African American men who have sex with men. *AIDS Education and Prevention, 10*(3), 278–292.

Strayhorn, T. L., Blakewood, A. M., & DeVita, J. M. (2008). Factors affecting the college choice of African American gay male undergraduates: Implications for retention. *NASAP Journal, 11*(1), 88–108.

Szymanski, D. M., & Gupta, A. (2009). Examining the relationship between multiple internalized oppressions and African American lesbian, gay, bisexual, and questioning persons' self-esteem and psychological distress. *Journal of Counseling Psychology, 56*(1), 110–118.

Teti, M., Bowleg, L., Rubinstein, S., Lloyd, L., Berhane, Z., & Gold, M. (2008). Present but not accounted for: Exploring the sexual risk practices and intervention needs of nonheterosexually identified women in a prevention program for women with HIV/AIDS. *Journal of LGBT Health Research, 3*(4), 37–51. doi:10.1080/15574090802226592

Thing, J. (2010). Gay, Mexican and immigrant: Intersecting identities among gay men in Los Angeles. *Social Identities, 16*(6), 809–831. doi:10.1080/1350463 0.2010.524787

Vidal-Ortiz, Salvador. (2005). *"Sexuality" and "gender" in Santería: Towards a queer of color critique in the study of religion* (Doctoral dissertation). New York, NY: The City University of New York.

Washington, H. A. (2002). Burning love: Big tobacco takes aim at LGBT youth. *American Journal of Public Health, 92*(7), 1086–1095.

Wilkerson, J. M., Rybicki, S., Barber, C. A., & Smolenski, D. J. (2011). Creating a culturally competent clinical environment for LGBT patients. *Journal of Gay & Lesbian Social Services, 23*(3), 376–394. doi:10.1080/10538720.2011.589254

Woodyard, J. L., Peterson, J. L., & Stokes, J. P. (2000). "Let us go into the house of the Lord": Participation in African American churches among young African American men who have sex with men. *Journal of Pastoral Care, 54*(4), 451–460.

Yip, A. K. T. (2008). Researching lesbian, gay, and bisexual Christians and Muslims: Some thematic reflections. *Sociological Research Online, 13*(1), 5.

3

Lesbian, Gay, Bisexual, and Transgender Public Health and Epidemiology

Randall Sell

Public health is the science and practice from a population perspective of promoting health through activities that either prolong life or improve quality of life by, for example, preventing disease or other threats to health. This differs from traditional clinical medicine that largely focuses on the health of the individual. Of course, public health and medicine are not mutually exclusive fields of study and practice but are complementary disciplines whose boundaries are often indistinguishable. Public health relies upon a number of disciplines in addition to medicine to accomplish its goals, including epidemiology, statistics, economics, management, engineering, law, sociology, anthropology, environmental studies, political science, zoology, and psychology, to name just some. Public health practice occurs through a combination of these disciplines working together.

The populations that are the focus of public health can be defined in many ways, including geography (for example, urban versus rural), race and ethnicity, age, income, or, in the case of what will be discussed here, sexual orientation and sex/gender identity. Focusing on lesbian, gay, bisexual, and transgender (LGBT) public health from a nonpathological perspective is a relatively new way of thinking within public health. Previously, public health and medicine focused on preventing, eliminating,

61

or "curing" lesbian, gay, and bisexual sexual orientations and making sure that gender identities matched sex assigned at birth (Katz, 1992).

WHY LGBT PUBLIC HEALTH?

Public health as an organized field has been in existence for more than a century, but there is a need within public health for a focus on LGBT health. This focus allows us to research, identify, and address specific health concerns in order to protect the overall health of LGBT populations. For public health workers, service providers, and government agencies or nonprofit organizations working with LGBT people, the need for LGBT public health was obvious but became glaringly so as the HIV/AIDS epidemic emerged (Schultz, 1988). However, an examination of funding (which is almost nonexistent) and educational opportunities at universities and schools of public health (also almost nonexistent) demonstrates that there is still a lack of concern or recognition for this field (Coulter, Kenst, Bowen, & Scout, 2014; Obedin-Maliver et al., 2011). Only very recently has the National Institutes of Health begun to recognize LGBT public health, even though it still actively excludes sexual orientation and gender identity from discussions of minority populations when not just overlooking them (Institute of Medicine Committee on Lesbian, Gay, Bisexual, and Transgender Health Issues and Research Gaps and Opportunities, 2011).

At its most basic, the answer to the question "Why LGBT public health?" is that LGBT people have: 1) documented or suspected *health disparities* (that is, increased or decreased risk of morbidity and mortality when compared to other populations), and 2) even where disparities are not known to exist, *health concerns that differ from other populations* in their causes or the methods that they need to be examined and remedied. This paper provides introductions to each of these two areas but first provides a discussion of the social construction of sexual orientation and gender (and the meaning of this for public health research and practice) and a brief introduction into the history of LGBT public health, followed by an introduction to several conceptual approaches/models that can be used to understand health and health disparities, including the *social ecological model* of health. The paper concludes with a discussion of existing and future challenges to the field of LGBT public health.

THE SOCIAL CONSTRUCTION OF SEXUAL ORIENTATION AND GENDER

As stated above, public health is about the study of populations, but as with all populations, the definitions that delineate who is included as a member of a population is evolving, with no single authority capable of providing an exact or standard definition and the very existence of a population dependent upon social prescriptions at the very least (Sell, 1997). Sexual orientation and gender are no more or less social constructions than race or ethnicity or even age in these matters (Fullilove, 1998). Recognizing how these populations are socially constructed is essential for researchers and public health practitioners. The social construction of LGBT populations influences not only how research studies are designed but also how we interpret the findings of studies, which in turn influences governmental and other organizational policies and programs.

Concerning sexual orientation, while women have undoubtedly been sexually attracted to other women and have been having sex with other women since women have existed (and likewise for men), the idea of lumping women with same-sex attractions or behaviors into categories that are labeled and thought of as those of a distinct population (currently commonly labeled "lesbians" in the United States, for example) has come and gone throughout the centuries and has been immensely influenced and constrained by geography and culture (Katz, 1983). With the creation of modern homosexuals in the mid-19th century, members of which category are referred to in this paper as "gays" and "lesbians," other categories to label everyone else became necessary. Those not labeled as gay or lesbian became known as "heterosexual" or "straight" (or sometimes "normal," indicating a social and medical preference for one category over all others), and people straddling these categories became known as "bisexual" (Katz, 1995). From these terms, which were largely created and promoted by the scientific and medical communities in Germany, England, and the United States, sprang individuals who took the terms on as identities. People with these identities congregated in parks or other outside locations and at parties in private homes and bars, eventually forming organizations to provide services to themselves and other people like them (very often providing legal representation against prosecution for same-sex sexual behavior but also sometimes for the detection and treatment of sexually transmitted infections) as well as to fight for civil rights (Chauncey, 1995). The rights fought for included the ability to keep jobs, not be subjected to legal persecution or mandated medical treatment, live together as same-sex couples in homes (many localities had provisions prohibiting unmarried adults from living together), adopt children, or even get married to same-sex spouses if they so choose (Bronski, 2012).

Like the categories of sexual orientation, the term "transgender" has a history rooted in the culture of science, medicine, and research. "Transgender" is used primarily to refer to anyone whose gender (for example, how a person identifies their gender—which can be an internal sense of being male or female, and also how their gender is expressed outwardly) diverges from the sex they were assigned at birth (which is largely based upon assessments of biological traits determined by parents or medical providers helping with delivery and early care) (Kaufman, 2008). The term "transgender," like the terms "lesbian" and "gay," has similarly been adopted by some in the community as a way of labeling themselves for coming together as an identifiable group. However, the term "transgender" can be problematic for many who find that their sex and gender diverge. For example, someone born appearing biologically male and labeled as male on their birth certificate but who has an internal sense of being female may prefer to identify as female rather than transgender. In fact, this individual may spend much of their life working to comfortably take on the label of "female" for themselves within their families and in broader society. These individuals do not necessarily want an additional label of transgender, which may be perceived by some as a "third sex." (Interestingly, the term "third sex" was commonly used in the early 20th century to identify homosexuals; Carpenter, 1908).

The central lesson here is that these terms do not mean the same thing to everyone. More specifically, they do not even mean the same thing to people within the populations the labels are used to describe, let alone to the public health workers and researchers attempting to understand and improve the health of these populations. While some public health service providers and researchers may see this as a reason to ignore LGBT public health, it can also be argued that this is a reason not to take these populations as fixed and unevolving but rather to see this as an opportunity to understand these populations at a much deeper level. How an individual chooses to label themselves or how researchers choose to label sexual minorities is influenced by many complicated interrelated factors that simultaneously impact the individual's ability to protect their health as well as factors that may possibly expose them to excess morbidity and mortality.

While it may not always be easy, one of the most important things that those working with these populations must do is identify who is a member of these populations. This may be done on an intake form for someone who is seeking health or social services of some type or may be done in the context of a research study or evaluation project. Much of my work has focused on how to ask sexual orientation in the context of research settings or evaluation projects where confidentiality or anonymity of responses is promised and an institutional review board approval solicited and received. The following are some questions that I have recommended using when sexual orientation or sex and gender identity data is being collected. The questions are by no means meant to be used in all settings and for all purposes, but they have been used successfully in various settings and are meant to serve as examples of the diversity of available questions.

Additional information about the questions and additional samples can be found at www.LGBTData.com, which is a Web site cataloging major surveys that have collected sexual orientation data.

> *Sexual Orientation Identity*: (From the National Epidemiological Survey on Alcohol and Related Conditions. Respondents are surveyed in their homes and given a card with the response options below and then asked this question):
>
> • **Which of the categories on the card best describes you? 1) heterosexual (straight), 2) gay or lesbian, 3) bisexual, 4) not sure.**
>
> *Sexual Behavior:* (From Vermont and Massachusetts BRFS. Respondents are surveyed by telephone and asked the following question):
>
> • **During the past 12 months, have you had sex with only males, only females, or both males and females?**
>
> *Sexual Attraction:* (From the National Survey of Family Growth. Respondents are surveyed in their homes with the following question asked using audio-CASI):
>
> • **People are different in their sexual attraction to other people. Which best describes your feelings? Are you . . . Only attracted to females, Mostly attracted to females, Equally attracted to females and males, Mostly attracted to males, Only attracted to males, Not sure.**

While these are certainly good questions, they may not be perfect for every need. For example, the identity question cannot be used over the telephone, since it requires the respondent to have a flash card with the available response options. The sexual behavior question may not provide the level of detail desired for some research studies or programs because it does not assess how many different male or female partners the respondent has had sex with, nor the frequency of that sex. When selecting questions, one must therefore carefully think about what the data will be used for as well as how the information will be collected (for example, through face-to-face interviews, mailed surveys, over the telephone, or using computer-assisted methods).

More recently, researchers at the National Center for Health Statistics have focused on evaluating sexual orientation identity questions and have recommended the following question, which is being asked on the National Health Interview Survey (Miller & Ryan, 2011):

• **Do you think of yourself as:**

[For men:]	[For women:]
Gay	Lesbian or gay
Straight, that is, not gay	Straight, that is, not lesbian or gay

Bisexual	Bisexual
Something Else	Something Else
Don't Know	Don't Know

Clearly there are many different questions that can be used reflecting the socially constructed nature of sexual orientation, but fortunately there is a fairly well-developed history of asking these questions (Sell & Holliday, 2014). Questions to assess sex and gender have not been equally subjected to evaluation, as most surveys have not attempted to identify transgender individuals, nor have they thought critically about how they collect sex data. Most surveys only assess one or the other (e.g., sex or gender), and most label variables and report results as "sex" (even if gender was what was assessed). But there are significant problems with how sex and gender are currently collected in most research studies, with the questions particularly problematic for assessing transgender status. For example, most surveys conducted by the federal government, including the U.S. Census, do not even ask sex or gender. If a survey is conducted face-to-face, the interviewer is instructed to select "male" or "female" as the sex of the person they are interviewing. This is how "sex" is collected in the National Health Interview Survey, for example. Other surveys conducted by the federal government that collect data over the telephone instruct the interviewer to select "male" or "female" for the respondent based upon the sound of their voice. In each of these cases (face-to-face or telephone), only a single assessment of sex is taken, and transgender status is impossible to determine. To further conflate sex and gender, some of these data sets label the data collected as "sex," while others label the data collected in the very same way as "gender." In reality, using appearance and voice to assess sex or gender is not a valid measure of either. And further complicating matters, researchers and policy makers utilizing data from the exact same data sets label and report it in conflicting ways (Conron, Landers, Reisner, & Sell, 2014).

For example, the National Health Interview Survey, on its Web site, tells respondents they will be asked about their sex; however, data is collected by visual inspection—which is more accurately an assessment of gender than sex. The variable is labeled in the National Health Interview Survey data set as "sex," while the researchers using this variable label it in published studies sometimes as "sex" and sometimes as "gender." There seems to be little, if any, interest on the part of leaders and survey administrators in the U.S. federal government of dealing with this confusion (Conron et al., 2014).

That said, the U.S. Department of Health and Human Services (HHS) has proposed some standards for the collection of data on sex. HHS recommends asking, "What is your sex?" with "male" or "female" as the only two response options (U.S. Department of Health and Human Services, 2011). As has already been discussed, this does not allow for the identification of individuals who are transgender, with the question making the assumption that sex is static across the life span and that current sex always corresponds to sex assigned at birth. To better assess gender and sex, the Centers for Disease Control has discussed using a "two-step approach" in which sex and gender are assessed sequentially. The Center of Excellence for Transgender Health offers an example of one such two-step approach that can be used to assess gender and sex (2014):

1. **What is your sex or current gender? (check all that apply)**
    Male
    Female
    TransMale/Transman
    TransFemale/Transwoman
    Genderqueer
    Additional Category (please specify) _____
    Decline to State
2. **What sex were you assigned at birth?**
    Male
    Female
    Decline to State

Clearly a two-step approach such as this is much better than previous methods of assessing sex and gender; however, two-step approaches have not been tested extensively enough to recommend their inclusion in most settings. With sexual orientation questions, one of the most problematic issues is how heterosexual or straight people comprehend and respond to such questions. Since heterosexual people make up the vast majority of the population, a small amount of reporting error (that is, people who are heterosexual misidentifying as gay, lesbian, or bisexual) can significantly skew results. Similarly, a small amount of reporting error (which can have many causes, including confusion over being asked what some people may consider the same question twice to simple errors in data entry) in the two-step approach to assessing sex and gender can totally obscure relationships between transgender status and health outcomes.

A BRIEF HISTORY OF LGBT PUBLIC HEALTH

The history of LGBT public health remains largely unacknowledged and unwritten. Consequently, public health researchers and practitioners as well as government officials, program providers, and clinicians work within environments uninformed of this history. The history should never be overlooked by those working in public health and related fields, because it explains the sometimes tenuous relationship between researchers, health care practitioners, and the community. For example, when thinking about the health of African Americans in the United States, it is important to understand the Tuskegee experiments from which a distrust of health care providers and researchers was fostered if not cemented (Jones, 1992). When a group of people has been abused, taken advantage of, or simply excluded and ignored, current interactions between service providers or researchers and the community are adversely impacted. Why should people who are LGBT ever trust service providers, public health workers, or researchers, given the history of mistreatment?

Focusing on LGBT public health since the field of public health first emerged over 100 years ago, two key points should be discussed. The first point is that there largely has not been such a thing as "LGBT public health" until recent times. Any recognition of the health of lesbian, gay, bisexual, and transgender people has largely (but not entirely) happened since the advent of the AIDS epidemic in the early 1980s. Prior to AIDS, there was some interest on the part of the Centers for Disease Control and drug companies concerning hepatitis as well as a few other sexually trans-mitted infections, but largely any interest from outside of the communities themselves focused on diseases spread through sex. This is not surpris-ing given that sexual behavior has been the defining characteristic of les-bian, gay, and bisexual people in the minds of most. Even within lesbian, gay, and bisexual communities, there was a focus on sexually transmitted infections, with possibly the first organized public health efforts to work within LGBT communities concerned with the treatment and prevention of these infections (Simpson, 1997). Clinics known to be sensitive to the issues faced by LGBT people, and often staffed by people who were lesbian, gay, bisexual, or transgender themselves, sprang up in many metropolitan areas. These clinics provided safe spaces for individuals to get treatment that was less judgmental and would not result in documentation in per-sonal medical records. Many of these clinics then transformed with the advent of the HIV/AIDS epidemic into more comprehensive centers for the provision of health care and the practice of public health (Schultz, 1988).

There are a number of moments one could select as the beginning of the modern LGBT public health movement, including but not limited to, the publication of Evelyn Hooker's paper in 1957 on "The Adjustment of the Male Overt Homosexual" (Hooker, 1957), the creation of the health clinics in the 1970s focused on the treatment of sexually transmitted infections discussed above, the removal of homosexuality from the Diagnostic and Statistical Manual of Mental Disorders in 1973 (Bayer, 1987), the creation of LGBT organizations within other professional organizations—such as the LGBT Caucus of Public Health Professionals at the American Public Health Association that was founded in 1975, or the creation of organizations to address the HIV/AIDS epidemic in the early 1980s such as Gay Men's Health Crisis (1982) and Act Up (1983) (Schultz, 1988). But these efforts, while essential for the development of a modern LGBT public health movement and supported by incredibly courageous and forward-thinking individuals, for the most part (with some notable rare exceptions) existed on the periphery of public health and were rarely given "seats at the table." Debatably, the beginning of the modern LGBT public health movement, defined as a moment in which LGBT health has been integrated into the broader field of public health in a meaningful way, was with the publication of Healthy People 2010 (HP2010) in 1999 (U.S. Department of Health and Human Services, 2000). HP2010 set a goal of "eliminating health disparities among different segments of the population. These include differences that occur by gender, race, ethnicity, education or income, disability, living in rural localities, or sexual orientation." Sexual orientation was modestly included in 29 of HP2010's 467 objectives (Sell & Becker, 2001). However, by including sexual orientation in these objectives, the U.S. government indicated in a very public way that it believed there was sufficient evidence to prove the existence of disparities based upon sexual orientation, and the government implicitly agreed to monitor progress toward eliminating these disparities. While the government failed to fund in any substantial way programs to address these health disparities or to fund research to understand their causes and cures, or to even monitor these objectives, this was a significant step forward.

The second point is that, prior to any truly modern conceptualizations of LGBT public health, public health and medicine's interaction with LGBT people was largely about the control of sexuality and gender and not about protecting the health of LGBT populations. The full extent of this history has not been explored in any depth. This is surprising given that public health and medical journals are filled with examples of "cures" for homosexuality. These documents are not hidden in old dusty file cabinets but in many cases are easily found online. Jonathan Ned Katz (1983), in his book *Gay/Lesbian Almanac: A New Documentary*, catalogs (but only begins to examine in any analytic way) a long list of publications and reports presenting the findings of studies on the treatment of homosexuality. Treatments documented in Katz's book include clitoridectomy, pudic nerve section, lobotomy, hypnosis, shock therapy (electric and chemical), aversion therapy, psychoanalysis (individual and group therapy), drug therapy (including hormones, LSD, sexual stimulants, and sexual depressants), primal therapy, vegetotherapy, and prolonged abstinence. This shadowy history of medicine's and public health's relationship to homosexuality deserves a very thorough examination. The hundreds, thousands, or maybe even hundreds of thousands of lives that were adversely impacted through these practices has yet to be quantified.

CONCEPTUAL APPROACHES TO UNDERSTANDING HEALTH AND HEALTH DISPARITIES

Even where health disparities have not been extensively documented, conceptual models can provide valuable insights into why there is a need for LGBT public health. These models can not only explain reasons for potential health disparities but also provide insight into how different causal pathways may result in particular health outcomes in LGBT populations (which may or may not result in disparities). One of the most popular models or approaches to understanding health is the social ecological model. Because this model has become so popular and has been written about in so many different fields of academic study and by so many different types of researchers trying to understand very diverse concerns, the model is often described and presented in very different ways. The version of the model presented here most closely resembles the model from Dahlberg and Krug (2002) as used to understand violence and currently used by the Centers for Disease Control. This model is a simplification of McLeroy et al.'s (1988) social ecological model. The social ecological model of health posits at its essence that there are multiple levels at which an individual's health may be impacted. These levels as delineated by McLeroy et. al. are (1) intrapersonal factors, (2) interpersonal processes and primary groups, (3) institutional factors, (4) community, and (5) public policy. The simplified model presented here recognizes all the complexities of the five-level McLeroy model but reorganizes them into four levels: (1) individual, (2) relationship, (3) community, and (4) societal (see Figure 3.1).

The first level, "individual," recognizes the role of biological influences, including genetic influences and personal history, on health. These factors

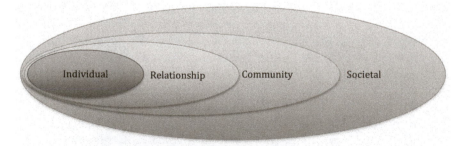

Figure 3.1 The Social Ecological Model of Health

can include demographic characteristics of the individual, including age, sexual orientation, sex, gender identity, race and ethnicity, educational attainment, and income. Some of these factors, such as race and ethnicity, are controversial and can be included at multiple levels (Shariff-Marco et al., 2011). This level also recognizes an individual's present status and history with specific health-related behaviors. Strategies to impact health at this level are often designed to change attitudes, beliefs, and behaviors that have the potential to impact health. The second level, "relationship," recognizes the immediate or close relationships an individual has with others and how these can expose them to risk as well as shield them from harm. These close relationships include a person's closest social circle, which can include peers, partners, and family members. Strategies to impact health at this level are usually designed to impact not just individuals but also those relationships around them. Peer programs are common examples of programs designed to help reduce interpersonal conflict and promote relationships that are healthy (Stangl, Lloyd, Brady, Holland, & Baral, 2013).

The third level, "community," recognizes the role that the settings an individual frequents, such as schools, workplaces, recreational centers, and bars or nightclubs, can play either positively or negatively on their health. This level recognizes that within these settings, ever-evolving communities exist within which an individual is a participant. Public health professionals often implement programs using social-marketing campaigns or other methods to impact social norms to influence the climate, processes, and policies within a given community. The ultimate goal, of course, is to improve health through influencing the relationships that exist within the community. And finally, the fourth level, "societal," recognizes the factors that extend beyond communities that can influence health. These factors can be formal policies and laws that are written and enforced publicly, or unwritten but still very powerful factors impacting health. Policies that impact education and economics and have the potential to reduce social inequalities are often targeted but also include very specific policies such as where a person may or may not smoke (or, even more specifically, what they may smoke).

The social ecological model of health is a helpful tool for understanding and assessing the many specific issues that are considered within the realm of LGBT health. For example, from a public health perspective, we are very interested in tobacco use by LGBT people. We can use the social ecological model to examine how each of these four levels can influence whether an individual smokes or whether they are more or less likely to smoke because of factors such as their sexual orientation or gender identity and consequently whether communities or populations are more or less likely to smoke—resulting in health disparities. This model is particularly helpful when designing research studies, because it recognizes the many complex factors that can influence health outcomes; however, the difficulty of practically specifying and measuring each of these factors is challenging, and only a few researchers have succeeded in doing it reputably.

Diez Roux (2012) does an excellent job of reviewing the most widely accepted conceptual approaches to the study of health disparities. While these conceptual approaches are relevant to any health disparity, they can be particularly helpful for understanding LGBT health disparities. The two conceptual approaches most relevant to LGBT health are the "fundamental cause model" and the "pathways model." Both of these models overlap with the social ecological model (and with each other) and in many ways are indistinguishable, but they are important to mention here because they provide different and sometimes conflicting perspectives from which to view health disparities. The fundamental cause model has been frequently used to explain racial and ethnic health disparities, and it emphasizes the "basic causes" of these disparities, which can be likewise applied to LGBT health. It is theorized that changes in these basic causes can impact particular health outcomes. The most interesting of these basic causes as outlined by Hatzenbuehler, Phelan, and Link include social conditions and, in particular, socioeconomic status (2013). They argue that when a program working at a level below the societal level fails to rectify health disparities, it may be because larger factors such as socioeconomic status have a greater influence on health. Hatzenbuehler, Phelan, and Link would argue that those with more resources have flexibility to ensure greater health. This model highlights the need for employment nondiscrimination laws for LGBT people.

The pathways model emphasizes the mediating pathways that influence health outcomes. This model largely differs from the fundamental causes model in emphasis. The pathways model focuses on identifying and measuring the specific mediating mechanisms that can influence health. For example, when looking at sexual orientation, this model may focus on experiences of sexual orientation that can include internalized homophobia or discrimination. What these two models and the social ecological model show us more than anything is the complex world within which health is produced and that oversimplified models of understanding health can produce findings that may mislead.

A final framework for understanding LGBT health comes from Sell and Silenzio (2006), who describe how the differing measures of sexual orientation described above (i.e., sexual orientation identity, sexual behavior, and sexual attraction) can each be expected to have different degrees of association with specific health outcomes (see Table 3.1). This model, which is slightly updated here, is not independent of the social ecological model or the fundamental causes model or the pathways model, but it is particularly helpful because it is the only model designed specifically to describe and

Table 3.1   A Framework for Lesbian, Gay, and Bisexual Health Research

Dimensions of Sexual Orientation	Associated Health Concerns
Sexual attraction	• Mental health concerns related to "coming out"
	• Suicide prevention interventions
	• Prevention interventions focusing on safer sexual behaviors predicted by sexual attractions
Behavior	• Sexually transmitted infections (e.g., hepatitis, syphilis, human papillomavirus, chlamydia, gonorrhea)
	• HIV/AIDS
	• Cancers (e.g., anal, rectal, Kaposi's sarcoma, breast, endometrial, ovarian)
Identity	• Access to care
	• Tobacco use
	• Cancers (e.g., lung, stomach)
	• Alcohol use
	• Drug use
	• Violence victimization
	• Teen suicide attempts
	• Eating disorders/nutrition
	• Parenting/marriage
	• Aging
	• Mental health
Cross-cutting	• Violence
	• Access to care (e.g., health insurance, sexual orientation history, cultural competence)
	• Sexual health
	• Public health education/media
	• Discrimination and prejudice
	• Legal protections (e.g., employment, marriage, adoption)

predict LGBT health. While it would be efficient if it were possible to measure a single dimension of sexual orientation and look for associations with health outcomes, each of the different dimensions can in theory be linked to different health outcomes to greater or lesser degrees. For example, people often develop their sexual orientation identities through interactions with other gay, lesbian, and bisexual people in settings and communities frequented by other gay, lesbian, and bisexual people. Many "gay" men came to label themselves as gay in the mid-to-late 20th century through interactions with other gay men in gay bars and bathhouses located in gay neighborhoods (Katz, 1995). These interactions with other gay men not only impacted the development of identities but also influenced health-related behaviors like smoking and alcohol and drug use. So there is a logical association between the development of some sexual orientation identities and some health outcomes. Table 3.1 attempts to categorize the various health outcomes that public health researchers often concern themselves with using this framework as a starting point. A lack of data has prevented many of the associations predicted in this framework from being examined empirically. Nonetheless, this framework provides a logical structure to further the understanding of LGBT health, as it provides insight into how there might be different pathways to the same health outcomes or how health disparities may be produced.

HEALTH DISPARITIES

The discussion of health disparities presented here is only a brief summary of some of the known public health concerns that the LGBT community faces. A full discussion of these concerns would require a large volume in and of itself, if not multiple volumes. LGBT public health has evolved from a discussion of mental health, body image, and sexually transmitted infections in the 1970s, to HIV/AIDS and cancers in the 1980s, to access to health care and mental health in the 1990s, to a comprehensive list of concerns with the advent of the 21st century. The topics listed here were chosen because they have been investigated empirically and/or because they provide insights into why LGBT public health is necessary; however, this is only a summary that does not attempt to address the comprehensive list of concerns that are now becoming better documented.

A list of LGBT health concerns should start with health care access. Health care access means many things. First and foremost, because there are so many LGBT-specific health concerns, if a health care provider does not know that a patient is LGBT, the patient has not had formal access to the health care system. This is particularly relevant for the primary care provider of an LGBT patient. But it can also be a concern to a provider who sees the patient only once in their lifetime, depending upon the service being rendered. Speaking in front of a large audience of physicians, I said there are many issues that one needs to be aware of if one is a provider to an LGBT patient, but if a patient comes with a broken arm to a doctor in the emergency room, they need the doctor and other staff to fix their broken arm. I argued that the LGBT status of the patient here is irrelevant to the provider. An emergency-room physician came up to me after one of the talks and told me that he needed to assess the LGBT status of many patients coming into the emergency room with broken arms. He mentioned the case of a woman with a broken arm who had presented herself in the emergency room with another woman. He was concerned about domestic violence and wondered what role, if any, the second woman might have played in the "accident" that had precipitated the first's condition. I, therefore, think that it is only in very rare situations where the LGBT status of the patient is irrelevant within the health care system. Therefore, if the status remains unknown, full access has not been achieved.

Access to health care goes beyond this example to include the health care provider's ability to know what to do if they know the LGBT status of the patient. Do they know that issues of domestic violence are of equal concern to people regardless of their sexual orientation or gender identity? And, access to the health care system can be obstructed in many other ways, such as by a fear of going to a provider. Many LGBT people, particularly older LGBT people, remember a time when a physician would recommend curing their homosexuality or the physician would not protect information about it from other family members or staff members who did not need to know it. They also worried about this information being recorded in medical records that an employer or insurer might have access to, or they remember physicians fearing to touch people who were gay because of HIV/AIDS (Schultz, 1988). And finally, concerning health insurance, the Affordable Care Act may level the ground somewhat in access to health insurance, but when health insurance is primarily obtained through employment, LGBT people have additional concerns. Because women are less likely to have insurance through the workplace, two women living together are less likely to have health insurance than a man and a woman living together (Patchias and Waxman, 2007). And if the two women are not able to marry, they may not be able to share health insurance with each other if only one is employed. If they can share insurance, there is significant tax penalty to doing so. And without job protections in many parts of the United States and the world, if you cannot obtain employment, you cannot obtain insurance economically.

There are many other health concerns beyond access that need to be included in the list of health disparity concerns, including cancers that may be more or less prevalent among LGBT people because of their association to viral causes (HIV and HPV, for example), or behavioral causes such as smoking, or taking or not taking oral contraception, or becoming pregnant (Boehmer, Miao, Maxwell, & Ozonoff, 2014; Burkhalter, Warren, Shuk, Primavera, & Ostroff, 2009). Mental health concerns have been shown to be more or less prevalent among LGBT people, including issues related to depression, suicide, body dysmorphic disorder, and eating disorders (Bostwick, Boyd, Hughes, West, & McCabe, 2014). The epidemiology of drug use and abuse of both illegal and prescribed drugs often differs between that of LGBT people and that of other populations, resulting in a host of physical and mental health disparities (Newcomb, Ryan, Greene, Garofalo, & Mustanski, 2014). Alcohol and tobacco use and the consequent health concerns similarly often show differential epidemiology between LGBT people and non-LGBT people (Reczek, Liu, & Spiker, 2014; Hatzenbuehler et al., 2014). Other issues such as homelessness and violence are of particular concern to LGBT people, who report higher rates of both within the myriad of health concerns that can result from them (Keuroghlian, Shtasel, and Bassuk, 2014; Oliffe et al., 2014).

Finally, it is important to mention sexually transmitted infections, which were once the only concerns recognized within the field of LGBT public health but are still of much concern today (Everett et al., 2014). The first books on LGBT health often had a chapter on each sexually transmitted disease focusing on its identification and treatment (Rowen & Gillette, 1981). Little attention was paid to prevention. Later, HIV became synonymous with the LGBT community, and particularly gay men, with AIDS first being named "gay-related immune deficiency" (GRID) (Kassler, 1983). HIV/AIDS still dominates the field of LGBT health, sometimes to the detriment of the many other health concerns but sometimes in warranted ways. While HIV/AIDS is no longer considered a "gay" disease, it still impacts the gay community at a much higher rate than any other community, with 63 percent of new infection among gay and bisexual men in 2010 (CDC, 2014).

HEALTH CONCERNS THAT DIFFER FROM THOSE OF OTHER POPULATIONS

In addition to the many health disparity issues discussed above, there are many concerns that may simply be experienced differently for someone who is LGBT than for someone who is not. Many of these issues involve disclosure of sexual orientation or transgender status in environments that may not be comfortable or, at worst, may be unsafe for the individual. For example, a lesbian or bisexual woman who has breast cancer and has had a mastectomy (or may be just considering getting one) may want to attend a support group to discuss concerns with other women who have also had cancer and have undergone similar medical procedures. Chances are, she will not be able to find a support group that includes other lesbians and bisexual women unless she is living in a large urban environment, and even then, such a group may be difficult to access. When confronted with a group that is entirely heterosexual, she has to decide whether to disclose her sexual orientation to the other women in the group. She may want to discuss how the cancer and medical procedures have impacted her emotional and sexual relationships with other women, including possibly a significant other or wife, or how she thinks they may impact these relationships. The woman in this case would first have to negotiate disclosing her sexual orientation to the other women in the group, which can be tricky and uncomfortable for both her and the other women participating in the group. It is easy to imagine situations in which lesbian or bisexual women may not even attempt to avail themselves of such support groups, or they may hide their sexual orientation and consequently not receive the full benefits of the group, or they may disclose their sexual orientation, resulting in unnecessary additional stress or stigma.

For a person who has transitioned from one gender to another or for a person who presents in a manner not socially congruent with their biological sex, there can be many instances where disclosing their biological sex may be of concern in a health care or public health setting. An extreme example is the case where an police officer refused to perform mouth-to-mouth resuscitation on a woman he discovered was biologically male (Dinkelspiel, 2014). This was certainly not the first or last case in which a health care provider refused to care for a transgender person. But even when care is provided, the patient should wonder if their care was equal to the care provided to others. In the past, the bar has often been set very low for what an LGBT person considered acceptable care. If the provider did not refuse to see them or did not attempt to fix their sexual orientation or gender identity, the provider may have been considered not just adequate but admirable or excellent. There are many problems with patients not knowing what acceptable or appropriate care should encompass.

As the number of openly LGBT people expands and ages, concerns related to their care at the end of life is becoming a greater concern in the community (Ramirez-Valles, Dirkes, & Barrett, 2014). For many individuals who have spent much of their lives "out of the closet," which is a relatively new phenomenon socially, decisions about how to present their sexual orientation or gender identity later in life, when they may not be able to care for themselves fully, is of great concern. An LGBT person needing any form of assisted living has to wonder if every employee providing services to them will feel comfortable doing so and, if they do not, how that may result in unequal care. And to some in the LGBT community who may have experienced abuse, discrimination, or stigma in the past, concerns of potential abuse, discrimination, and stigma while they lose the ability to care and protect themselves are real and frightening (Leyva, Breshears, & Ringstad, 2014).

In addition, other large policy concerns that may at first appear to be beyond the scope of public health actually have important public health ramifications and should be dealt with within public health. For example, the "don't ask, don't tell" policy that prevented lesbian, gay, and bisexual people from serving openly in the military had important public health ramifications related to job protection and stigma and discrimination; it still impacts transgender people (Yerke & Mitchell, 2013). Same-sex marriage laws—both those preventing same-sex marriage and those allowing for such marriages—have important public health concerns (Buffie, 2011). And, of course, nondiscrimination laws in the workplace have important implications for health both through the access to insurance or other services provided through employment, as well as the ability to earn a living and the consequent health protections that income provides (Bailey, Wallace, & Wright, 2013).

DISCUSSION AND FUTURE CHALLENGES

In summary, LGBT public health is an important specialization within public health that has slowly struggled to emerge from a time when medicine and public health invested extensive resources in curing homosexuality and aligning the sex and gender of transgender people. While LGBT people benefit from most aspects of public health, they experience disparities in health outcomes as a direct and indirect result of their LGBT status and have health concerns that may not result in disparities with heterosexual populations but differ from those of heterosexuals in a meaningful ways nonetheless. The ecological model of public health provides an informative model for understanding these concerns. The ever-expanding mission of LGBT public health is to understand the public health concerns of the LGBT community as summarized here through interdisciplinary research, through the development of public health policies that recognize the needs of LGBT communities, and through the education of health care providers and those in related fields to the needs of LGBT people.

However, there are many challenges to the practice of LGBT public health, including but not limited to funding and the marginalization and stigma that still exist for researchers working in this field (Comfort, 2010). With progress being made socially for LGBT people, and particularly related to same-sex marriage and employment protections, one can hope that the field of public health will advance simultaneously with the concerns of LGBT people being fully considered, investigated, and addressed.

REFERENCES

Bailey, J., Wallace, M., & Wright, B. (2013). Are gay men and lesbians discriminated against when applying for jobs? A four-city, Internet-based field experiment. *Journal of Homosexuality, 60*(6), 873–894.

Bayer, R. (1987). *Homosexuality in American psychiatry: The politics of diagnosis.* Princeton, NJ: Princeton University Press.

Boehmer, U., Miao, X., Maxwell, N. I., & Ozonoff, A. (2014). Sexual minority population density and incidence of lung, colorectal and female breast cancer in California. *BMJ Open, 26*(3), e004461.

Bostwick, W. B., Boyd, C. J., Hughes, T. L., West, B. T., & McCabe, S. E. (2014). Discrimination and mental health among lesbian, gay, and bisexual adults in the United States. *American Journal of Orthopsychiatry, 84*(1), 35–45.

Bronski, M. (2012). *A queer history of the United States.* Boston, MA: Beacon Press.

Buffie, W. C. (2011). Public health implications of same-sex marriage. *American Journal of Public Health, 101*(6), 986–990.

Burkhalter, J. E., Warren, B., Shuk, E., Primavera, L., & Ostroff, J. S. (2009). Intention to quit smoking among lesbian, gay, bisexual, and transgender smokers. *Nicotine & Tobacco Research, 11*(11), 1312–1320.

Carpenter, E. (1908). *The intermediate sex.* London: Allen and Unwin.

Center of Excellence for Transgender Health. (2014). Recommendations for inclusive data collection of trans people in HIV prevention, care and services. Retrieved from http://transhealth.ucsf.edu/trans?page=lib-data-collection

Centers for Disease Control. (2014). HIV among men in the United States. *World Wide Web.* Retrieved from https://www.cdc.gov/hiv/group/gender/men/index.html

Chauncey, G. (1995). *Gay New York: Gender, urban culture, and the making of the gay male world, 1890–1940.* New York, NY: Basic Books.

Comfort, J. (2010). LGBTI Health research: Challenges and ways forward. *Gay and Lesbian Issues and Psychology Review, 6*(3), 132–138.

Conron, K. J., Landers, S. J., Reisner, S. L., & Sell, R. L. (2014). Sex and gender in the US Health Surveillance System: A call to action. *American Journal of Public Health, 104*(6), 970–976.

Coulter, R. W., Kenst, K. S., Bowen, D. J., & Scout. (2014). Research funded by the National Institutes of Health on the health of lesbian, gay, bisexual, and transgender populations. *American Journal of Public Health, 104*(2), e105–e112.

Dahlberg, L. L., & Krug, E. G. (2002). Violence—A global public health problem. In E. Krug, L. L Dahlberg, J. A. Mercy, A. B. Zwi, & R. Lozano (Eds.), *World report on violence and health* (pp. 1–56). Geneva, Switzerland: World Health Organization.

Diez Roux, A. V. (2012). Conceptual approaches to the study of health disparities. *Annual Review of Public Health, 33,* 41–58.

Dinkelspiel, F. (2014). Berkeley slapped with lawsuit over Kayla Moore's death. *Berkelyside.com,* February 14.

Everett, B. G., Schnarrs, P. W., Rosario, M., Garofalo, R., & Mustanski, B. (2014). Sexual orientation disparities in sexually transmitted infection risk behaviors and risk determinants among sexually active adolescent males: Results from a school-based sample. *American Journal of Public Health, 104*(6), 1107–1112.

Fullilove, M. T. (1998). Comment: Abandoning "race" as a variable in public health research—An idea whose time has come. *American Journal of Public Health, 88*(9), 1297–1298.

Hatzenbuehler, M. L., Keyes, K. M., Hamilton, A., & Hasin, D. S. (2014). State-level tobacco environments and sexual orientation disparities in tobacco use and dependence in the USA. *Tobacco Control, 23*, e2. doi:10.1136/tobaccocontrol-2013-051279

Hatzenbuehler, M. L., Phelan, J. C., & Link, B. G. (2013). Stigma as a fundamental cause of population health inequalities. *American Journal of Public Health, 103*(5), 813–821.

Hooker, E. (1957). The adjustment of the male overt homosexual. *Journal of Projective Techniques, 21*(1), 18–31.

Institute of Medicine Committee on Lesbian, Gay, Bisexual, and Transgender Health Issues and Research Gaps and Opportunities. (2011). *The health of lesbian, gay, bisexual, and transgender people: Building a foundation for better understanding.* Washington, DC: National Academies Press.

Jones, J. H. (1992). *Bad blood: The Tuskegee syphilis experiment.* New York, NY: Free Press.

Kassler, J. (1983). *Gay men's health: A guide to the AID Syndrome and other sexually transmitted diseases.* New York, NY: Harper and Row.

Katz, J. N. (1983). *Gay/lesbian almanac: A new documentary.* New York, NY: Harper & Row.

Katz, J. N. (1992). *Gay American history: Lesbians and gay men in the USA.* New York, NY: Meridian, 1992.

Katz, J. N. (1995). *The invention of heterosexuality.* Chicago: The University of Chicago Press.

Kaufman, R. (2008). Introduction to transgender identity and health. In H. Makadon, K. H. Mayer, J. Potter, & H. Goldhammer (Eds.), *Fenway guide to lesbian, gay, bisexual, and transgender health* (pp. 331–363). Philadelphia: American College of Physicians.

Keuroghlian, A. S., Shtasel, D., & Bassuk, E. L. (2014). Out on the street: A public health and policy agenda for lesbian, gay, bisexual, and transgender youth who are homeless. *American Journal of Orthopsychiatry, 84*(1), 66–72.

Leyva, V. L., Breshears, E. M., & Ringstad, R. (2014). Assessing the efficacy of LGBT cultural competency training for aging services providers in California's central valley. *Journal of Gerontological Social Work, 57*(2–4), 335–348.

McLeroy, K. R, Bibeau, D., Steckler, A., & Glanz, K. (1988). An ecological perspective on health promotion programs. *Health Education Quarterly, 15*(4), 351–377.

Miller, K., & Ryan, J. M. (2011). *Design, development and testing of the NHIS sexual identity question.* Questionnaire Design Research Laboratory, Office of Research Methodology, National Center for Health Statistics. Retrieved from http://lgbttobacco.org/files/Final%20Report%20Sexual%20Identity.pdf

Newcomb, M. E., Ryan, D. T., Greene, G. J., Garofalo, R., & Mustanski B. (2014). Prevalence and patterns of smoking, alcohol use, and illicit drug use in young men who have sex with men. *Drug & Alcohol Dependence, 141,* 65–71. doi:10.1016/j.drugalcdep.2014.05.005.

Obedin-Maliver, J., Goldsmith, E. S., Stewart, L., White, W., Tran, E., Brenman, S., ... Lunn, M. R. (2011). Lesbian, gay, bisexual, and transgender-related content in undergraduate medical education. *Journal of the American Medical Association, 306*(9), 971–977.

Oliffe, J. L., Han, C., Maria, E. S., Lohan, M., Howard, T., Stewart, D. E., & MacMillan, H. (2014). Gay men and intimate partner violence: A gender analysis. *Sociology of Health and Illness, 36*(4), 564–579.

Patchias, E. M., & Waxman, J. (2007). *Women in health coverage: The affordability gap.* The Commonwealth Fund issue brief. Retrieved from https://www.commonwealthfund.org/publications/issue-briefs/2007/apr/women-and-health-coverage-affordability-gap

Ramirez-Valles, J., Dirkes, J., & Barrett, H. A. (2014). GayBy boomers' social support: Exploring the connection between health and emotional and instrumental support in older gay men. *Journal of Gerontological Social Work, 57*(2–4), 218–234.

Reczek, C., Liu, H., & Spiker, R. (2014). A population-based study of alcohol use in same-sex and different-sex unions. *Journal of Marriage and Family, 76*(3), 557–572.

Rowen, R. L., & Gillette, P. J. (1981). *The gay health guide.* London: TBS The Book Service.

Schultz, R. (1988). *And the band played on.* New York: St. Martin's Press.

Sell, R. L. (1997). Defining and measuring sexual orientation: A review. *Archives of Sexual Behavior, 26*(6), 643–658.

Sell, R. L., & Becker, J. B. (2001). Sexual orientation data: Inclusion in health information systems used to monitor HP2010. *American Journal of Public Health, 91*(6), 876–882.

Sell, R. L., & Holliday, M. L. (2014). Sexual orientation data collection policy in the United States: Public health malpractice. *American Journal of Public Health, 104*(6), 967–969.

Sell, R. L., & Silenzio, V. M. B. (2006). Lesbian, gay, bisexual, and transgender public health research. In M. D. Shankle (Ed.), *The handbook of lesbian, gay, bisexual, and transgender public health: A practitioner's guide to service* (pp. 33–56). Binghamton, NY: The Haworth Press.

Shariff-Marco, S., Breen, N., Landrine, H., Reeve, B. B., Krieger, N., Gee, G. C., ... Johnson, T. P. (2011). Measuring everyday racial/ethnic discrimination in health surveys. *Du Bois Review, 8*(1), 159–177.

Simpson, L. A. (1997). History of gay and lesbian physician groups. *Journal of the Gay and Lesbian Medical Association, 1*(1), 61–63.

Stangl, A. L., Lloyd, J. K., Brady, L. M., Holland, C. E., & Baral, S. J. (2013). A systematic review of interventions to reduce HIV-related stigma and discrimination from 2002 to 2013: How far have we come? *Journal of the International AIDS Society, 16*(3 Suppl 2), 18734.

U.S. Department of Health and Human Services. (2000). *Healthy People 2010: Understanding and improving health* (2nd ed.). Washington, DC: U.S. Government Printing Office.

U.S. Department of Health and Human Services. (2011). Implementation guidance on data collection standards for race, ethnicity, sex, primary language, and disability status, October. Retrieved from http://aspe.hhs.gov /datacncl/standards/aca/4302/index.pdf

Yerke, A. F., & Mitchell, V. (2013). Transgender people in the military: Don't ask? Don't tell? Don't enlist! *Journal of Homosexuality, 60*(2–3), 436–457.

4

Transgender Medical Care in the United States: A Historical Perspective

Madeline B. Deutsch, Marci L. Bowers, Asa Radix, and Tamar C. Carmel

Transgender care programs began to develop in the 1950s in the United States at a number of universities (Stryker, 2008). Transgender care was the subject of research and was covered by insurance plans. After researchers started to question the utility of surgery in improving psychological outcomes and some controversial cases, most university programs had closed by the early 1990s (Diamond & Sigmundson, 1997; Meyer & Reter, 1979; Wise & Lucas, 1981). At the same time and for similar reasons, insurance companies effectively excluded transgender coverage wholesale.

The movement of transgender health care out of universities had benefits and drawbacks. Once transgender health care was no longer restricted to universities, community clinics and private practitioners moved in to fill the void. Decentralized and unencumbered by the complexities of research and academia, the field was able to evolve at a much more rapid and creative pace. Transgender health care in the United States today is fairly flexible compared to in other Western nations, such as those in Europe, where more rigid and structured guidelines exist as a result of centralized, university-based programs.

However, there are drawbacks to this shift as well. Funding the change from university-based to community care has fallen by and large on transgender persons themselves, who often must pay out of pocket for their own care. While stepping away from insurance plans frees transgender people to work with their providers in more flexible ways, it also puts an undue financial burden on them. Additionally, the loss of university-based programs has all but eliminated large-scale transgender health care research in the United States; most current research is from Europe, where funding still exists (Reisner et al., 2016). Additionally, the decentralization of care led to a lack of standardized practices. In recent years, several best practices guidelines have been developed and made available to the general public (Vancouver Coastal Health, 2015; Center of Excellence for Transgender Health [CoE], 2016). Optimally, over time more practitioners will begin to standardize their practices to be in line with current research and standards of care.

Recently, important changes have occurred in the insurance landscape related to transgender care. The National Coverage Determination (NCD) that had previously denied Medicare coverage of all "transsexual" surgery was determined to be invalid, allowing access to gender-affirming surgeries for the first time since the ban was introduced in 1981 (Department of Health and Human Services Departmental Appeals Board, 2013). Several states have introduced legislation mandating coverage of transgender-related care by both commercial insurances and Medicaid (Human Rights Campaign, 2015). Health care plans under the Affordable Care Act are required to cover sex-specific preventive health services for transgender persons, ending a practice that often prevented transgender persons from accessing needed preventive screenings. Long-awaited changes have also occurred in funding since the release of the Institute of Medicine (IOM) report with increases in National Institutes of Health (NIH) funding directed toward transgender-related research (Coulter, Kenst, Bowen, & Scout, 2014; Institute of Medicine, 2011).

A COMMENT ON TERMINOLOGY

The terminology used to describe and define the transgender community is a constantly evolving subject of intense debate and discussion and is not cut and dried. For the purposes of this medical discussion, the umbrella term "transgender" will be used in general reference to persons seeking medical or surgical interventions to somehow alter their secondary sex characteristics. It is recognized that great diversity exists among transgender and gender-variant persons in both identity and preferred terminology. (See Table 4.1.)

Table 4.1   Transgender Terminology

Cisgender	Individuals whose gender identity aligns with their assigned sex at birth.
Gender identity	A person's inherent sense of being male or female or something else.
Gender nonconformity	Refers to the extent to which a person's gender identity, role, or expression differs from the cultural norms prescribed for people of a particular sex.
Nonbinary/genderqueer	A term for people who embrace a gender identity that is not exclusively male or female and therefore outside of the binary.
Transgender	An umbrella term for people whose gender identity, expression, or behavior is different from those usually associated with their gender assigned at birth. It includes a wide variety of identities. Transgender people may undergo medical or surgical treatments to change secondary sex characteristics.
Transition	The process by which a person begins to live as the gender they identify with instead of the gender they were assigned at birth. Transition may include social, medical, or surgical changes.
Transsexual	A medical term, currently infrequently used, that refers to individuals who have undergone hormonal or surgical interventions to transition from their sex assigned at birth to their affirmed gender.

TRANS-COMPETENT AND AFFIRMING HEALTH CARE ENVIRONMENTS

In addition to taking care with language, it is important that health care agencies be safe spaces for transgender people from the moment a transgender person enters until they leave. Every provider and staff person should utilize the transgender individual's preferred name and pronouns, regardless of what is on their legal documents. Intake forms should provide the space and language for transgender identities. Documentation in the medical chart should also be consistent with the individual's identity.

One caveat is when treating transgender youth and young adults, as families may not be supportive or even know about the patient's transgender identity. Unintentionally outing a transgender person can potentially set them up for verbal abuse, physical violence, and homelessness. Outing of one's transgender identity can be done accidentally in person, via obtainable documentation in the medical record, or through insurance billing. Thus it is important that young adults are involved in conversations about how they want to be identified in the medical chart, what diagnoses should be used for billing purposes, and how to keep them safe.

The above holds true for treating transgender individuals in an inpatient setting as well. It is important to make sure all staff, providers, and fellow patients use the correct name and pronouns as identified by the transgender patient. Safety is a huge concern on inpatient units. Care and diligence should be used in rooming accommodations to be respectful of the person's gender identity while remaining mindful of the risk of physical and sexual violence against the trans patient. Bathroom accommodations should be similarly approached and gender-neutral bathrooms utilized for all patients when possible. Rather than make these decisions *for* the transgender patient, discussions and decisions about rooming and bathrooms should be made *with* the trans patient.

PREVENTIVE HEALTH IN TRANS POPULATIONS

Transgender people have two broad areas of concern with respect to preventive health. General health issues such as diet and exercise; screening of cholesterol, blood pressure, and blood sugar; immunizations; and malignancies unrelated to gendered body parts (such as colon cancer) are often dealt with in a similar way in cisgender people. Detailed discussion of these matters is beyond the scope of this text. However, up-to-date preventive health guidelines for transgender people can be accessed through the online University of California at San Francisco (UCSF) Transhealth Protocols (CoE, 2016). Another area of preventive health for transgender people, to be discussed here, concerns transgender-specific matters and, for the most part, involves awareness of the particular anatomy of a transgender individual. In addition, mental and social health issues such as substance abuse, depression, and anxiety tend to have a higher prevalence in the transgender population due to the inherent stress of living in the world as a transgender person. Mental health and substance abuse screening is part of preventive health for all populations.

In general, practitioners should follow the axiom, "If you have it, check it," referring to the organs a person has. When establishing a relationship with a new patient, practitioners should take an inventory of exactly what organs a patient has. This may not always be straightforward, as often patients themselves may not know exactly what organs they do and do not have.

Cervix: Trans men and genderqueer persons with a cervix require screening in line with current recommendations for cervical cancer screening in cisgender women. The screening pelvic exam generally involves using a gloved hand inside the vagina and another hand on the abdomen to evaluate the uterus and ovaries, and then placing a speculum inside the vagina to allow the provider to visualize the cervix and obtain a Pap smear, a test for changes to the cervix that may be signs of cervical cancer.

Trans men may find this exam to be emotionally or physically challenging or painful and are less likely than cisgender women to undergo cervical cancer screening (Peitzmeier, Khullar, Reisner, & Potter, 2014). In some cases, it may be impossible to complete the exam due to a partially or completely intact hymen. Using one and then two fingers at the vaginal opening to apply gentle pressure while the patient bears down as if to urinate can help relax pelvic musculature. Using a small speculum and an appropriate amount of lubricant can also help minimize discomfort. Contrary to what some believe, it is possible to use a lubricant for a pap smear when using a liquid-based pap test. The manufacturer can provide a list of approved compatible lubricant brands. The lubricant should be applied on both sides of the speculum.

Many trans men and providers wonder if a pap is needed in persons who have not had any penetrative penile-vaginal activity. Cervical cancer is caused by the human papillomavirus (HPV), which can be transmitted sexually. Very limited research suggests that cisgender women with no history of penile insertion have a low risk of cervical cancer in the short to medium term (Johnson, Smith, & Guenther, 1987). Given the technical limitations of performing a pap smear in some trans men, it is within reason for trans men who have had no penile-penetrative activity to have a discussion of this subject with their providers, particularly if they plan on a hysterectomy (removal of the uterus), with possible removal of the cervix, in the medium-term future. Another option is to try to obtain a specimen by blindly inserting a swab and sending it for high-risk HPV testing. This option for cervical cancer detection is being investigated but is not currently the standard of care (Virtanen, Anttila, & Nieminen, 2015).

Because the shape of the cervix changes when someone is on testosterone, providers may find a high percentage of pap specimens are inconclusive due to a lack of cells of the crucial transitional zone within the cervical canal (Peitzmeier, Khullar, Harigopal, & Potter, 2014). This and the above-described technical difficulties may lead providers to perform a blood test for high-risk HPV as a surrogate marker of cervical risk. This practice has not been studied or validated but may play a role in the context of harm reduction.

For those up to age 26, an HPV vaccine (Gardasil) is available and should be offered if it has not already been received.

Uterus: While it is believed that testosterone causes atrophy (decrease in the amount of tissue) of the endometrium (uterine lining), a precancerous overgrowth known as hyperplasia is still a theoretical, though rare, possibility. In general, once menstruation stops with testosterone, any return of vaginal bleeding or menstruation while still on testosterone warrants an investigation with at least an ultrasound. A missed or changed dose of testosterone, or the addition of a medicine that affects testosterone levels, may cause bleeding. Providers should use clinical judgment in these cases to guide the decision for ultrasound evaluation.

Some patients may experience pelvic pain or cramping when on testosterone. Ongoing pelvic pain or vaginal bleeding may suggest persistently elevated estrogen levels, increased sensitivity to estrogen, or some combination of the two. Since estrogen is synthesized by the body from testosterone, trans men taking testosterone may suffer these symptoms of persistent estrogen function. Potential remedies include the use of progestagens such as depo-medroxyprogesterone that stabilize the endometrium and shut down pituitary gonadotropin (FSH/LH) release. Another more experimental option would be to add an aromatase inhibitor such as anastrozole, which blocks the synthesis of estrogen. Both of these medications can increase the risk of osteoporosis and require ongoing bone health screening and care.

Trans men may have or develop uterine fibroids, endometriosis, or other gynecologic conditions. Continued vaginal bleeding, cramping, or other symptoms not responsive to basic interventions or that is severe should be evaluated by a gynecologist.

Ovaries: It is believed that testosterone causes changes in the ovaries similar to polycystic ovarian syndrome (PCOS). This may predispose trans men to ovarian pain syndromes, and may interfere with fertility, even if testosterone is stopped; however, there is no link between polycystic ovaries and increased risk of ovarian cancer. Ovarian cancer is a somewhat rare condition that is difficult to detect in early stages. Most people are diagnosed with ovarian cancer at a later stage, and five-year survival is less than 50 percent. The well-known story of Robert Eads (a trans man diagnosed with ovarian cancer who had difficulty finding a provider willing to treat him) may mislead some to believe that he died only because of his difficulties in finding care. In fact, his cancer was diagnosed at an already terminal stage. No screening tests or recommendations exist for ovarian cancer. Regular pelvic exams can help providers detect pelvic masses as early as possible to facilitate further testing and, if needed, referral to a gynecologist.

Prostate: The prostate is left intact after vaginoplasty, so prostate cancer remains possible in transgender women after this surgery. Prostate cancer, in many cases, is so slow growing that it may go undetected and without symptoms for decades or even a lifetime. The incidence of prostate cancer in trans women has not been studied, and data is limited to isolated case reports. It is important to note that in most cases of prostate cancer, the treatment is estrogen and/or testosterone blockade. As such, one would expect a low incidence of prostate cancer in trans women, who often take these medications routinely as part of hormone therapy. However, given that prostate cancer typically grows slowly and can go undetected for decades, it is possible that a trans woman could have undetected prostate cancer when she begins estrogen treatment. Prostate masses, or symptoms of benign prostatic hypertrophy (BPH, an increase in the size of the prostate), or prostatitis (infection of the prostate), such as urinary retention or pain, in trans women should be approached as they would be in cisgender men, with urine studies, ultrasound, or biopsy as indicated and, if appropriate, consultation with a urologist.

The use of prostate-specific antigen (PSA) testing should be discussed on an individual basis with a provider. There are some instances where this test can be useful, but it is no longer recommended for routine screening for prostate cancer. A PSA test in a patient undergoing estrogen therapy will be unreliable and lack sensitivity due to a false lowering effect of estrogen.

Breast: Breast cancer in trans women is a seemingly rare occurrence, with only a few reports in the medical literature (Brown, 2015; Brown & Jones, 2015; Gooren, van Trotsenburg, Giltay, & van Diest, 2013). That said, trans women may lack access to medical care and have cases that go undetected until these women die of other causes. Lacking any scientific data, because breast cancer risk can be related to estrogen exposure, intuitively it makes sense that a trans woman's risk of breast cancer is dependent on the age at which she started hormone replacement therapy (HRT), how long she has been on HRT, and other risk factors such as family history or smoking. In general, it is a good idea to begin to consider screening after a trans woman has both been on hormones for five years and after she has reached the age to begin screening in cisgender women.

The screening for breast cancer in trans women may have several special considerations. First, the smaller and more dense and fibrous breasts found in trans women can make mammograms and their interpretation more technically difficult and could increase the risk of a false positive test; false negatives would also be possible from increased density. False positives can lead to stress, and invasive tests such as biopsies and are no small matter. Some trans women have breast abnormalities related to injection of street silicone. In these instances, providers may consider using ultrasound or MRI screening as available and in consultation with a breast radiologist.

Trans women with breast implants may require specialized mammography equipment and techniques. Currently, the two silicone breast implant manufacturers in the United States recommend periodic specialized MRI screening every two to three years to assess the integrity of the breast implant. This recommendation is controversial since it is expensive, and some sources suggest it can be more harmful to remove a leaking implant than to simply leave it in place. Large studies have shown that silicone breast implants do not increase the risk of autoimmune disease or breast cancer (Noels, Lapid, Lindeman, & Bastiaannet, 2015). However, several recent case reports have been published documenting anaplastic large-cell lymphoma in women with silicone breast implants (Berlin et al., 2018).

Especially in the early stages of hormone therapy, trans women may develop small, firm nodules under the nipple known as breast buds. This is a normal stage of breast development and in general should not warrant further investigation. Some trans women may periodically have a thick white nipple discharge, usually in connection with a high or sudden change in estrogen dose. In most cases this is a benign process, but it could signify a problem with the pituitary gland (see below).

Trans men who have not had top surgery (or who had a partial mastectomy or liposuction only) require continued breast cancer screening in accordance with age-matched recommendations for cisgender women. Trans men with residual breast tissue may encounter similar technical difficulties in mammogram interpretation. As with trans women, ultrasound or MRI may be useful adjuncts. Limited data suggest that testosterone treatment does not increase a trans man's risk of breast cancer above where it was before HRT, but it is unclear if testosterone reduces breast cancer risk. Clinicians should discuss these unknowns with transgender men both before and after chest surgery, and consider clinician breast exams yearly in the absence of any other feasible screening method.

Pituitary gland: The pituitary is a pea-sized gland at the base of the brain. A rare tumor known as a prolactinoma can develop on its own or in response to estrogen treatment. This benign tumor is not life-threatening, but because of its location next to the optic nerve can lead to vision changes or blindness. High estrogen levels can cause prolactin levels to climb, which may be a marker of an enlarging pituitary gland. Since prolactin is the hormone involved in breast milk production, people with elevated prolactin levels may notice some breast milk discharge. In most cases, breast milk is minimal and not due to a prolactinoma but to changing or high estrogen levels. Because the Endocrine Society guidelines for management of an incidentally found asymptomatic pituitary adenoma is to do nothing, routine screening for prolactin levels is not indicated. Diagnostic prolactin should be tested in patients with suggestive symptoms such as galactorrhea, new-onset headaches, or visual changes.

Bones: Sex hormones are involved in maintaining bone integrity and strength. Cisgender women who have gone through menopause are at increased risk of osteoporosis, or weakening of the bones. Low or absent levels of estrogen or testosterone can lead to osteoporosis (severe bone degeneration) or a less severe condition known as osteopenia. Both conditions predispose individuals to an increased risk of fractures, particularly of the hip and spinal column. The exact roles of estrogen, testosterone, and other factors in preventing osteoporosis are somewhat unclear. Research on cisgender men with prostate cancer who are on androgen blockers suggests that healthy bones require maintaining enough sex hormone to keep FSH and LH levels in the normal range through feedback inhibition. Providers may consider periodic checks of LH and FSH in trans persons who are on low doses of hormones or off hormones after gonadectomy (removal of the testes or ovaries) to be sure bone health is optimized. If FSH/LH are elevated, increased sex hormone dosage (and other prevention measures such as vitamin D supplementation or exercise) should be considered. All trans persons should be evaluated for vitamin D deficiency and should be supplemented with calcium and vitamin D according to current published guidelines. Weight-bearing exercise such as light weight lifting/muscle toning is important in maintaining bone health and is appropriate for transgender men and women.

MENTAL HEALTH AS PREVENTIVE HEALTH

Mental health screening is as important as general health screening for all people, including transgender people. Due to a number of factors, in large part societal stigma and violence, transgender people are at higher risk than the general population for a number of mental health issues.

Society's Effect on Transgender Mental Health

Transgender individuals disproportionately experience microaggressions and institutionalized discrimination in their daily lives, and worse, overt discrimination and violence, predisposing the population to negative mental health outcomes.

Transgender individuals are subject to daily reminders of their stigmatized identity, including misgendering; lack of inclusion in nondiscrimination policies; harassment when using public restrooms; hiring discrimination or firing from jobs; bullying and violence; lack of legal protections; and trans care exclusions in insurance coverage. Fifty to eighty percent of trans individuals report violence and victimization, including sexual assault (Clements-Nolle, Marx, & Katz, 2006; Kenagy, 2005;

Lombardi, Wilchins, Priesing, & Malouf, 2001). Transgender women of color are at particularly increased risk of violence, victimization, and murder.

As we know from general psychiatric research, a trauma history increases risk for depression, post-traumatic stress disorder (PTSD), self-harm, suicidal thoughts and attempts, and substance use problems. The societal microaggressions, discrimination, and violence add up, increasingly taking a toll on trans people's mental health. Because of this, the trans community has disproportionate rates of depression, anxiety, self-harm, suicidal thoughts, suicide attempts, and substance use disorders, even more so than that experienced by their gay, lesbian, and bisexual peers (de Vries, Doreleijers, Steensma, & Cohen-Kettenis, 2011; Office of Disease Prevention and Health Promotion, 2018; Roberts, Rosario, Corliss, Koenen, & Austin, 2012).

Mental Health Disparities

The prevalence of depression in the trans community is estimated to be approximately 50 to 60 percent and believed to be directly linked to discrimination and violence (Nuttbrock et al., 2010; Rotondi et al., 2011).

Although theoretically there is a link between hormone use and mood symptoms, this is not typically seen in trans people taking hormones as prescribed. Mania or aggression on testosterone is rare, as is depression on feminizing hormones. In fact, trans individuals who begin hormones may experience *lessening* of preexisting depressive and anxiety symptoms related to their gender dysphoria as their bodies and social roles align more with their internal gender and sense of self. Transgender individuals with anxiety, depression, or other mental illnesses not related to their gender identity/dysphoria are unlikely to experience changes in their mental illness on hormones. Cases of increased mood symptoms are sometimes linked to taking more than prescribed doses of hormones.

Trans and gender-nonconforming (GNC) individuals experience an undue burden of compounding psychosocial stressors (such as bullying, harassment, violence, lack of legal protections, unemployment, homelessness, etc.) that negatively impact their mental health. Trans patients may express their psychic pain through self-injury, generally through superficial cutting behavior, similarly to the general population. In rare, yet severe cases, trans individuals may engage in mutilation of their chest or genitals. Trans individuals are also at a heightened risk of suicidal thoughts and attempts, with larger studies showing astounding lifetime rates of suicide attempts of approximately 40 percent (National Center for Transgender Equality, & National Gay and Lesbian Task Force, 2010; American Foundation for Suicide Prevention, & Williams Institute, 2014). It is thus very important to screen for self-harm and suicidal ideation in trans people and explore psychosocial stressors, supports, and the individual's personal strengths and resilience factors to make an informed risk assessment.

Given the high rates of trauma, PTSD and anxiety disorders are likely to be increased in trans populations. Trans individuals also have higher rates of substance misuse. They may utilize drugs and alcohol for various reasons, such as to self-medicate their mental health issues and numb their pain, or as a social lubricant to feel more comfortable with their body and identity. In some, alcohol and illicit substances may be used to facilitate sex work for self-preservation. Substance use correlates with negative mental health outcomes and increased risk of sexually transmitted infections (STIs).

Transgender people are not thought to be at increased risk of bipolar disorder or schizophrenia compared to the general population, likely because these illnesses have a significant genetic basis. However, similarly to the larger population, there are small percentages of transgender people with these illnesses. Trans people with severe and persistent mental illness (SPMI) often have difficulty accessing needed services due to the double stigma of being transgender and having a major mental illness.

Resilience

Despite the somber tone and statistics noted above, a sizable portion of the trans community does not have mental health issues. Research done by the Family Acceptance Project and others has shown that social and familial support has a strongly positive impact on transgender people's lives. In fact, a recent study on trans youth showed that familial support and social transition mitigated negative mental health outcomes (Olson, Durwood, DeMeules, & McLaughlin, 2016).

Discrimination in Healthcare Settings

Similar to what they experience in society at large, trans individuals face remarkable challenges when trying to obtain medical and mental health care (CoE, 2016). Trans individuals may lack insurance coverage or not have access to trans-competent and affirming providers. Of those who have been able to access care, many trans patients have experienced institutionalized and/or targeted discrimination in health care settings, further traumatizing trans patients and the broader community and leading to postponement of needed care (Reisner et al., 2015). It is important for health care providers to understand, validate, and positively support trans patients in order to provide a safe environment for healing. Providers must consciously work to avoid triggers and retraumatizing the trans patient. Trans patients may seek mental health care to address challenges faced during their gender transition and other trans-related themes, or they may enter care to address mental health issues unrelated to their gender identity. It is important *not* to assume that all of a trans person's issues are related to their gender identity and instead to listen to the person and allow them to identify their areas of concern.

Gender Dysphoria as a Diagnosis

The Diagnostic and Statistical Manual (DSM) published by the American Psychiatric Association is the diagnostic bible, so to speak, of psychiatrists and psychologists practicing in the United States. Trans-related mental health diagnoses first appeared in the DSM-II (1968) as "Transvestitism." In the DSM-III (1980), the diagnosis morphed into two separate diagnoses of "Transsexualism" and "Gender Identity Disorder of Childhood." In further editions, the diagnosis remained as "Gender Identity Disorder" with designations of "in children" or "in adolescents or adults," until the most recent edition, DSM-5 (2013), changed to the less stigmatizing language of "Gender Dysphoria."

To be diagnosed with gender dysphoria, there must be a "marked incongruence" between one's identified gender and sex assigned at birth, of at least six months duration, as well as significant distress or impairment in one's life, thereby removing well-adjusted trans persons from this mental health diagnosis. The diagnosis also includes specifiers for "disorders of sex development" (DSDs, also known as intersex conditions) and those who are "post-transition."

To Diagnose or Not to Diagnose?

There is controversy within the trans community as well as among providers as to whether a trans-related mental health diagnosis should exist. Some assert that having a mental health diagnosis pathologizes trans identities and individuals regardless of whether they are having difficulties in their lives or not. Some further assert that trans mental health disparities are due to societal stigma and discrimination and not inherent problems within trans people themselves. Others argue for a trans diagnosis to justify the fight for insurance coverage of transition-related therapy, hormones, and surgeries. Still others argue that if a diagnosis is to exist, it should be a medical diagnosis, not a mental health one, since the treatments needed are medical and surgical in nature.

The breadth and nuances of this debate are beyond the scope of this chapter. However, trans people and providers should have frank conversations about the use of these diagnoses. Some mental health providers choose to avoid trans-related diagnoses altogether, instead utilizing traditional mental health diagnoses such as depressive disorders or anxiety disorders, when applicable, or adjustment disorder when the issue is primarily related to transition. On the medical side, providers may opt to use the diagnosis "Unspecified Endocrine Disorder" rather than the trans-related ICD code to avoid stigmatization and to attempt to obtain insurance coverage of needed hormones.

World Professional Association for Transgender Health (WPATH) Mental Health Recommendations for Hormonal and Surgical Transition

WPATH is an international association composed of physical and mental health providers with an expertise in transgender care. It produces the Standards of Care (SOC), a consensus guideline that sets forth recommendations for transition-related care (Coleman et al., 2012). The SOC no longer requires therapy, mental health care, or "real-life experience" before one can obtain hormones for a gender transition. It is recommended that the prescribing practitioner screen for mental illness and provide mental health referrals when indicated.

Though not required, trans individuals may benefit from therapy before and during their transition to address such areas as coming out to family, approaching social transition and disclosure, dealing with societal discrimination, maintaining physical and emotional safety, developing realistic expectations of physical transition, living in a body incongruent with one's gender identity, and navigating dating and romantic relationships.

The WPATH Standards of Care do recommend that transgender individuals obtain one letter of support from a mental health provider in order to obtain top surgery (male-contoured chest reconstruction or breast augmentation) and two letters from two different providers in order to obtain bottom surgery (genital surgeries). These letters are to confirm the individual's trans identity, identify any other mental health concerns, attest to the individual's emotional stability for undergoing the surgical intervention, and affirm that the individual understands the procedure and that it is in line with their transition goals. It is helpful for the individual and the surgeon to identify the individual's support system and coping mechanisms. If the individual has mental illness or concerns, this does not preclude them from surgery. However, it is important that these concerns are addressed and relatively stable prior to surgery so as to allow for a safe and emotionally stable postoperative period. Most surgeons who perform transgender-related surgeries follow the WPATH Standards of Care and will not schedule a surgery without obtaining the aforementioned letter(s).

TRANSITION-RELATED MEDICAL CARE

Transition-related medical care can be broken up into three broad categories; medical (hormonal) care, surgical care, and additional care and procedures.

Hormone therapy (also known as hormone replacement therapy, cross-gender hormone therapy, or hormonal therapy) involves administering hormones of the affirmed gender, perhaps in conjunction with hormone blockers to minimize or eliminate the effects of circulating hormones. The use of hormone therapy in transgender persons dates back to the middle of the 20th century; however, there has been limited research to evaluate its effectiveness in improving the quality of life of transgender persons. Anecdotally, most medical providers observe that patients tolerate hormone therapy very well and that quality of life is significantly improved once hormone therapy is initiated; several recent studies have indeed begun to demonstrate just that.

The use of hormones for medical transition is an "off-label" practice in the United States. In other words, it involves using medications for purposes other than those approved by the U.S. Food and Drug Administration (FDA). This does not mean that use of these drugs is illegal or that it increases a provider's risk of malpractice suits (Deutsch, 2012). It simply means that providers must acknowledge that they are using a treatment that has not been fully evaluated by the U.S. FDA for that purpose. Obtaining FDA approval for a specific indication is a costly process that requires extensive research testing under very specific guidelines; given the lack of transgender research funding, this kind of large-scale testing is unlikely to happen in the near future. However, there does exist a large body of published evidence supporting the use of various hormone and related treatments in transgender persons (Asscheman et al., 2008; Asscheman, Gooren, & Eklund, 1989; Gooren, 2011; Gooren, Giltay, & Bunck, 2008; Hembree et al., 2009; van Kesteren, Asscheman, Megens, & Gooren, 1997).

Basic Hormone Physiology

A hormone is a chemical that is used by the body to relay a message. Hormones are generally secreted by glands in response to instructions by either the brain or larger nervous system or by other hormones. These chemical messengers then travel through the blood (or directly through tissues) to reach their receptors. Receptors are special locations inside or outside a cell that, when stimulated by contact with a specific hormone, will relay a message to the cell machinery. This message may tell the cell to make more estrogen, grow less hair, burn more calories, etc.

The endocrine system is controlled by the pituitary gland, the body's "master gland." The pituitary is responsible for regulation of sex hormones, stress hormones, thyroid function (control of overall metabolic rate and energy use), growth hormones, lactation, menstruation, and salt and water balance. The pituitary itself is controlled by the hypothalamus, the part of the brain responsible for interfacing between the nervous and endocrine systems. In fact, the endocrine system can be thought of as functioning similarly to the nervous system but using hormones instead of nerves to send messages to target organs. The nervous and endocrine systems are closely linked. The endocrine system, under the control of the brain, is responsible for the regulation of metabolism and many body functions.

Sex hormones (such as estrogen and testosterone) are produced when the gonads (testicles or ovaries) are instructed to do so by the pituitary gonadotropin hormones follicle-stimulating hormone (FSH) and luteinizing hormone (LH). The pituitary makes these hormones in response to signals from the hypothalamus. In addition to stimulating the production of sex hormones, FSH and LH are responsible for directing the production of sperm, ovulation (maturation and release of eggs), and controlling the lining of the uterus (endometrium) and the menstrual cycle.

FSH and LH levels are controlled via a feedback inhibition loop. In this system, rising sex hormones cause falling FSH/LH levels, and low sex hormone levels cause FSH and LH to climb. The system is somewhat like driving a car. As you notice your speed climbing, you let up on the accelerator pedal. As your speed falls, you press on the accelerator. This feedback loop allows the brain to control sex hormone levels within a set range. Additionally, the brain is able to make changes in the set range, such as the fluctuations involved in the menstrual cycle. You might think of this as driving in different speed limit zones, where the brain makes adjustments to the parameters of the feedback loop.

Sex hormones belong to a larger category known as steroid hormones. Other steroids include cortisol (involved in regulation of the immune system, sugar balance, and the "fight-or-flight" sympathetic response), aldosterone (involved in water and salt balance), and vitamin D. All steroid hormones are derived from cholesterol in a complicated series of interconnected interactions. Because of their common origin and regulation by the pituitary, the actions of all steroid hormones are interconnected, and making changes in one hormone axis might have effects on others. It should be noted that the anabolic steroids discussed in the setting of bodybuilding are only one small group of steroid hormones and that not all steroid hormones cause muscle growth and related side effects. It is also noteworthy that in almost all cases, dietary cholesterol and serum cholesterol levels do not have a significant effect on sex steroid production.

While a detailed discussion of this subject is beyond the scope of this chapter, it is important to remember that cross-gender hormone therapy might have effects on other hormone systems. For example, "cross-talk" may exist between the receptors for thyroid hormone and estradiol. As such, maintaining one's balance of thyroid hormone (through diet and replacement if needed), cortisol (through exercise, diet, and stress management), and vitamin D (through sunlight, diet, and supplementation) is important to anyone undergoing cross-gender hormone treatment.

Feminizing Regimens

The biggest issue in the transition from male to female is the elimination of the past and present effects of the hormone testosterone on the body. Second is the administration of female hormones (estrogens, and in some cases, progestins). All humans make some degree of estrogen in fat tissues; a baby born without gonads will develop female secondary sex characteristics by default. Trans women have a varying degree of "virilization" (the effects of testosterone and other androgens—male hormones—on the body) depending on individual factors such as genetics and the age at which hormone therapy is begun.

Testosterone causes many physical changes to begin at puberty, with some changes continuing across the life span. It is important for trans women to maintain reasonable expectations about what to expect in their medical transition. A 50-year-old body that is just beginning hormone therapy has experienced 35-plus years of the effects of testosterone and is at an age when cisgender women are entering menopause. The changes with respect to breast development and fat redistribution will be more modest than would be seen in a 20- or 30-year-old. Taking higher doses of hormones to obtain a more dramatic effect or to help overcome the effects of testosterone often comes with increased risks. Cisgender women of all ages struggle with body image and the aging process as well (Lombardi et al., 2001; Nuttbrock et al., 2010; Rotondi et al., 2011). (See Table 4.2.)

1. Estrogen Therapy

Estrogens are responsible for the development of female secondary sex characteristics (Table 4.2). Estrogens are made in the ovaries in cisgender women and in body fat in all humans. They act directly on individual cells and tissues and also act to suppress the release of LH and FSH from the pituitary gland, thereby having some effect on reducing the production of

Table 4.2   Effects of Masculinizing and Feminizing Regimens

Testosterone Therapy	Estrogen Therapy
Increased muscle strength	Decrease in muscle mass and strength
Clitoral enlargement	Decreased libido
Deepening of the voice	Breast growth
Increase in skin oiliness/acne	Decreased sperm
Androgenetic hair loss (male-pattern baldness)	Reduced erections
Male body and pubic hair distribution (beard growth)	Reduced testicular volume
Minimization of subcutaneous (under the skin) fat layer, depositing of fat in the abdomen area	Redistribution of fat to the hips and buttocks

(Adapted from Hembree et al., 2009)

testosterone as well. "Estrogen" is an umbrella term for a family of hormones that include estradiol (the most common estrogen in the body), estrone, and estriol. Synthetic estrogens also exist and include ethinyl estradiol, which is used in some oral contraceptives. Nonhuman estrogens such as conjugated equine estrogens (Premarin) are also available.

All estrogens are not created equal. Because estrogen therapy is widely used in the fields of menopause and contraception, large bodies of data exist on its use. Estrogens can be broken down both by compound and by route of administration. In general, estrogens administered by a transdermal (through the skin) route are the safest with respect to risk of venous thromboembolism (blood clot), the most common serious side effect seen in estrogen therapy in trans women (Canonico et al., 2007). Transdermal estradiol is absorbed directly into the blood at a constant rate and therefore closely approximates secretion of estrogen by the ovary. Oral estrogens undergo what is known as a "first pass" metabolism, whereby they are first digested and then processed by the liver before entering the bloodstream. As the liver processes these oral estrogens, it has a side effect of interfering with the normal production of various blood-clotting factors in the liver that leads to the increased risk of blood clots.

Oral estrogens are not all the same. Recent studies show that the real culprits when it comes to increased risk of blood clots are nonnatural estrogens. Though manufactured from yam extract, oral estrogens such as estradiol are "bioidentical" to the estrogens secreted by the human ovary. It makes sense that hormones designed for humans are safer than those that were not. Ethinyl estradiol is a scientific creation that was designed to maintain very predictable levels needed for contraception. These tightly controlled levels are not relevant in menopausal or cross-gender hormonal therapy. In effect, the increased risk of blood clots associated with ethinyl estradiol is accepted in exchange for reliable contraception. Conjugated equine estrogens are obtained by keeping a horse pregnant with a urinary catheter in place, collecting the horse's urine, and isolating a variety of estrogens called equillins. Conjugated equine estrogens have been shown to bring a higher risk of blood clots when compared to oral estradiol and should generally be avoided (Smith et al., 2014; Blondon et al., 2014).

Some providers recommend using oral estrogen preparations via a sub-lingual (under the tongue) route. In this method, the oral estrogen pill is placed under the tongue and allowed to dissolve. The theory is that this estrogen is absorbed directly into the blood rather than going through the digestive system and liver. Therefore, one avoids the "first pass" effect and delivers the estrogen directly to the blood as with transdermal routes. Limited evidence, some of which is unpublished, suggests that this is a safe route with respect to blood clots. It is important to mention that this route will only work with estrogen preparations that are micronized (prepared specially for better absorption). Not all estrogen preparations are micron-ized; the dispensing pharmacist should research this prior to beginning sublingual administration of a particular brand or generic. Ethinyl estra-diol and conjugated equine estrogens cannot be administered via a sublin-gual route.

Estrogen also exists in an injectable form. In the past, before antiandro-gens were in use, this form was used because of the high levels of estrogen needed to prevent testosterone production via suppression of pituitary LH. In addition to high estrogen levels, injections tend to bring varying blood levels over the injection interval, which can cause mood swings, hot flashes, migraines, and other unwelcome symptoms. Intuitively, it seems concerning to maintain high (sometimes pregnancy-range) estrogen levels over the long term. With the current use of antiandrogens, high doses of injected estrogen are no longer needed to suppress testosterone produc-tion. More and more providers are moving away from injected estradiol for these reasons. Estrogen pellet skin implants have also been used in the past and have fallen out of favor for the same reasons.

A detailed discussion of hormone dosing and therapeutic ranges (hor-mone levels) is beyond the scope of this chapter. There are several hormone protocols available that outline both optimal dosing and monitoring (CoE, 2016; Hembree et al., 2009). However, it is important to remember that the most important factor in feminization is the lowering of testosterone levels to the normal female range, which is usually accomplished using androgen blockers. Higher estrogen doses and levels may bring temporary improve-ments in feminization but at the cost of increased risk of blood clots, high blood pressure, weight gain, mood swings and depression, migraines, and perhaps other conditions. High estrogen levels put the body into a pregnancy-like state; pregnancy is something that is supposed to happen for just a few months under very specific circumstances and is hard on the body. It is best to maintain healthy estrogen doses and levels and maintain reasonable and realistic expectations for a medical transition.

2. Testosterone Blocking (Anti-Androgen) Therapy

As mentioned above, blocking the synthesis and/or action of testosterone (a member of the androgen family of virilizing hormones) is the most important factor in the feminization process. Testosterone is synthesized in the testicle, with smaller amounts as well as weaker androgens such as dihydroepiandrosterone (DHEA) synthesized in the adrenal gland of all people. The adrenal gland is the source of all androgens after an orchiectomy (removal of the testicles) that may be performed on its own or as part of a vaginoplasty (genital surgery) procedure. Approaches to blocking testosterone include preventing its production or blocking its action in cells and tissues. Below are descriptions of several testosterone blockers commonly used in trans women.

Spironolactone is the most commonly used anti-androgen in the United States. It acts both by blocking testosterone action at target tissues, and to some degree by preventing androgen synthesis. Spironolactone is actually a blood pressure medicine that works by causing the kidneys to make excess urine (known as a diuretic medicine), and it was found that antiandrogen activity was a side effect. As such, people taking spironolactone may become dehydrated or notice excessive urination, thirst, and salt craving. It is important to prevent dehydration and drink plenty of fluids when taking spironolactone. People with kidney disease or who are taking certain other medications can have a dangerous reaction that causes an increase in blood potassium levels, which can cause cardiac arrest and be fatal. Most of the blood pressure effects of spironolactone level out after a few weeks of therapy. For most people who have no kidney disease or interacting medications, there is no need to limit the dietary intake of potassium or high-potassium foods such as bananas. Periodic blood tests to evaluate potassium levels and kidney function are vital when taking spironolactone.

5-Alpha reductase inhibitors (finasteride, dutasteride) are members of a newer antiandrogen class that were developed for the management of prostate disorders and later used in lower doses for male-pattern baldness. These medications prevent the conversion of testosterone into dihydrotestosterone (DHT), a much more powerful androgen that has effects on the skin, hair, and prostate. There are two pathways for the production of DHT. Finasteride blocks one of these pathways, and the more powerful dutasteride blocks both pathways. These medicines are useful in people who cannot take or cannot tolerate spironolactone, but they are in general less effective because they do not block testosterone itself, only DHT. It is unclear if 5-AR medicines are of any benefit to scalp hair regrowth in people who already have a full androgen blockade. These medicines tend to be somewhat expensive. The side effects are minimal.

Cyproterone acetate is a member of the progestagen family (see below). In addition to suppression of pituitary gonadotropins, this synthetic progestagen has very strong anti-androgen properties. Cyproterone acetate may precipitate significant mood disorders such as depression and may cause liver toxicity or damage. Cyproterone is not FDA approved for sale in the United States for *any* indication and as such is not available for prescription. Cyproterone is used widely outside of the United States.

Flutamide is an older anti-androgen that has been used in the treatment of prostate cancer. It carries a high risk of liver injury and should not be used in trans women.

GnRH Analogs (leuprolide, histrelin, goserelin, and others) work at the level of the pituitary gland. They cause massive release of gonadotropins, which temporarily cause the gonad to secrete a surge of sex hormones. After this initial surge (lasting 7 to 14 days), the gonads effectively stop making sex hormones through a process of receptor downregulation. In effect, the gonads become so flooded with gonadotropins that they simply shut down. These medicines are very expensive and are generally used in pubescent transgender youth as "puberty blockers."

3. Progestagens, Another Class of Sex Hormones

The prototypical hormone found in humans is progesterone, and numerous synthetic progestagens have been developed. Progesterone has many roles in female physiology. It is responsible for preparing and maintaining the endometrium (uterine lining) for pregnancy and for breast growth. It also contributes to libido, mood, and likely to overall brain health. Progesterone is present in cisgender men and women and likely plays many important roles, some of which have not yet been defined. Progestagens as a class have a range of anti-androgen activity through direct action and through pituitary suppression. Though solid evidence is lacking, some providers believe that progesterone is important for breast and nipple development and maturation.

Many providers choose to prescribe medroxyprogesterone acetate, a synthetic progestagen that is less expensive and more readily available than natural progesterone. Medroxyprogesterone has been implicated in an increased risk of breast cancer and, as such, usage in the general population has dropped sharply (Chlebowski et al., 2015). However, the study linking medroxyprogesterone to breast cancer had numerous design flaws and involved patients also taking conjugated equine estrogens. It is unlikely that progestagens increase the risk of breast cancer in transgender men or women, especially if bioidentical estrogens are used.

As discussed above, cyproterone is a commonly prescribed progestagen outside of the United States that also has strong anti-androgen activity; however, use may be associated with the issues listed above, as well as an increased risk of meningioma (Gil et al., 2011).

Masculinizing Regimens

On the surface, the female-to-male transition is somewhat straightforward. A body that has not undergone a male puberty will respond quickly and drastically to the addition of androgens (male hormones), specifically testosterone. This process is known as virilization. Changes can be so rapid that in the course of just a few months, it is possible for some trans men to become unrecognizable as having been assigned female at birth. This consideration is important because, unlike trans women, who can in some cases remain on hormone treatment for years without socially transitioning, trans men beginning testosterone treatment in many cases must be prepared for a social transition within as little as three months after beginning treatment. Trans men should also be prepared for an at times awkward period where they are perceived as a much younger male than they actually are. This may occur because they are seen as a male going through puberty, even if they are in actuality in their 30s or 40s. As such, some trans men choose to begin with lower doses of testosterone and move more slowly through their social transition.

Besides the administration of testosterone, it is unusual that a trans man will require any additional hormone treatments or blockers. Testosterone effectively shuts down the complex cycles of pituitary activity that cause menstruation, and the overriding effects of testosterone on secondary sex characteristics such as skin, muscle, body hair, odors, and voice tend to mask any remaining background estrogen activity. Specific circumstances where estrogen activity is still of concern or other treatments are needed are discussed below.

Testosterone is the mainstay cross-gender hormone treatment for trans men. Testosterone is available in several forms such as an injection, a patch, a gel, a cream, or a troche (a small adhesive square applied to the inner cheek). Long-term pellets and injections are also available, lasting up to six months. While many synthetic androgens exist, there is no benefit to using one of these instead of bioidentical testosterone. In fact, many synthetic androgens (i.e., anabolic steroids used by bodybuilders) have been associated with liver damage. No oral form of testosterone is available. In general, testosterone injections are required for life in order to maintain muscle mass and other masculine secondary sex characteristics.

Injection is the most common route of testosterone administration in trans men. The most frequently prescribed preparations are testosterone cypionate and testosterone enanthate. Injections are generally given every one to two weeks; most men find that weekly injections result in fewer mood swings by keeping testosterone levels more even. Maintaining even testosterone levels is also helpful in preventing a dangerous climb in the amount of red blood cells (hematocrit) sometimes seen in people on androgen treatment, which can increase the risk of stroke. Injection every one to two weeks into the muscle over many years can lead to scarring and pain; a subcutaneous injection technique that involves injecting into the fat just below the skin (similar to injecting insulin) is now an acceptable route to deliver injectable testosterone (Hembree et al., 2017). This technique is believed to be equally effective and avoids the long-term consequences of repeated muscle injection.

Transdermal testosterone is another option for trans men. Products include patches and gels or custom-compounded testosterone creams. These products in general work well and are very useful for those who respond poorly to the cyclic nature of injections or who do not want to inject. Those using gels and creams must be sure to avoid any contact with females or children until dry. Other options include a subcutaneous skin pellet implant that lasts three to six months but is very expensive and may not achieve a therapeutic blood level in men who produce effectively no testosterone on their own, and a long-term injection (testosterone undecanoate) that lasts two to three months. Testosterone undecanoate is difficult to access in the United States due to regulatory requirements for in-clinic administration and monitoring. The oral-adhesive troche form is expensive and not commonly used.

Estrogen is made from testosterone in the ovary and in body fat. As such, an excess of testosterone will cause an excess of estrogen. Some trans men are able to tolerate the continued presence of estrogen while on testosterone. Others will develop symptoms of mood swings, pelvic cramping, or bleeding. In these cases, it may be useful to check estrogen and testosterone levels. If both estrogen and testosterone levels are high, try a reduction in the testosterone dose. If estrogen is high but testosterone is normal, a provider might consider using an aromatase inhibitor that blocks the conversion of testosterone to estrogen and will help lower estrogen levels. Aromatase inhibitors can cause a loss of bone density that can lead to osteoporosis; bone density should be monitored while on these medications. Most trans men will not need this type of medicine.

Progestagens (discussed in detail in the section on feminizing regimens) are sometimes used for trans men having vaginal bleeding or with persistent menstruation. Progestagens help to stabilize the uterus and can stop the menstrual cycle. It is rare that a trans man will need a progestagen at all, and it is even rarer that it will be needed in an ongoing manner. Progestagens should not interfere with the virilization process.

Hormone Blood Levels

There is no consensus across hormone guidelines regarding the optimal frequency of hormone level monitoring. There are relatively standard doses of hormones that are used, and most people respond well to these doses. In general, hormone levels are checked every three months for the first year and then annually or as needed depending on the guideline followed. Hormone levels are worth checking when transition is not progressing as expected or when unusual or uncomfortable symptoms are experienced (mood swings, persistent menses, or continued erections). Hormone levels are usually done mid-cycle between injections; however, some clinicians check trough and peak levels. It is useful to check free *and* total testosterone. Total testosterone includes free testosterone (unbound to proteins) and bound testosterone, which is bound to sex-hormone-binding globulin (SHBG) and albumin. SHBG levels vary from person to person and are related to the amount of estrogen in the body as well as other hormones (insulin, growth hormone, etc.), some medical conditions, and drugs. The total testosterone level will give you a big-picture idea of how levels are responding to dosing. The free testosterone, about 0.1 to 0.3 percent, will tell you how much testosterone is available and biologically active. The bioavailable testosterone includes free testosterone plus testosterone weakly bound to albumin, which is also biologically active. Because of this, bioavailable testosterone monitoring may be superior to free testosterone measurement. Some people may have a normal total testosterone but a low free or bioavailable testosterone and would benefit from an increase in dose, or vice versa. Total estrogen levels usually suffice, since as long as they are relatively consistent, estrogen levels are less critical and have a wider "normal" range than testosterone.

Bioidentical Hormones

There has been much recent discussion on the subject of bioidentical hormones. In their purest form, bioidentical hormones are human, naturally occurring substances such as estradiol, estrone, progesterone, DHEA, and testosterone. Pharmaceutical-grade bioidentical hormones are made in a lab from yams and other substances and are identical in structure and function to natural human hormones. Intuitively it would make sense that supplementing or replacing human hormones with bioidentical hormones is ideal. There has been little research in this area, in part because natural substances are difficult to patent, and therefore there is little interest on the part of the pharmaceutical industry to conduct this research.

In practice, many people discuss bioidentical hormone therapy as a method of using custom-blended creams, gels, capsules, and other forms to deliver bioidentical products. This practice is somewhat more controversial, as these custom blends are prepared at local compounding pharmacies and are not regulated by the FDA. Doses may vary from product to product. Practitioners of this method tend to rely more on checking blood hormone levels in order to achieve an appropriate dose. The use of these hormones will likely continue to be an area of debate. Many providers and patients stand firmly by bioidentical hormone therapy as a way to achieve an individualized hormone regimen, arguing that a person's individual genetic makeup determines their hormonal needs and balance points.

A complete discussion of bioidentical hormone therapy is beyond the scope of this chapter. In general, compounded creams of varying concentrations of estradiol, estrone, estriol, progesterone, DHEA, and testosterone are used alone or in combination with certain FDA-approved bioidentical products such as oral estradiol or progesterone.

One example of a use for bioidentical hormone therapy would be in patients who have a difficult time tolerating transdermal estradiol patches. The human body normally has a balance between estradiol and estrone sulfate. Estrone sulfate is a substance that serves as an "estrogen reserve." The body uses a specific enzyme to convert between estrogen and estrone sulfate as a way of keeping up with estradiol demand and, at the same time, avoiding having too much of it. In women with functional ovaries, this is less of an issue because the ovaries can help keep up with demand.

However, in women without functional ovaries taking estradiol replacement, the conversion into estrone sulfate may not be fast enough, and so instead the liver removes excess estradiol. Later (for example, on day five of a seven-day patch), when estradiol levels are falling, there is not enough estrone sulfate to be converted back into estradiol, and the woman will feel hot flashes, anxiety, or fatigue. Adding a component of estrone sulfate to a compounded estradiol cream can help maintain this "reserve" and prevent these cyclic symptoms. Interestingly, oral estradiol tablets result in a higher blood level of estrone sulfate than sublingual or transdermal. This occurs due to the processing by the liver that takes place when taking oral estradiol as opposed to other routes. While this route may be appropriate for the management of some estradiol-related symptoms, it is important to consider the risks and benefits of taking oral versus other forms of estradiol, as discussed previously. Ultimately, each patient may respond differently based on route of administration due to differences in individual metabolic phenotypes; to simplify, if a patient has physiologic hormone levels and is experiencing hormone-attributed symptoms, consider changing the route of administration.

Genderqueer and Other Gender Nonconforming/Nonbinary Persons

Not all gender-diverse people identify as transgender or transsexual, and not all fit into a gender binary system. Gender identity and expression exist on a spectrum (Kuper, Nussbaum, & Mustanski, 2012). Transgender and gender-diverse people may have a range of gender expressions, which can include butch trans women or effeminate trans men. The World Professional Association for Transgender Health Standards of Care, 7th Edition, reminds providers to approach each gender-diverse person as an individual rather than trying to fit people into molds (Coleman et al., 2012).

With the increasing visibility of a wide range of gender-diverse identities comes a new set of medical dilemmas. For example, some female-assigned genderqueer persons may wish to take low-dose testosterone or only take testosterone for a period of time and then stop. Little is known about the long-term effects of sex hormones on the body, and even less is known on the long-term effects of low or intermittent dosing of these hormones.

Long-Term Considerations in Hormone Therapy

There have been few publications on the long-term effects of cross-gender hormonal therapy; however, data suggest that the practice is safe (Asscheman et al., 2011; Gooren et al., 2008).

For trans women, it would seem appropriate for those who have had an orchiectomy or vaginoplasty to consider stopping estrogen therapy at or around age 50 (the average age of menopause in cisgender women). The decision to stop hormone therapy at this point should be driven by patient preferences, the age at which hormonal therapy was begun, and a discussion of the known and unknown risks and benefits of continuing hormonal therapy after this age. If hormonal therapy is discontinued, ongoing osteoporosis prevention measures should be undertaken as would be done with menopausal cisgender women.

For trans men, it seems intuitive that continuing testosterone for life is appropriate, given that cisgender men continue to produce testosterone across the life span. That said, cisgender male testosterone levels peak in their 20s and slowly decline thereafter. One might consider tapering down the testosterone dose in trans men over age 50, again based on patient preference, length of time on testosterone, and consideration of the long-term risks (such as the above-mentioned unquantified risk of ovarian or endometrial cancer). In addition to increasing the risk of osteoporosis, lowering or stopping testosterone may lead to depressed mood, decreased muscle mass and libido, increased body fat ratio, and softening of the skin. If the ovaries are still present, these effects will be more pronounced, and depending on age and time on testosterone, menstruation may resume in those who still have a uterus.

Issues Relating to Medication Administration

Patches are designed to be applied to hairless skin and to remain on during bathing or exercise. People who perspire excessively or are very physically active may find them to be less suitable. While testosterone patches are designed to be changed daily, estrogen patches remain on for up to seven days, depending on the product. In these cases, if a patch begins to fall off, become soiled, or cause irritation, it may be changed earlier. Using a small amount of prescription triamcinolone cream (or over-the-counter hydrocortisone cream) on the area 15 to 30 minutes before applying the patch may help prevent this reaction. It is important to rotate the skin location of patches between several sites.

Gels and creams require that the area not get wet for a certain period of time after application. Of particular importance is to be sure that testosterone creams or gels do not come into contact with anyone who does not desire their effects (Stahlman et al., 2012).

Sublingual pills are placed under the tongue and dissolve directly into the bloodstream, bypassing the intestines and therefore the liver. Sublingual medicine must be micronized, a special way of packaging the medicine within the pill that is not standard across all brands and generic manufacturers. Your pharmacist should be able to tell you if the product they carry is micronized.

Injections may be intramuscular ("IM"—into the muscle) or subcutaneous ("SQ" or "sub-Q"—into the fat just below the skin). While the FDA label route for estrogen and testosterone injections is intramuscular, this route can be painful and over many years of two to four injections per month can cause muscle scar tissue to build up. As such, some providers are beginning to experiment with subcutaneous testosterone with reports of high patient satisfaction, less pain, and adequate medication effect (Olson, Schrager, Clark, Dunlap, & Belzer, 2014). Most evidence is moving away from estrogen injections altogether due to fluctuating, sometimes high levels of estrogen, in addition to issues directly related to injections. Furthermore, there has been an ongoing shortage of availability of injected forms of estrogen in the United States.

If injecting into the muscle, the outer thigh or upper, outer buttock area are best. Neither of these areas contains bone or important blood vessels or nerves. Sometimes when injecting, one might see a small amount of blood or feel a shooting pain up the leg. While this is alarming, it is likely that the needle has run into minor local nerves or vessels that are not of clinical concern. Some people may have irritation, redness, or inflammation at the injection site. If this becomes a recurrent problem, consider changing to another preparation or another type of oil (e.g., cottonseed instead of peanut). Occasional bruises after injection are due to leaking from an injured minor vessel and can be treated with ice and pain medication.

Miscellaneous Conditions of Interest

Male-pattern baldness (MPB) in trans women will usually stop progressing and may reverse somewhat once hormones are begun. MPB in trans men should be approached similarly to baldness in cisgender men, with Rogaine, finasteride, and other current treatments, as well as work on self-acceptance and understanding that balding is something that *all* men (not just trans men) may struggle with and is part of the natural aging process. A healthy, balanced diet with a good multivitamin and B-complex supplement may help with thinning hair or balding.

Just as with menopausal women, some trans women may notice general hair thinning after orchiectomy, vaginoplasty, or a reduction in hormone levels. This is usually transient. However, many women do experience gradual hair thinning across the life span.

Migraines have a strong hormonal component and may be experienced by trans men or women. In addition to typical migraine remedies, transgender people may benefit from switching to a more constant route of hormone administration such as a patch. Keeping a log of migraine symptoms as they relate to diet, sleep patterns, exercise, stress, and hormone dosing may help determine triggers so that lifestyle changes may be made to minimize migraine frequency and intensity.

Acne is common during transition and may relate to excessive testosterone dosing. In addition to typical remedies, if severe, it should prompt checking testosterone levels.

SEXUAL HEALTH

Transgender persons are sexual beings and may be eager to (and are encouraged to) explore sexuality from the perspective of a physical body that matches their gender identity. Given the anatomical particulars of transgender bodies, several unique issues may present themselves and are discussed here. Furthermore, working with a therapist may help address psychological issues and trauma surrounding sexuality.

Transgender people may be heterosexual, homosexual, bisexual, pan-sexual, or asexual. Health care providers and others should use the affirmed gender when defining sexuality. For example, a gay trans man is a trans man who is attracted to other men.

Trans men who enjoy receptive vaginal penetrative sex may experience vaginal dryness, irritation, or difficulty with penetration due to hormone-related changes in vaginal structure and function. Trans women who have had penile-inversion vaginoplasty require an external source of lubrication and may have difficulty with penetration if they have not remained active with dilation or penetrative sex. Possibly helpful interventions include lubricants, masturbation with sex toys and dildos, or vaginal estrogen creams.

Vaginal discharge or odor in trans men might relate to shifts in natural bacterial and yeast balances that occur with hormonal reassignment. Trans women often experience vaginal discharge, irritation, or odor. Given that a penile-inversion vagina is a skin-lined pocket (as opposed to a mucous membrane), infectious vaginitis in trans women is somewhat rare; instead, irritation is more likely due to accumulation of dead skin cells, sweat, oils, semen, lubricant, and other debris that is unable to clear natur-ally as in a vagina that is made up of mucous membrane. Recently postop-erative trans women may notice excessive discharge that is due to actively healing (granulation) tissue and, in most cases, will resolve over time. Trans women who have undergone surgery to create the vagina using a section of bowel (colovaginoplasty) have naturally occurring discharge with a mixed microflora of aerobic and anaerobic bacteria.

People who have had genital or breast procedures are encouraged to masturbate and explore new areas, sensations, and activities that promote pleasure. Post-vaginoplasty trans women are encouraged to locate and explore their clitoris (sensitive organ/area located outside of the vagina and just above the urinary opening) and their prostate, which can be stim-ulated through the upper inside wall of the vagina.

Some transgender persons may experience low libido or difficulty in achieving orgasm. While a psychoemotional component should always be considered, changes in nerve connection, hormone balances, and other physical factors can have significant effects on sexual function. Trans women who have had an orchiectomy or vaginoplasty may benefit from low-dose testosterone or dihydroepiandosterone (DHEA) supplementation to maintain blood levels in the female range, although these approaches have not been found to be beneficial in studies; and progesterone may be helpful in supporting libido as well. Trans women who have difficulty achieving orgasm should remain encouraged and should remember that up to 50 percent of cisgender women have difficulty or are unable to achieve orgasm.

Discussions of fertility and reproductive potential are extremely important when initiating hormone therapy. Estrogen therapy and androgen blockers reduce spermatogenesis (the production of sperm) and can result in azoospermia (the termination of sperm production), though trans women who are unsure if they are still producing sperm should use pregnancy prevention techniques if having penile-vaginal penetrative sex (Schulze, 1988). Testosterone treatment will inhibit ovulation and reduce fertility in transgender men but is not guaranteed to prevent pregnancy, so other forms of protection should be used. Long-acting reversible contraception such as intrauterine devices and depot medroxyprogesterone (DMPA) may be acceptable methods for transgender men wanting to avoid pregnancy.

Options for transgender people to have biological offspring include sperm, oocyte, or embryo cryopreservation ("banking"); however, these methods are expensive and may not be covered under insurance plans. Successful pregnancies have occurred in trans men after stopping testosterone but may not be possible in everyone (Light, Obedin-Maliver, Sevelius, & Kerns, 2014).

OTHER NONSURGICAL TRANSITION-RELATED TREATMENTS

Most transgender women will require some degree of facial hair removal. Hormone therapy and testosterone blockage causes some facial hair thinning, but often not enough for a feminized facial appearance. Electrolysis and laser hair removal are the two most common methods, and a combination of the two may be used as needed. Electrolysis is the only proven form of permanent facial hair removal, while laser hair removal is FDA approved for facial hair reduction. Laser tends to bring quicker results initially, with electrolysis providing more reliable long-term results. Both processes are costly and generally painful, in many cases requiring topical or regional anesthetics as well as pain medication.

Trans women will not experience any voice feminization when on hormone therapy. Speech modification of some kind is needed in most cases if and when voice feminization is desired. Speech therapy using prerecorded or online materials, or in consultation with a speech-language pathologist experienced in voice feminization, can yield impressive results. Trans men may also desire voice virilization training, as testosterone causes vocal cord changes but does not change the shape of the larynx or size of the head and sinus cavities and may be insufficient to satisfactorily virilize the voice. Speech modification techniques for transgender men and women include vocal health training as well as changes in pitch, resonance (head for women, chest for men), word usage, speech rhythms, and nonverbal communication. Some transgender people have used mobile apps to assist with voice training.

The illicit use of silicone injections has been on the rise, particularly among sex-working trans women and trans women of color (Wilson, Rapues, Jin, & Raymond, 2014; Herbst et al., 2008). In this procedure, silicone or other compounds are injected directly into the breasts, face, hips, buttocks, or elsewhere with the goal of achieving a rapid and striking degree of feminization. In addition to peer and societal pressures, women may be driven to this process out of necessity. Sex workers can earn more money with a more strikingly feminized body, and women in some cultures or regions may be in physical danger if they are visibly transgender and unable to blend into mainstream society.

Silicone injections are usually performed by unlicensed or unscrupulous practitioners under varying degrees of sterility. If medical-grade silicone is unavailable, substances such as industrial silicone lubricant or adhesives/sealants, cooking oil, or even motor oil may be used. There may be migration and calcification of injected substances leading to deformity and pain. This procedure can also result in complications and death due to overwhelming infection or inflammatory response—or to entrance into the bloodstream, causing pulmonary embolism or stroke. Treatment options are limited and are mostly supportive and focused on symptom and pain management. Two recent reports suggest the immune-modulating drug etanercept may be effective in reducing chronic inflammatory symptoms related to silicone injections (Desai, Browning, & Rosen, 2006).

HISTORY OF TRANSGENDER SURGERY

Although Lili Elbe later died from complications of her procedure, she is credited as the first transgender woman to undergo formal genital reassignment surgery. Popularized in the film *The Danish Girl*, Ms. Elbe's surgical endeavor in 1930s Berlin was the culmination of years of transgender research (Stryker, 2008). Many years later, with surgical innovations from unlikely geographic locations including Casablanca (Dr. Georges Borou), Copenhagen, Trinidad (Dr. Stanley Biber), Neenah (Dr. Eugene Schrang), Belgrade (Drs. Perovic/Djordjevic), Scottsdale (Dr. Toby Meltzer), and Ghent, the field has advanced. Professional organizations such as the World Professional Association for Transgender Health (WPATH) have ensued. Owing to these early pioneers and others, WPATH now provides orderly and scientific guidelines for the dissemination of transgender services, including surgery (Coleman et al., 2012).

Sex Reassignment Surgery (SRS), now known as "gender-confirming sur-gery" (GCS) or "gender-affirming surgery" (GAS), was formerly a bastion of university-based surgical programs in the United States. Following Dr. Burou's 1950s description of the penile inversion technique for vagino-plasty, American university gender clinics abounded. Similar advances in phalloplasty allowed for universities, including Virginia-Norfolk; Univer-sity of Texas-Galveston; University of California, Los Angeles; University of Washington; University of Minnesota; Johns Hopkins; and others to flourish within the United States. Sex change was progress and paralleled efforts to reach the moon. The sky was the limit. Then, in 1977, political reality emerged as conservative thinking began to question the ethics of sex change.

Despite evidence to the contrary, Jon Meyer's 1979 article in the Archives of General Psychiatry titled "Sex Reassignment: Follow-Up," sanctioned by Paul McHugh, the chair of psychiatry at Johns Hopkins, purported to show that transsexual patients were no happier after comple-tion of surgery than prior and resulted in ongoing misery and suicide for these "victims" of surgery (Meyer & Reter, 1979). Subsequent studies affirming positive outcomes aside, McHugh's work played a major role in university programs' subsequent decisions to close doors against the pleas of transgender patients whose numbers had not diminished. Simultan-eously, Dr. Biber ascended, working in private practice in remote Trinidad, Colorado (Rossi Neto, Hintz, Krege, Rubben, & Vom Dorp, 2012). As the preeminent remaining U.S. surgeon, Dr. Biber understood both the need and the validity of surgery for transgender people.

Today, gender-confirming surgery for the management of gender dys-phoria has become an accepted final stage of gender transition. Patients consistently report high levels of satisfaction with whichever procedural approach is chosen, regardless of complications and whomever the sur-geon (Eldh, 1993; Reed, 2011). That said, there is correlation between over-all happiness and quality of the surgical result (Lawrence, 2003). This fact places emphasis on establishing standards for surgical care, improvement in surgical training, and proper management of complications. Complica-tions, while comparatively minor and relatively rare, can lead to chronic problems and long-term medical needs including multiple subsequent sur-gical procedures, pain, and disappointment.

The Choice to Undergo Gender-Confirmation Surgery

Although it is true that the affirmation and recognition of one's gender identity does not require genital or other surgery, surgery remains a fixa-tion for many and an important goal for some—but not all—transgender people. When discussing surgery, it is important to be open to those who, for whatever reasons, do not wish to or cannot pursue surgery. When *genitalia* are discussed, consider that genitalia are not public commodities and not something that strangers would learn about in an informal encounter. Society makes assumptions about genitalia unconsciously in virtually every social interaction. When we see someone who appears to be a man, we assume he has a penis and scrotum—and vice versa. Thus, it is the individual's *gender expression* (what we wear, how we talk and act) that society judges and sees as being the essentials that make someone male or female. Genitals are personal and private.

Difficulty with financing is a reason that many people do not to undergo GCS as part of the gender transition process. While U.S. states (11 at this time) increasingly mandate insurance coverage for transgender individuals, many people work for smaller companies, companies with an out-of-state corporate structure, or in states where insurance coverage is not mandatory. Medicare, while it has removed its exclusion on transgender surgical coverage, has not yet taken an affirmative step in addressing transgender patients' surgical needs. Medicaid coverage remains spotty and local, with some states providing coverage—but most not. Furthermore, low reimbursement for surgical services affords a further reason that surgeons often refuse Medicare or Medicaid as a means of payment. Thus, cost remains a considerable obstacle for many without coverage. Various organizations, such as the Jim Collins Fund, have arisen to help with funding but only address a tiny portion of the need. Creative funding sources such as crowdsourcing and projects like GoFundMe can offer some hope.

Some transgender people, for personal reasons, do not wish to pursue surgery at all. These reasons can include a fear of surgical complications, worry in regard to sexual or reproductive function, family or partner-related dissuasion, or simply that they do not feel that surgical alterations are needed to feel gender affirmed.

Surgical regret remains a much-talked-about but very rare outcome. Most incidences of regret are related to social issues, intimacy factors, specific surgical complications, or discrimination-based problems rather than an outright change of heart or the result of an inaccurate diagnosis of gender dysphoria. Feelings of being wrongly gendered are long and deep for most trans individuals, making outright regret very rare. In fact, the observation that *should* be made is that for something as traumatic and difficult as gender transition, the relative lack of regret among trans people is astounding.

Ability to orgasm after GCS, fortunately, is highly likely (Rehman & Melman, 1999). For trans men, testosterone has an additive effect on libido. While many trans women are orgasmic after genital surgery, still others find orgasm challenging to achieve following GCS. Anatomically, this makes sense given the reduction of exposed erectile tissue. During GCS, the penile head is not only reduced in size but partially buried beneath skin and the clitoral hood. On the other hand, many trans women find the added stimulus of the post-op internal G-spot to more than compensate for the reduced clitoral size. The G-spot is technically the original erectile tissue surrounding the urethral tract located along the front of the neovagina, virtually identical to that which exists for cisgender women. A reduced sexual frequency for trans women is consistent with the lowered hormonal milieu, as is the highly enhanced incidence of sexual thoughts for trans men due to increased testosterone levels.

Fertility concerns for those choosing GCS can be crucial. Financial issues may preclude gamete (egg or sperm) storage for some. However, ethically, the subject of fertility must be addressed prior to initiation of hormonal therapy and again prior to GCS. If fertility is a consideration, GCS must not include hysterectomy, gonadectomy, or vaginectomy. Successful pregnancies following metoidioplasty have been reported. Pregnancy following phalloplasty is generally discouraged and technically unlikely.

The decision to undergo GCS is a deeply personal decision. Many factors parlay into pros and cons for each surgical procedure and need to be considered individually. Regardless, each surgical step must be considered permanent. Quick fixes or return to something original are simply not possible and should not be considered as options. Additionally, any surgery, however well planned, cannot replicate nature and cannot be guaranteed in its outcome. At best, outcomes come with compromises, including scarring and changes in function or aesthetics. Ultimately, it is the personal, private moment of adjustment during transition where a person decides that what they knew must be traded for something that better affirms their gender identity, however imperfect that surgery. With reasonable expectations, surgery can live up to its hopeful potential for most patients.

GCS and the WPATH Standards of Care

Surgeons who perform GCS are expected to follow the WPATH Standards of Care (SOC) (Coleman et al., 2012). Although reasonable exceptions to the SOC are permitted in the current Version (7), insurance companies who preauthorize surgery do so now with the SOC firmly in hand. Similarly, those who wish for surgery on demand—as is common for other nontransgender surgical procedures—will find themselves up against the preapproval process and the SOC. For now, it is best to view these as semirigid safeguards that are put in place with well-intentioned ideals. Briefly, the SOC require a person to live in their desired gender role (DGR) while taking appropriate cross-sex hormones for a period of one year prior to surgery. Psychological support is also a component of the SOC, with final approval requiring letters of support from two licensed mental health specialists for genital surgeries. Lesser standards, and sometimes no letter at all, depending on the procedure, are required for nongenital surgeries.

Preoperative Requirements

Patients preparing for surgery should be in the best possible *physical condition*. It may be necessary to lose weight prior to surgery. Patients that are either too heavy or too thin put themselves at risk for poor healing. The same is true of tobacco smoking. Marijuana use remains equivocal and is likely acceptable if done in moderation. For those with a *medical condition* of any kind, clearance from a specialist is necessary at least 6 to 12 weeks prior to surgery. Physically active individuals, in general, recover more quickly, but extreme changes in exercise just prior to surgery are not advised. *Payment* issues should be dealt with early to avoid last-minute stress. *Hotel and transportation* should be confirmed as soon as surgery is scheduled. It is advisable to check with the surgeon's office immediately prior to booking, because scheduling can change. *Hormones* are often, but not always, discontinued or reduced weeks prior to surgery due to potential blood-clotting risk, so the surgeon should be consulted. *Herbal supplements* can have powerful medicinal properties that can adversely impact surgery and need to be discontinued or approved by the surgeon. *Aspirin* and anything aspirin-like must be discontinued at least one week prior to surgery.

Transfeminine Spectrum Surgery Options

Nongenital Surgery

Feminization surgery (FFS), arguably the *most* feminizing of all GCS procedures, does *not* currently require a letter of support per the SOC. Facial features that create an appearance of maleness or femaleness vary across a spectrum, not surprisingly, with relatively masculine features sometimes found among cisgender females and vice versa. Visual maleness and femaleness of facial features is a sum of bony differences, soft tissue differences, hormonal status, hairline, skin quality, and beard presence or absence, in addition to societal input including makeup, jewelry, hairstyle, and other gender cues. FFS should be viewed as a means to add or subtract physical features that push a face visually into one gender camp or the other.

FFS can include one or a number of surgical procedures. Each should be considered independently, with attendant consequences of each surgical procedure weighed. Often, less is better when it comes to FFS. Frequently, a good forehead contouring with rhinoplasty and additional beard removal can work wonders. Surgical procedures that offer the most in terms of feminization, in general, include forehead contouring, rhinoplasty, and tracheal shaving (chondrolaryngoplasty). Additional procedures that may be very useful on an individual basis include cheek enhancement (implants), jaw contouring or genioplasty (advancing or reducing jaw prominence), hairline advance, chin implants, hair transplantation, and lip procedures or injections. Results vary greatly in terms of surgeon approach, aggressiveness, and technique. It is important to review or interview FFS surgeons to assure that there is a suitable match between physical needs, financial reality, and expectations. Private payers are beginning to recognize that FFS can be not only cosmetic but lifesaving and medically necessary for individuals in their attempt to live in a world that applies great scrutiny to the female face. As a result, insurance coverage for FFS is increasing. Coverage may require a letter of medical necessity from the surgeon or referring medical provider. Most FFS procedures can be performed as single procedures or in combination with others, including vaginoplasty.

Thanks to superb blood flow, the face heals remarkably well. Unsightly scars, asymmetry, residual tissue from a less aggressive surgical approach, or even infection or implant expulsion are contained within the list of potential surgical complications. While rare in good hands, voice coarsening can occur as a result of tracheal shaving, although its incidence remains rare. Cost for FFS can exceed $100,000, although piecemeal and selected procedural choices often suffice for a fraction of that expense.

Breast augmentation (BA) does require a single (1) letter of support per the WPATH SOC. Breast augmentation is technically easier and less individual than FFS, but surgeons can have important differences in perspective. It can be helpful to investigate the reputation of a surgeon for a particular procedure, as well as to understand how the staff generally interacts with trans patients. Like FFS or tracheal shaving, not all transgender women will require BA. A minimum of (2) years on HRT is recommended before assessing for BA.

Due to the improved safety profile for silicone implants combined with less likelihood of leaking or necessity for replacement, silicone implants are generally favored over saline implants. *Surgical incision choices* are less debatable for silicone implants, as the size of the implants preclude axillary (armpit), periareolar (around the nipple), or navel incisions. With rare exception, an incision below the breast is necessary to place the silicone implant. Residual controversy surrounds the issue of subpectoral (below the chest muscle) or prepectoral (in front of the chest muscle) placement of the implant. In general, a very thin patient with little breast development and little subcutaneous fat will be considered for a subpectoral implant placement in order to avoid creating an externally visible implant edge. However, it should be noted that breast tissue occurs naturally in a prepectoral location in cisgender women.

Implant choice is personal and subject to considerations of age (breasts get bigger and sag more as one ages), lifestyle (large breasts can impede exercise), and fashion (small tops do not accommodate larger breasts). Plastic surgeon offices commonly use software that can simulate various surgical options. *Contoured implants* (as opposed to unshaped silicone that simply pushes the breasts forward) can be helpful for those with smaller chests. Trans women are typically advised to choose larger implants than similarly sized cis women due to having broader chests. Larger implants can also offset relative hip narrowness and offer the suggestion of curviness.

Transgender women are increasingly seeking body contouring. Alternatives do exist to the dangerous injections of nonmedical silicone mentioned earlier. *Liposuction* from other body areas and injection of the suctioned fat into the buttocks region can be helpful in adding to the right places (butt, face, or breasts) while subtracting from others (low abdomen, arms, or thighs). The procedure does require meticulous aftercare, a period of immobilization, and no sitting for weeks.

Vocal cord surgery is a delicate procedure performed by surgically narrowing the vocal cords to create a higher resonance in hopes of *raising pitch*. However, the surgery has many caveats. For one, the voice has several components—pitch, resonance and inflection—that sum to create a female-sounding voice. There are many examples of women who have a deep, smoky voice that is still unmistakably feminine. Thus, raising pitch alone affects only one of the three necessary components of the gendered voice. Voice experts, as mentioned previously, can provide nonsurgical techniques to develop a more feminine voice. Seeking voice surgery alone without a first undergoing a successful course of speech therapy will almost universally lead to unsatisfactory outcomes.

Genital Surgery

Orchiectomy (bilateral removal of testicles) is a time-honored surgical procedure normally performed as an outpatient surgery or even office procedure. Orchiectomy is a short procedure, relatively uncomplicated (rare instances of bleeding, infection, or pain), and very effective in reducing testosterone. The procedure leaves the individual infertile and with a markedly reduced libido (unless previously on HRT, in which case it may already be low). Orchiectomy is chosen as an interval procedure (to lower testosterone and increase feminization while reducing hormone risk and expense) or as an end-stage procedure for those who are either too medically risky or who choose not to pursue vaginoplasty at the time, or ever. Undergoing orchiectomy without previously experiencing chemical suppression of testosterone into the female range may produce surprising and potentially problematic symptoms; performing this procedure in such patients should occur only after a detailed discussion and mental health evaluation to ensure clear goals and expectations.

Scrotectomy (removal of the scrotum) at the time of orchiectomy is rare but may be chosen by those who do not wish ever to pursue vaginal surgery and who wish a completely smooth contour. In the vast majority of cases, patients with desire for vaginoplasty must retain their scrotum, as it is the graftable material that will line the future vagina.

Vaginoplasty: The prototype vaginoplasty via "penile inversion" was invented and popularized by Dr. Georges Burou, a French gynecological surgeon working in Casablanca. His technical drawings eventually surfaced at Johns Hopkins University, where they were sought in 1969 by a young Stanley Biber, MD, in order to help a local trans woman who was a social worker in the small town of Trinidad, Colorado. Eventually, surgeons around the globe went still further to utilize the penile glans in order to create a truly functional clitoris and aesthetic modeling of the perineal skin to simulate a more realistic vulva. Dr. Donald Laub, practicing at Stanford in the 1980s, popularized a vaginoplasty technique that utilized the lower rectum in the creation of a neovagina. This latter technique, while highly effective in providing vaginal lubrication (from active colonic mucosa), was less aesthetically similar to cisgender women's vaginas and had higher rates of complications. This so-called *colovaginoplasty* has been relegated to current status as a salvage technique for those who have failed prior operations.

Vaginoplasty techniques today, in general, are variations of the penile inversion technique. Although surgeons at times claim exception to penile inversion (by relying on scrotal skin exclusively to line the vagina), techniques do not vary appreciably. The testicles are removed, the scrotum becomes labia and portions of the vagina, and the glans of the penis becomes the clitoris. Still, results vary wildly due to differences in cosmetic treatments, choice of sensory regions, incisional approach, depth created, sensory retention, and overall technical proficiency.

Vaginoplasty outcomes have evolved markedly since the early days of Lili Elbe. So too have patient expectations. In some locales, surgery is still performed in two stages. Increasingly, though, patients are demanding shorter hospital stays, one-stage procedures, and seamless outcomes. This puts further demand upon the providers of those services to utilize contemporary technique and expertise in offering these services.

Depending upon surgeon, costs for vaginoplasty range from USD $8,000 overseas (particularly Thailand, where currency valuations magnify cost differential) to the United States and Europe, where vaginoplasty can exceed USD $40,000. Travel costs, risks of blood clotting or complications, and surgeon-mandated recuperation time do remain in the financial equation.

In general, expectations for outcomes should include adequate depth (15 cm), acceptable sensory function to allow orgasm, and a realistic cosmetic internal and external appearance with minimal scarring. Meeting those objectives is not always possible. Limitations on depth or vaginal caliber may limit penetration and cannot always be predicted prior to surgery. Sensation should be a given, although the incidence of clitoral necrosis is not negligible. Direct stimulus to the penis is often less than pleasurable, and it thus makes sense that direct stimulus of the neoclitoris may be uncomfortable. Internal sensation is often intact, largely due to the homologous structures of the G-spot, which are nearly identical to that region in cis females. However, not all patients enjoy penetration or stimulation of these regions following GCS. The vaginal lining is considerably thinner than that of cis females. In addition, lubrication is minimal across the vaginal walls. However, considerable lubrication with arousal is reported for many due to the external glands and structures that do remain intact and appear to produce lubrication qualitatively similar to cis-gender women. These contributing structures include the Cowper's glands, prostate, and, probably, seminal vesicles. The prostate is not and cannot be removed at the time of vaginoplasty. Attempts to line the neovagina with urethral, buccal (mouth), or colonic mucosa in hope of providing lubrication are risky, suspect, and do not align with how vaginal lubrication is produced physiologically. Interestingly, there are some who have observed that the newly created vaginal lining appears to adopt a remarkably similar appearance to that of cisgender vaginas, possibly as a result of *metaplasia* (change of one cell type to another). Often, the neovaginal appearance after one year is remarkable.

Because the lining of the vagina is created with the same epithelial skin type (squamous), the *bacterial population of the neovagina* also adopts a somewhat similar makeup to that of the cis female. However, there are major deficits in the number of lactobacilli due to the lack of neovaginal wall glycogen. Lactobacilli normally predominate in the vagina of cis females, metabolize glycogen stores, and consequently acidify the cis-gender vagina. Transgender neovaginas are alkaline with a mixed bacterial flora but are qualitatively similar to the vaginas of cis females (smell, taste, touch).

After vaginoplasty, dilation is very important. At rest, all vaginas, trans or not, lie with walls in contact with one another. Neovaginas differ in risking agglutination (sticking together) and scarring of the walls that can potentially narrow or scar the vagina closed. Risk is highest over the first 18 months following vaginoplasty. Dilation is a mechanical expansion of the vagina that prevents this scarring or narrowing of the vagina. Various dilation schedules exist, and various dilators are prescribed following surgery. Dilator composition can be silicone, acrylic, or plastic. Rigidity must be sufficient to forcefully but gently allow the dilator to advance. No dilation frequency is too often, but each dilation puts additional strain on sutures, at least in the first three weeks following surgery, so lubrication should be used liberally. For those who cannot or will not dilate, particularly early on, there is risk for narrowing and closure (stenosis) of the vaginal opening. This is an unfortunate outcome that cannot be easily remedied outside of an operating theater.

Secondary operations to regain depth exist but vary from an outpatient vaginal-reopening procedure (opening the original neovagina along internal scar lines) to the essentially do-over vaginal-deepening procedure with skin grafting (usually grafted from lower abdominal skin). Costs for vaginal deepening are close to those of a primary operation. Following dilation instructions can assist in avoiding repeat procedures.

Scar creams such as Mederma and others can reduce scar visibility externally. Minimizing scars by avoiding secondary operations and obscuring scars by hiding them along groin creases can be even more helpful.

Complications of vaginoplasty are uncommon but can be significant. Acute problems (within two weeks of surgery) can include infection, bleeding, asymmetry, hematoma, numbness, wound separation, tissue necrosis, or fistula. Aside from bleeding or wound separation, these problems each require their own approach and each require communication with the surgeon and/or primary care provider. That said, most problems will resolve simply if given time. Full recovery after vaginoplasty requires at least 8 to 12 weeks. It is difficult to assess cosmetic appearance until one is fully healed and recovered. Any incision can be accompanied by numbness. Major nerve injury is unlikely, and much of the numbness, if any, will generally resolve in time. Fistula can be caused by faulty dilation (poor angle) or self-injury (sharp instrumentation) but is typically a result of surgical injury. Fistula is a leak or passageway from one structure (such as the rectum) to another (e.g., the vagina). Passage of stool, gas, or urine should prompt medical attention and can indicate fistula. Fistula can be repaired but often requires multiple operations and, occasionally, diversions (such as a colostomy—a medical bag for stool evacuation) in order for the body to heal.

Urinary difficulties following vaginoplasty remain possible but related primarily to technique and the avoidance of complications or injury to either the bladder or urethra, which lie in close proximity during surgery. Incontinence due to disruption of the urinary sphincter mechanism is unlikely.

Chronic problems (present more than two weeks after surgery) include pain, scarring, fistula, dilation difficulties, poor cosmetic appearance, inability to orgasm, and ongoing bleeding or discharge due to granulation tissue. *Granulation tissue* is easily recognized as fleshy, red tissue that can follow any surgical treatment, particularly where there is a gap in the epithelial edges. Granulation tissue is the most common chronic problem experienced following vaginoplasty and is best treated with excision at its base and treatment with silver nitrate. Operative approaches for chronic granulation can include electrocautery or even laser vaporization.

For the foreseeable future, vaginoplasty remains a highly artistic endeavor with a wide range of surgical strategies and outcomes. Consensus seems unlikely. Those considering vaginoplasty should beware of shameless self-promotion and expediency, do research, and not fall for catchy nomenclature and marketing gimmicks. Surgeons should be able to provide photos of results. There should be evidence that the surgeon has consistent competency. Some surgeons offer a number of different procedures, so it is important to know how often they do each procedure. Being in a rush to find a surgeon can lead to poor results.

Labiaplasty is largely a cosmetic secondary operation following vaginoplasty. It can be performed as either a planned procedure (in two-stage vaginoplasties) or as a cosmetic surgery to improve a prior result. It is performed no earlier than three months following initial vaginoplasty in order to allow the surgical site to have fully healed. Labiaplasty can include revisions of the surgical scars, creation of a clitoral hood, further definition of the labia, removal of granulation tissue or excess erectile tissue, and correction of urinary spray ("urethroplasty") to improve the final result. It is normally performed as an outpatient procedure, and full recovery is short (one to two weeks); typically, it is uneventful. Costs for labiaplasty range from USD $4,000 to $7,000. If insurance coverage is possible for vaginoplasty, labiaplasty is normally a covered procedure.

Transmasculine Spectrum Surgery Options

Nongenital Surgeries

Chest surgery (simple mastectomy) is the most common surgical option for trans men. The vast majority of trans men seek a masculine chest contour in favor of inconvenient and uncomfortable breast binding. Surgical approaches in removal of breast tissue include a keyhole incision or traditional ("anchor") incision. Unless minimal tissue exists (A cup), the anchor incision yields a better cosmetic result. Free nipple grafting is often necessary, particularly for large areolae. Scar creams can be helpful as can selective tattooing of surgical scars.

Chest surgeons are more easily found than genital surgeons, with quality results available regionally. However, chest surgery is artistic, and individual approaches vary. Those considering surgery will want to compare before-and-after photos and talk to others, especially to ask how complications or "dog ears" (leftover flaps of skin) are handled.

Complications of chest surgery include poor cosmetic outcome (including scarring and "dog ears"), residual breast tissue, hematoma or seroma (serous fluid or blood beneath the incision), or loss of nipple graft. Complications, aside from scarring and "dog ears," fortunately, are rare.

Facial masculinization surgery, the analog of FFS for trans men, is normally not necessary due to the powerful effects of testosterone. That said, the Adam's apple, even with testosterone, does not change appreciably in trans men.

Adam's Apple Augmentation (AAA) is a surgical procedure chosen occasionally by trans men who seek a more masculine neck profile. The Adam's apple is a hallmark masculine prominence of the thyroid cartilage. It can be augmented by insertion and fixation of a plastic insert. The incision is normally hidden beneath the jawline. *Pectoplasty* (insertion of chest implants to enhance pectoral musculature) is also considered by occasional transmasculine individuals.

Genital Surgeries

For trans men, choices in genital surgery are less definitive and, frankly, chosen less often than for trans women. Some put the number of trans men proceeding with "bottom surgery" in the United States at less than 10 percent. Costs, risks associated with surgery, and donor site morbidity (in the case of phalloplasty) are major reasons that misgivings regarding genital surgery exist. However, increasingly covered by insurance, genital surgeries are becoming more in demand.

Before proceeding with bottom surgery, trans men must consider expectations of each considered procedure, financial resources, tolerance for complications or morbidity, and lifestyle. Many surgeries are staged procedures, meaning multiple visits and recovery times. Costs of surgery can vary. Because genital surgery will have a major impact on sex life, it is also imperative that the trans-masculine individual understand their sexuality in terms of orgasm, self-pleasure, and intimacy with their partner(s). Phalloplasty leaves genitalia that are markedly different in form and function in comparison to metoidioplasty. Although with enough time and money, one can move from meta to phallo (but not vice versa), it is ideal to match preferences with postoperative anatomy and proceed with one surgical direction. Goals of genital surgery for trans men are construction of a male-appearing phallus, maintenance (or enhancement) of sexuality, and (optionally) the ability to stand while urinating.

Metoidioplasty (in Latin, "becoming male") is a surgical procedure that creates a neophallus from the testosterone-enlarged clitoris. The meta procedure creates a penis by releasing the tethered-down clitoris from the labia minora underneath and allowing the potential penis to spring forward by dividing ligaments that lie deeply beneath the clitoris skin above and below the shaft. These ligaments give the unaltered clitoris a curved shape prior to release. After release, the penis is straighter and longer. Labial skin is then drawn around to the front and surgically sewn closed.

For the *ring meta (RM)*, a urethral tube is additionally closed within the meta skin by sewing the labial skin (ring flap) around a urinary tube. An additional patch of mucosa obtained from the vagina completes the urinary tube.

For any genital procedure chosen by a trans man, the difficulties lie in creation of a watertight urethra suitable for conducting urine and allowing the man to stand while urinating. As a result, complications can exceed 10 percent but are often addressed at *scrotoplasty*, performed as a secondary procedure in three months or later. Complications of ring meta can include urinary stricture (narrowing) or fistula (leaking) of the urinary tract. When fully healed, the ability to stand with urination is possible. The penis, when engorged, has penetrative potential although lacks the cismale tunica, meaning erections are less rigid. The procedure is considered relatively contraindicated for larger men (BMI > 30) or for those with a large amount of mons fat due to the subtraction of length that accompanies the surrounding extra fat.

The *simple meta* (SM) creates a neophallus but does not elongate the urethral tube. It is created from the body of the clitoris, closure of the perineal skin, and midline approximation of the levator muscles. Urinary flow is not appreciably affected, and standing to urinate is not possible without using a device. The ventral chordae and suspensory ligaments are often but not always included to add length to the phallus. Complications aside from basic wound healing are rare. It can be performed in just one stage even if combined with vaginectomy and/or scrotoplasty.

The *classical meta (CM)* utilizes buccal mucosa rather than the ring flap mucosa, labial mucosa, or both to extend the urinary tract. Other aspects of the procedure are similar to the RM above.

Phalloplasty involves sophisticated techniques of tissue mobilization and arterial and nerve preservation to create a male phallus in a single or staged procedure. Pieces of skin taken from the inner arm (radial forearm graft), lower flank (latissimus dorsi flap), front and side of the thigh (anterolateral thigh flap), lower abdomen (inferior epigastric flap) or other locations are rounded and secured to the front of the pelvic bone.

A *simple phalloplasty (SP)* retains tactile sensation but not erogenous sensation and does not extend the urinary tract. *Free flap phalloplasty* assumes the additional goals of erogenous sensation as well as ability to stand to urinate. The latter procedure is normally performed in multiple procedures. Both urinary connections to the urethra and nervous connections to the dorsal nerves of the clitoris/phallus are considered. A microsurgical team is typically utilized. Complications include flap necrosis, infection, and urinary stricture or fistula. Complications typically exceed 10 percent but are manageable in most cases.

Results, particularly after *glansplasty*, can be quite excellent. Glansplasty involves surgically delineating the distal tip of the phalloplasty in the shape of a male glans as a secondary procedure. *Intercourse* is achievable with placement of an inflatable pump or thin rod that must be inserted prior to sexual engagement.

Vaginectomy is removal or destruction of the vaginal lining. Concurrent or prior hysterectomy is mandatory. True vaginal lining removal is arduous and bloody. Most contemporary surgeons opt to perform a version of colpocleisis: obliteration and surgical closure of the vagina. The result is a male perineum (bottom). Vaginectomy is possible but incomplete when performing simple meta. This is due to the remaining presence of periurethral glands that will continue to produce mucus and discharge near the urethra. Although undocumented, some argue that *urinary fistula* (leak) incidence is higher when urethral lengthening is performed without vaginectomy. Although rare, risks of vaginectomy include retention of viable vaginal lining and consequent internal mucus buildup or discharge.

Scrotoplasty involves creating a male scrotum from the labia majora (large labia). There is variability among surgeons in unification of the labia versus persistent clefting in this area. With simple meta, a unified scrotum is not possible due to the need to preserve urinary outflow. Testicle implants of silicone or saline of various sizes may be optionally inserted at scrotoplasty. Some surgeons wait to perform the scrotoplasty and implants as a secondary procedure. Because the implants are foreign bodies, risks of scrotoplasty in particular include infection and implant expulsion. The larger the implant, the greater the chance of expulsion. Thigh musculature (bulk), scrotal skin volume, amount of skin stretching, and other factors make selection of proper implant size imperative.

Monsplasty can be thought of as a very low tummy tuck/abdominoplasty. The goal, however, is not solely to flatten the stomach but rather to reduce the profile of the mons region in hopes of drawing the meta/phallus upward and forward. Subcutaneous fat inferior to the incision can be removed as well in achieving a more masculine contour in this region. Aside from scarring or the possibility of asymmetry, complications are minimal.

Surgical Aftercare

Although patients may remain or live within proximity of their surgeon, indefinite follow-up is not possible, and care is eventually transferred back to the patient's primary care provider (PCP). This model of providing after-care, particularly with discrimination and lack of provider knowledge as obstacles, is particularly troublesome. Clear handoff to a PCP is essential with guidance available should complications arise. Fortunately, most complications that do arise are of the chronic variety, meaning emergency services are only rarely required. Urgent situations that can lead to presentation in the emergency room include bleeding, hematoma, tissue necrosis, wound breakdown, or thromboembolism (blood clots). Intra-abdominal bleeding is not a realistic concern for any GCS. If there is bleeding or a tissue problem, it should be readily evident. The attending surgeon should be available for at least verbal consultation with emergency or primary care providers. Some surgeons choose to insist upon follow-up visitation after healing has completed. For most, resumption of normal life activities effectively diminishes the role of the surgeon.

The PCP is essential in surgical follow-up. In the short term, the PCP can be helpful in establishing a new hormone regimen, evaluation of healing, and diagnosis of possible complications. Evaluation of emotional status is also important. Surgery can be draining, both physically and mentally. Some period of follow-up is clearly beneficial with a postsurgical visit ideally scheduled no later than four weeks after any GCS. So, too, it is wise not to disregard the role of the mental health specialist in aftercare. Once surgery is past, there can be a bit of a letdown as the anticipation fades. There can also be a period of adjustment, particularly if there are complications or frustrations associated with the GCS process.

Gender-Confirmation Surgery for the Gender-Nonconforming Individual

Increasingly, gender is being viewed in its components, segments, and pieces. For some, gender identity and anatomy are separate pieces, where some portions fit and others do not. For others, gender valuation of any kind is intolerable. Sexuality may or may not be a part of that mix. The rules are changing, and for some, no rules is the new normal. The fact is that many today are self-identifying outside of binary gender designations.

These genderqueer, agender, neutrois, or undesignated individuals seek gender-neutralizing surgeries (e.g., top surgery, castration) or selective cross-gender surgeries (e.g., metoidioplasty, vaginoplasty) and appear happy with their respective decisions in the vast majority of cases.

Offering GCS or gender-neutrality surgeries to the diverse population of gender-nonconforming individuals will remain controversial and pits ethical considerations against the ideals of individual choice and autonomy. In general, if appropriate consultation and letters of evaluation are in place, it is unethical to deny care. The WPATH Standards are silent on GCS for gender-nonconforming persons or gender neutrality. A longer period of preoperative counseling may be helpful.

REFERENCES

Asscheman, H., Giltay, E. J., Megens, J. A., de Ronde, W. P., van Trotsenburg, M. A., & Gooren, L. J. (2011). A long-term follow-up study of mortality in transsexuals receiving treatment with cross-sex hormones. *European Journal of Endocrinology/European Federation of Endocrine Societies, 164*(4), 635–642.

Asscheman, H., Gooren, L. J., & Eklund, P. L. (1989). Mortality and morbidity in transsexual patients with cross-gender hormone treatment. *Metabolism: Clinical and Experimental, 38*(9), 869–873.

Berlin, E., Singh, K., Mills, C., Shapira, I., Bakst, R. L., & Chadha, M. (2018). Breast implant-associated anaplastic large cell lymphoma: Case report and review of the literature. *Case Reports in Hematology, 2018,* 2414278. doi:10.1155/2018/2414278

Blondon, M., van Hylckama Vlieg, A., Wiggins, K. L., Harrington, L. B., McKnight, B., Rice, K. M., . . . Smith, N. L. (2014). Differential associations of oral estradiol and conjugated equine estrogen with hemostatic biomarkers. *Journal of Thrombosis and Haemostasis, 12*(6), 879–886.

Brown, G. R. (2015). Breast cancer in transgender veterans: A ten-case series. *LGBT Health, 2*(1), 77–80.

Brown, G. R., & Jones, K. T. (2015). Incidence of breast cancer in a cohort of 5,135 transgender veterans. *Breast Cancer Research and Treatment, 149*(1), 191–198.

Canonico, M., Oger, E., Plu-Bureau, G., Meyer, G., Lévesque, H., Trillot, N., . . . Estrogen and Thromboembolism (ESTHER) Study Group. (2007). Hormone therapy and venous thromboembolism among postmenopausal women: Impact of the route of estrogen administration and progestogens: The ESTHER study. *Circulation, 115*(7), 840–845.

Center of Excellence for Transgender Health. (2016). *Guidelines for the primary and gender-affirming care of transgender and gender nonbinary people* (2nd ed.). San Francisco: Deutsch, M. B.

Chlebowski, R. T., Rohan, T. E., Manson, J. E., Aragaki, A. K., Kaunitz, A., Stefanick, M. L., . . . Prentice, R. L. (2015). Breast cancer after use of estrogen plus progestin and estrogen alone: Analyses of data from 2 Women's Health Initiative randomized clinical trials. *JAMA Oncology, 1*(3), 296–305.

Clements-Nolle, K., Marx, R., & Katz, M. (2006). Attempted suicide among transgender persons: The influence of gender-based discrimination and victimization. *Journal of Homosexuality, 51*(3), 53–69.

Coleman, E., Bockting, W., Botzer, M., Cohen-Kettenis, P., DeCuypere, G., Feldman, J., . . . Zucker, K. (2012). Standards of care for the health of transsexual, transgender, and gender-nonconforming people, version 7. *International Journal of Transgenderism, 13*, 165–232.

Coulter, R. W., Kenst, K. S., Bowen, D. J., & Scout. (2014). Research funded by the National Institutes of Health on the health of lesbian, gay, bisexual, and transgender populations. *American Journal of Public Health, 104*(2), e105–e112.

Dahl, M., Feldman, J. L., Goldberg, J., Jaberi, A., & Vancouver Coastal Health. (2015). *Endocrine therapy for transgender adults in British Columbia: Suggested guidelines.* Vancouver, BC: Vancouver Coastal Health. Retrieved from http://www.phsa.ca/transcarebc/Documents/HealthProf/BC-Trans -Adult-Endocrine-Guidelines-2015.pdf

de Vries, A. L., Doreleijers, T. A., Steensma, T. D., & Cohen-Kettenis, P. T. (2011). Psychiatric comorbidity in gender dysphoric adolescents. *Journal of Child Psychology and Psychiatry, and Allied Disciplines, 52*(11), 1195–1202.

Department of Health and Human Services Departmental Appeals Board. (2013). *Transsexual Surgery* (Docket No. A-13-47 NCD, Ruling No. 2). Washington, DC: Department of Health and Human Services. Retrieved from https://www.hhs.gov/sites/default/files/static/dab/decisions/board-deci-sions/2014/dab2576.pdf

Desai, A. M., Browning, J., & Rosen, T. (2006). Etanercept therapy for silicone granuloma. *Journal of Drugs in Dermatology, 20*(4), 757–790.

Deutsch, M. B. (2012). Use of the informed consent model in the provision of cross-sex hormone therapy: A survey of the practices of selected clinics. *International Journal of Transgenderism, 13*(3), 140–146.

Diamond, M., & Sigmundson, H. K. (1997). Sex reassignment at birth. Long-term review and clinical implications. *Archives of Pediatrics & Adolescent Medicine, 151*(3), 298–304.

Eldh, J. (1993). Construction of a neovagina with preservation of the glans penis as a clitoris in male transsexuals. *Plastic and Reconstructive Surgery, 91*(5), 895–900; discussion 901–903.

Gil, M., Oliva, B., Timoner, J., Macia, M. A., Bryant, V., & de Abajo, F. J. (2011). Risk of meningioma among users of high doses of cyproterone acetate as compared with the general population: Evidence from a population-based cohort study. *British Journal of Clinical Pharmacology, 72*(6), 965–968.

Gooren, L. J. (2011). Clinical practice. Care of transsexual persons. *The New England Journal of Medicine, 364*(13), 1251–1257.

Gooren, L. J., Giltay, E. J., & Bunck, M. C. (2008). Long-term treatment of trans-sexuals with cross-sex hormones: Extensive personal experience. *The Journal of Clinical Endocrinology and Metabolism, 93*(1), 19–25.

Gooren, L. J., van Trotsenburg, M. A., Giltay, E. J., & van Diest, P. J. (2013). Breast cancer development in transsexual subjects receiving cross-sex hormone treatment. *Journal of Sexual Medicine, 10*(12), 3129–3134.

Gorin-Lazard, A., Baumstarck, K., Boyer, L., Maquigneau, A., Gebleux, S., Peno-chet, J. C., . . . Bonierbale, M. (2012). Is hormonal therapy associated with better quality of life in transsexuals? A cross-sectional study. *Journal of Sexual Medicine, 9*(2), 531–541.

Grant, J. M., Mottet, L. A., & Tanis, J. (2010). *National transgender discrimination survey report on health and health care.* Washington, DC: National Center for Transgender Equality & National Gay and Lesbian Task Force.

Haas, A. P., Rodgers, P. L., & Herman, J. L. (2014). *Suicide attempts among transgender and gender non-conforming adults: Findings of the national transgender discrimination survey.* Los Angeles, CA: American Foundation for Suicide Prevention & Williams Institute.

Hembree, W. C., Cohen-Kettenis, P., Delemarre-van de Waal, H., Gooren, L. J., Meyer, W. J., III, Spack, N. P., . . . Endocrine Society. (2009). Endocrine treatment of transsexual persons: An Endocrine Society clinical practice guideline. *The Journal of Clinical Endocrinology and Metabolism, 94*(9), 3132–3154.

Hembree, W. C., Cohen-Kettenis, P., Gooren, L., Hannema, S. E., Meyer, W. J., Murad, M. H., . . . T'Sjoen, G. G. (2017). Endocrine treatment of gender-dysphoric/gender-incongruent persons: An Endocrine Society clinical practice guideline. *The Journal of Clinical Endocrinology & Metabolism, 102*(11), 3869–3903.

Herbst, J. H., Jacobs, E. D., Finlayson, T. J., McKleroy, V. S., Neumann, M. S., Cre-paz, N., & HIV/AIDS Prevention Research Synthesis Team. (2008). Estimating HIV prevalence and risk behaviors of transgender persons in the United States: A systematic review. *AIDS and Behavior, 12*(1), 1–17.

Human Rights Campaign. (2015). *Finding insurance for transgender-related healthcare.* Retrieved from http://www.hrc.org/resources/finding-insurance-for-transgender-related-healthcare

Institute of Medicine. (2011). *The health of lesbian, gay, bisexual, and transgender people: Building a foundation for better understanding.* Washington, DC: The National Academies Press.

Johnson, S. R., Smith, E. M., & Guenther, S. M. (1987). Comparison of gynecologic health care problems between lesbians and bisexual women. A survey of 2,345 women. *The Journal of Reproductive Medicine, 32*(11), 805–811.

Kenagy, G. P. (2005). Transgender health: Findings from two needs assessment studies in Philadelphia. *Health & Social Work, 30*(1), 19–26.

Kuper, L. E., Nussbaum, R., & Mustanski, B. (2012). Exploring the diversity of gender and sexual orientation identities in an online sample of transgender individuals. *Journal of Sex Research, 49*(2–3), 244–254.

Lawrence, A. A. (2003). Factors associated with satisfaction or regret following male-to-female sex reassignment surgery. *Archives of Sexual Behavior, 32*(4), 299–315.

Light, A. D., Obedin-Maliver, J., Sevelius, J. M., & Kerns, J. L. (2014). Transgender men who experienced pregnancy after female-to-male gender transitioning. *Obstetrics and Gynecology, 124*(6), 1120–1127.

Lombardi, E. L., Wilchins, R. A., Priesing, D., & Malouf, D. (2001). Gender violence: Transgender experiences with violence and discrimination. *Journal of Homosexuality, 42*(1), 89–101.

Meyer, J. K., & Reter, D. J. (1979). Sex reassignment. Follow-up. *Archives of General Psychiatry, 36*(9),1010–1015.

Meyerowitz, J. (2002). *How sex changed: A history of transsexuality in the United States.* Cambridge, MA: Harvard University Press.

Newfield, E., Hart, S., Dibble, S., & Kohler, L. (2006). Female-to-male transgender quality of life. *Quality of Life Research, 15*(9), 1447–1457.

Noels, E. C., Lapid, O., Lindeman, J. H., & Bastiaannet, E. (2015). Breast implants and the risk of breast cancer: A meta-analysis of cohort studies. *Aesthetic Surgery Journal, 25*(1), 55–62.

Nuttbrock, L., Hwahng, S., Bockting, W., Rosenblum, A., Mason, M., Macri, M., & Becker, J. (2010). Psychiatric impact of gender-related abuse across the life course of male-to-female transgender persons. *Journal of Sex Research, 47*(1), 12–23.

Office of Disease Prevention and Health Promotion. (2018). Lesbian, gay, bisexual, and transgender health. *Healthy People 2020.* Retrieved from https://www .healthypeople.gov/2020/topics-objectives/topic/lesbian-gay-bisexual -and-transgender-health

Olson, J., Schrager, S. M., Clark, L. F., Dunlap, S. L., & Belzer, M. (2014). Subcutaneous testosterone: An effective delivery mechanism for masculinizing young transgender men. *LGBT Health, 1*(3), 165–167.

Olson, K. R., Durwood, L., DeMeules, M., & McLaughlin, K. A. (2016). Mental health of transgender children who are supported in their identities. *Pediatrics, 137*(3), 1–8.

Peitzmeier, S. M., Khullar, K., Reisner, S. L., & Potter, J. (2014). Pap test use is lower among female-to-male patients than non-transgender women. *American Journal of Preventive Medicine, 47*(6), 808–812.

Peitzmeier, S. M., Reisner, S. L., Harigopal, P., & Potter, J. (2014). Female-to-male patients have high prevalence of unsatisfactory Paps compared to non-transgender females: Implications for cervical cancer screening. *Journal of General Internal Medicine, 29*(5), 778–784.

Reed, H. M. (2011). Aesthetic and functional male to female genital and perineal surgery: Feminizing vaginoplasty. *Seminars in Plastic Surgery, 25*(2), 163–174.

Rehman, J., & Melman, A. (1999). Formation of neoclitoris from glans penis by reduction glansplasty with preservation of neurovascular bundle in male-to-female gender surgery: Functional and cosmetic outcome. *The Journal of Urology, 161*(1), 200–206.

Reisner, S. L., Deutsch, M. B., Bhasin, S., Bockting, W., Brown, G. R., Feldman, J., . . . Goodman, M. (2016). Advancing methods for US transgender health research. *Current Opinion in Endocrinology, Diabetes, and Obesity, 23*(2), 198–207.

Reisner, S. L., Hughto, J. M., Dunham, E. E., Heflin, K. J., Begenyi, J. B., Coffey-Esquivel, J., & Cahill, S. (2015). Legal protections in public accommodations settings: A critical public health issue for transgender and gender-nonconforming people. *The Milbank Quarterly, 93*(3), 484–515.

Roberts, A. L., Rosario, M., Corliss, H. L., Koenen, K. C., & Austin, S. B. (2012). Childhood gender nonconformity: A risk indicator for childhood abuse and posttraumatic stress in youth. *Pediatrics, 129*(3), 410–417.

Rossi Neto, R., Hintz, F., Krege, S., Rubben, H., & Vom Dorp, F. (2012). Gender reassignment surgery—A 13 year review of surgical outcomes. *International Brazilian Journal of Urology, 38*(1), 97–107.

Rotondi, N. K., Bauer, G. R., Scanlon, K., Kaay, M., Travers, R., & Travers, A. (2011). Prevalence of and risk and protective factors for depression in female-to-male transgender Ontarians: Trans PULSE Project. *Canadian Journal of Community Mental Health, 30*(2), 135–155.

Schulze, C. (1988). Response of the human testis to long-term estrogen treatment: Morphology of Sertoli cells, Leydig cells and spermatogonial stem cells. *Cell and Tissue Research, 251*(1), 31–43.

Smith, N. L., Blondon, M., Wiggins, K. L., Harrington, L. B., van Hylckama Vlieg, A., Floyd, J. S., . . . Psaty, B. M. (2014). Lower risk of cardiovascular events in postmenopausal women taking oral estradiol compared with oral conjugated equine estrogens. *JAMA Internal Medicine, 174*(1), 25–31.

Stahlman, J., Britto, M., Fitzpatrick, S., McWhirter, C., Testino, S. A., Brennan, J. J., & Zumbrunnen, T. L. (2012). Serum testosterone levels in non-dosed females after secondary exposure to 1.62% testosterone gel: Effects of clothing barrier on testosterone absorption. *Current Medical Research and Opinion, 28*(2), 291–301.

Stryker, S. (2008). *Transgender history.* Berkeley, CA: Seal Press.

van Kesteren, P. J., Asscheman, H., Megens, J. A., & Gooren, L. J. (1997). Mortality and morbidity in transsexual subjects treated with cross-sex hormones. *Clinical Endocrinology, 47*(3), 337–342.

Virtanen, A., Anttila, A., & Nieminen, P. (2015). The costs of offering HPV-testing on self-taken samples to non-attendees of cervical screening in Finland. *BMC Women's Health, 15*, 99.

Wilson, E., Rapues, J., Jin, H., & Raymond, H. F. (2014). The use and correlates of illicit silicone or "fillers" in a population-based sample of transwomen, San Francisco, 2013. *The Journal of Sexual Medicine, 11*(7), 1717–1724.

Wise, T. N., & Lucas, J. (1981). Pseudotranssexualism: Iatrogenic gender dysphoria. *Journal of Homosexuality, 6*(3), 61–66.

5

Exploring the Health Issues of LGBT Adolescents

Travis A. Gayles and Robert Garofalo

Being an adolescent and teenager can be challenging as a time of physical, social, and emotional adjustment. Adolescence is a time of self-exploration and identity construction. Adolescents learn to navigate the physical changes of puberty, deal with budding physical attractions to others, and begin to explore future career choices as an adult. Adolescents are at an "in-between" age neither fully in the pediatric nor adult worlds. As such, they are given increasing responsibility, such as participating more in their health care decisions, but must continue to rely on adults to provide financial, social, and logistical support, including transportation and housing. Their health is significantly influenced by family and neighborhood environments and recently, more heavily influenced by social media and expanding technology such a cell phones and text messaging.

For LGBT youth, though, there can be a number of additional challenges to achieving traditional adolescent developmental milestones as they navigate the growth and maturity process in the context of increased homophobia, victimization, and largely discriminatory social policies (e.g., opposition to gay marriage and adoption as but two examples). No doubt, there have been great strides made in advancing LGBT rights over the past decade, including increasing political support for gay marriage and adoption rights, the repeal of "don't ask, don't tell" (a military policy preventing openly gay and lesbian soldiers from serving in the military), and a greater presence of diverse LGBT characters in pop media and culture. These progressive changes are helping to create a social environment where LGBT adolescents may be more comfortable with themselves and choosing to come out at an earlier age compared to previous generations. However, in spite of this progress, LGBT adolescents continue to encounter homophobic messages from many segments of society that can make coming out and growing up healthy difficult and challenging, as evidenced by the increased publicity of bullying and victimization of children based on sexual and gender identity. They may not be equipped to handle the emotional stresses that these challenges present or to handle societal pressures while constructing their own unique support systems and identities.

There has been much written previously about the lives and experiences of LGBT adolescents—most recently a summary of the existing research in this area by the Institute of Medicine (IOM). The aim of this chapter is to build on these previous efforts in the setting of changing political and social dynamics. We will highlight the overall experience of LGBT adolescents through their developmental and expression of sexual identity and the broader health and social challenges they face in relation to their heterosexual peers. The chapter will next examine the historical context of research opportunities and key findings on this population as highlighted in the IOM report. We will conclude with a discussion of important clinical and policy implications for health care providers dedicated to caring for LGBT youth.

WHO ARE LGBT ADOLESCENTS?

For the purposes of this chapter, "adolescents" are defined as people between the ages of 10 and 21. Adolescents and young adults comprise approximately 22 percent of the U.S. population (CDC, 2016a). Adolescent health represents a critical transition from childhood to adulthood and is marked by an increasing number of developmental milestones. Adolescents are typically healthy compared to other age groups, with the leading causes of morbidity and mortality related to unintentional injuries, homicides, and suicides that vary across demographic indicators such as gender, race, and age. The Healthy People 2020 initiative identified 21 critical areas of attention for adolescent health that disproportionately affect this age group, including lack of physical activity, unintentional injuries, violence-related injuries and death, drug and alcohol usage, teenage pregnancy, suicide rates, and the impact of diminished self-esteem and sexually transmitted infections. Significant health disparities by racial category exist, as adolescents and young adults who are African American, American Indian, or Hispanic are disproportionately impacted by many of the above-mentioned health areas (CDC, 2016b). LGBT adolescents encounter these same health issues, but as we will discuss later in the chapter, several additional health concerns have the potential to affect healthy development in this population.

It is difficult, if not impossible, to quantify the exact number of LGBT adolescents; there is scant national data available on the number of LGBT adolescents in the United States. A recent report by the Safe Schools Coalition of Washington analyzed several state studies that attempted to quantify the percentage of LGBT youth; the ratio ranged from 0.2 percent of self-identified LGBT adolescents in a sample of San Francisco high school students to 5.3 percent of young men and 3.4 percent of young women in Vermont having engaged in same-gender sexual activity (Reis & Saewyc, 1999). The study further found that uncertainty about sexual orientation declined with age, from 25.9 percent of 12-year-olds being uncertain to 5 percent of 17-year-old students. A separate national survey of college students (Mulye et al., 2009) found that 48 percent of self-identified gay and bisexual college students reported becoming aware of their sexual identity in high school, while 26 percent found their true sexuality in college. Twenty percent of self-identified gay and bisexual men knew that they were gay or bisexual in junior high school, and 17 percent said they knew in grade school. Six percent of self-identified gay or bisexual women knew that they were gay or bisexual in junior high school, and 11 percent knew in grade school. These studies as well as a cadre of others suggest that adolescence is often the most likely time of acknowledgment and development of sexual identity.

HISTORICAL PERSPECTIVES

The hallmark of the adolescent LGBT experience is the initial formation and further development of sexual identity. The first models that examined identity construction were based on retrospective accounts from white adult patients (IOM, 2011) and were constructed during a period when social stigma and homophobia were much more prevalent than today. The Cass (1979) model was the first to normalize homosexual behavior and is based on the belief that identity construction is a stepwise process. As pointed out, however, by Kaufman and Johnson (2004), the model failed to include an adequate representation of racial minority youth and did not fully address the impact of sociocultural factors that shape identity development or the impact of increased public perception and acceptance.

There has been extensive literature on sexual identity development but less regarding gender identity. This is especially significant given the increasing prevalence of children expressing gender variance and the new changes in the DSM-V manual that replace gender identity disorder with gender dysphoria. Brill and Pepper (2008) provided the first comprehensive guide to gender variance from birth through college. Unlike sexual orientation, gender identity begins to emerge as early as children learn to speak—as toddlers begin to assert their identity behaviorally and/or verbally (Brill & Pepper, 2008). Table 5.1 shows the developmental states and the transgender child in comparison with LGB youth. Similar to the coming-out process, expression of gender identity is a fluid process heavily influenced by social norms, peer pressure, and level of familial support.

Table 5.1   Developmental States of Gender and Sexual Identity Minorities

Age	Transgender Child	LGB Child
Ages 2–3	Gender identity emerges. Child can identify men/boys and girls/women by external appearances. Children seek cues for how to act from same-sex models based on their internal gender identity and may begin to announce to caregivers their sense of difference between their internal gender identity and what they are told they are.	No clear data.
Ages 3–4	Child is aware of their gender identity, become aware of anatomical differences, and incorporate info about the sexes into stereotypes. Gender segregation begins. Child struggles to express gender variance (e.g., "I want to be a girl when I grow up"; "My heart is girl, but my body is boy"; "God made a mistake with me.")	No clear data.
Ages 4–6	Children associate gender with specific behaviors using gender scripts (e.g., girls wear makeup, so anyone with makeup on is a girl; all doctors are men) and understand behaviors as applying only to one gender or the other. Exposure to tolerance of gender differences in school and at home can help	No clear data.

(continued)

Table 5.1   **(continued)**

Age	Transgender Child	LGB Child
	children adapt their constructs. Indicators of gender variance clearly emerge with boys repeatedly playing dress-up and making dresses out of towels, tablecloths, etc. Children often believe they can grow up to become the opposite sex. Consistent and persistent cross-gender identity for several years now.	
Ages 5–7	Children understand gender consistency and stability. Children gravitate toward dress and behaviors that express their internal gender identity or, depending on the safety of their environment, may choose not to express their identity. Gender-variant children who are forced to limit their expression may develop behavioral problems at school and may express suicidal ideation.	No clear data.
Ages 9–12	Gender identity continues to stabilize. However, because of increasing social pressure, gender-variant children may attempt to enact more stereotypically gendered behavior and dress of their birth sex. As pubertal changes begin, gender dysphoria may emerge, and transgender children may resist body changes. Depression can emerge and manifest in displays of self-neglect and/or self-harm. These children may realize they are transgender and may need therapeutic guidance to determine causes of stress.	(Ages 10–14) Peers begin to influence interests and clothing styles. Sexual curiosity may lead to the initiation of sexual experimentation with masturbation or early sexual activity with same-gender or opposite-gender partners. For boys who are gender atypical, this may be a period of heightened psychological turmoil, as they may be harassed by peers. Secondary sexual characteristics appear in early adolescence and, consequently, accentuated gender differentiation.

(*continued*)

Table 5.1 (continued)

Age	Transgender Child	LGB Child
		Young girls, particularly those who are athletic, may be somewhat uncomfortable with breast development.
Ages 12–18	Gender identity fully develops. Hormonal and concurrent physical changes of puberty clarify for the child that they are going through the "wrong" puberty. Teens may withdraw socially or experience depression. They may communicate with urgency regarding their gender identity as their changing body takes them further from their true nature. They may internalize shame around being transgender, especially if they lack family support. Contact with other transgender teens is an important psychological and social support.	
Late adolescence– young adulthood	Adolescents may continue to question their identity and mental health. They may overcome their shame and guilt, bringing their mind and body more closely in alignment through gender-affirming social and medical transition.	(Ages 14–17) Physical changes of puberty are completed during middle adolescence. Adolescents begin to have more romantic relationships, typically characterized as dating or serial monogamy. They begin to distance themselves from parents and place emphasis on peers. LGB youth experience the same physical changes as their heterosexual peers. These changes warrant open discussions about normal breast development in young women and increased penile and

(continued)

Table 5.1   (continued)

Age	Transgender Child	LGB Child
		testicular size in males. While middle adolescents often engage in risk-taking behaviors such as substance use and sexual activity, they may not yet fully understand the consequences of their actions. This may lead to heightened risk for HIV and STIs among sexually active middle adolescents.

(Brill & Pepper, 2008; Garofalo & Church, 2007)

Development of both sexual and gender identity for LGBT youth is further complicated by the fact that many of these adolescents are more likely to reside in environments that lack familial and otherwise readily available social support. Lack of accessible role models has been shown to increase psychological stress among LGBT adolescents (Bird, Kuhns, & Garofalo, 2012). A Human Rights Campaign (HRC, 2012) survey found that 56 percent of LGBT youth reported being out to their immediate family and 25 percent to their extended family. They found that only 37 percent of LGBT youth were happy with their lives compared to 67 percent of non-LGBT youth. Additionally, 29 percent reported that they had an adult that they could talk to about personal problems. Approximately 47 percent of LGBT youth say they do not fit in in their environment compared to only 16 percent of non-LGBT youth. Forty percent do not feel that their community is accepting of them. They were also more likely to report being less confident in obtaining success as an adult, such as having a good job, going to college, or raising children with a long-term partner in the same community. When asked to describe the one thing that they would like to change, LGBT youth reported they wanted to increase tolerance, parental/familial support, and change the location where they lived. Non-LGBT youth were more likely to focus on money/finance and appearance and weight. The same youth identified issues such as nonaccepting families, school bullying, and fear of being outed, while non-LGBT youth were more worried about academic performance and college and career choices. The most common place for negative messages about LGBT peers was school

(74 percent), the Internet (70 percent), and peers (69 percent). Conversely, the most common place where LGBT youth heard positive messages were the Internet (88 percent), peers (69 percent), and movies, TV, and radio (59 percent).

A small number of empirical studies have collected descriptive data on the demographic background and behavior of LGBT adolescents. The 1987 Minnesota Adolescent Health Survey was the first to include LGBT youth demographic data in behavioral analysis, specifically sexual history. They found that female respondents were more likely to express attraction to both genders, while a higher percentage of younger (defined as 14 years of age or younger) male respondents reported having had a sexual experience with another male (45.2 percent versus 8.2 percent) (Saewyc, Bearinger, Heinz, Blum, & Resnick, 1998).

As a result of these early studies, in 1989, the American Academy of Pediatrics (AAP) released its first statement on homosexuality encouraging pediatricians to provide comprehensive medical treatment for LGBT adolescents, including a thorough sexual history and education about sexually transmitted infections (STI). Additionally, the AAP statement firmly stated that therapies aimed at changing sexual orientation, commonly referred to as reparative or conversion therapy, were contraindicated in adolescent youth. The AAP reaffirmed this statement in 1993 and 15 years later partnered with 11 other organizations, including the American Psychological Association, to write a primer for school officials about the needs and issues of LGBT adolescents (AAP, 1993).

The first developmental study of adolescent LGBT sexual identity was conducted by Herdt and Boxer in 1993. Their study concluded that the development of sexual identity is an evolving process, with gay males developing awareness of same-sex attraction at age nine, a year earlier than lesbian females. Research on LGBT adolescent behavior and sexual identity expression has increased slightly over the past decade, as evidenced by several large-scale studies such as the Youth Risk Behavior Surveys (YRBS) across a number of states, including Illinois and Massachusetts. These surveys include sexual identity items while also asking adolescents a broad range of questions on behavioral activities such as bullying and victimization, sexual activity, alcohol and drug use, and self-esteem. A number of subsequent studies continued exploring sexual identity as a developmental milestone heavily influenced by internalized homophobia and external stigmas. More recently, the Massachusetts YRBS data (1995) reported that LGB orientation was associated with having had sexual intercourse before 13 years of age, having sexual intercourse with four or more partners both in a lifetime and in the past three months, and having experienced sexual contact against one's will (Garofalo, Wolf, Kessel, & Palfrey, 1998). There continues to be a disparity, however, in the inclusion of racial and ethnic minorities and adequate sampling in comprehensive research studies.

Coker, Austin, and Schuster (2010) chronicled the lack of recent comprehensive data for LGBT youth, noting a lack of national studies with identifying markers for sexuality, lack of standardized data sets, stigmatization of identification, lack of certain measures of degree of sexual identity, and lack of inclusion of transgender youth. As a result, the IOM report further recommended collection of sexual orientation and gender identity data on federally funded surveys concerned with health and social and economic conditions (IOM, 2011). Additionally, it encourages the National Institutes of Health to support development and standardization of sexual orientation and gender identity measures, encouraging grant applicants to address inclusion and exclusion of LGBT populations in their research samples.

Increased data would help inform clinical care and specifically help construct health behavior models better applied to LGBT youth that may better explain behaviors such as sexual activity and risk taking. For example, there is a growing body of literature exploring health risk behavior into STI rates and condom usage (Brown et al., 2008) and the impact of social media on sexual development, interpersonal violence, and early initiation behaviors. Improvements in research and data will help clinicians better understand the health concerns facing the adolescent LGBT population. They may also better equip health care providers to serve as conduits for obtaining vital health information and identifying potential research participants.

HEALTH ISSUES AND CONCERNS

Adolescents are typically healthier than older age groups. As mentioned, adolescents are most affected by unintentional injuries and behavior-related health concerns such as smoking, obesity, and drug use. LGBT adolescents share these concerns but also are disproportionately affected by a number of other health conditions. According to the 2015 CDC Youth Risk Behavior Survey (YRBS) data across 25 states and 19 large urban districts, LGB students had higher prevalence rates for risk in behaviors that contribute to violence, tobacco use, alcohol use, drug use, weight management, sexual behaviors, and behaviors related to attempted suicide. There were no significant differences in risks associated with behaviors that contributed to unintentional injuries, dietary behavior, and physical activity. LGBT youth have consistently also identified as highest ranked regarding health concerns like depression, risky sexual behavior, and harassment as well as general health prevention and nutrition (CDC, 2015).

Violence/Bullying

Bullying and interpersonal violence against LGBT adolescents is not a new phenomenon but has received significantly more attention over the past several years due to a number of high-profile suicides and violent episodes. Evidence of bullying directed at gay and lesbian adolescents was first reported by Pilkington and D'Augelli (1995); 83 percent of youth sampled had experienced some form of harassment and victimization. Over a decade later, 81 percent of LGB youth reported having been verbally abused, 15 percent had been physically assaulted, 38 percent had been threatened with physical violence, 16 percent were victims of sexual assault, and 6 percent had been assaulted with a weapon (D'Augelli, 2002; Espelage & Swearer, 2008).

Emerging data suggests that schools are a frequent site of bullying and victimization of LGBT youth. The 2011 National School Climate Survey conducted by the Gay, Lesbian and Straight Education Network (GLSEN) reported that out of over 8,500 teens surveyed, 8 out of 10 LGBT students experienced harassment at school in the past year because of their sexual orientation, and three-fifths felt unsafe at school because of their sexual orientation (GLSEN, 2012). Thirty-three percent of all adolescents reported that they had witnessed others frequently harassed because of their perceived or actual sexual orientation, and 52 percent reported hearing homophobic remarks. Among LGBT high school students, 86 percent reported experienced verbal harassment, 76 percent were often called derogatory terms like "faggot" or "dyke," and 64.3 percent reported feeling unsafe at school. Sexual minority youth, as a result of this harassment, reported that they had also missed school more often than their heterosexual peers because they felt unsafe (CDC, 2015).

Persistent exposure to bullying can potentially lead to a host of negative health outcomes. As a result of bullying, some LGBT youth may develop anxiety and depression, decreased self-esteem, and engage in otherwise risky behaviors such as smoking, underage alcohol use, and unprotected sex. LGBT bullying victims are two to three times more likely to commit suicide than their heterosexual peers and more likely to experience suicidal ideation. Additionally, these adolescents are three times more likely to drop out of school and skip school due to safety concerns (CDC, 2016a).

There is little information about transgender youth in the context of victimization, as evidenced by the lack of inclusion in surveys such as the YRBS, which, to date, lack a survey item measuring anything other than a binary (e.g., male or female) gender identity. Like LGB youth, though, empirical studies suggest that transgender youth are at increased risk of victimization and harassment. The first study in 1997 by Wilchins was the first to examine transgender violence, finding that 78 percent had been verbally harassed and 48 percent were victims of assault. Most recent statistics, published by GLSEN (2003), are consistent, as 55 percent of transgender respondents had been attacked, 74 percent had been harassed, and 90 percent felt unsafe at school due to their identity expression. Literature also suggests that transgender male-to-female are at increased risk of HIV and other sexually transmitted infections. Consistent with other LGB youth, over 33 percent of transgender youth have attempted suicide (Clements-Nolle, Marx, & Katz, 2006).

Smoking

Forty percent of adolescent smokers in a National Youth Advisory Committee study were self-described LGBT (Mulye et al., 2009). Closer inspection reveals that smoking in this cohort is heavily tied to social settings such as bars and clubs, with 20 percent of respondents self-reporting as social smokers. Initial studies such as the National Longitudinal Study on Adolescent Health suggested no statistical significance between LGBT adolescence and smoking rates, but more recently, studies suggest that smoking is disproportionately high here, as 40 percent of adolescents in one sample were LGBT. Interestingly, 50 percent of these adolescents thought that LGBT youth smoked at comparable or higher rates than their heterosexual peers (Marshall et al., 2008; CDC, 2015).

Alcohol

The national alcohol survey showed greater alcohol dependence among LGBT, specifically women, and underscored the need for inclusion of sexuality as a subpopulation for observation. A meta-analysis of 18 previous studies showed higher rates of substance abuse, including of alcohol, tobacco, marijuana, and illicit drugs (e.g., cocaine, methamphetamines, and IV drugs) among LGB youth. Overall, LGB youth were 190 percent more likely to use and abuse an illicit substance. Within this group, bisexual youth and lesbians (340 and 400 percent respectively) had much higher rates of alcohol usage (Coker et al., 2010). Bisexual youth, additionally, had an illicit drug rate consistently higher than other sexual minority peers.

Sexual Health and STIs

Sexually transmitted infections (STIs) remain a concern for all adolescents as rates of diseases, such as chlamydia, gonorrhea, syphilis, and HIV have increased in the past decade (CDC, 2016a).

- In 2016, there were 1,008,403 cases of chlamydia among youth ages 15 to 24, representing 63.1 percent of all reported cases; this represented a 4 percent and 1.9 percent increase from the previous year for those ages 15 to 19 and 20 to 24, respectively. Young women (15 to 19 years old) represented the most impacted group;

- Gonorrhea cases increased during 2015 to 2016: 11.3 percent for persons age 15 to 19 and 10.9 percent for those age 20 to 24; the rate for women 15 to 24 was 540.8 cases per 100,000 females, and among men aged 15 to 24, the rate was 455.3 cases per 100,000 males;

- Primary and secondary syphilis rates increased 13 percent among persons aged 15 to 19 and 8.1 percent among persons 20 to 24 between 2015 and 2016.

There are no specific large-scale data sets that distinguish the above STI rates by sexual identity, as there is scant literature on the incidence or prevalence of STIs other than HIV among this population.

With regard to HIV, young persons (ages 13 to 24) accounted for more than one in five new HIV infections while composing only approximately 21 percent of the total U.S. population.; 81 percent of the new diagnoses among youth occurred among gay and bisexual males (CDC, 2015). Black youth, in particular, accounted for 55 percent of new HIV infections in young persons in 2015. Sexual minority youth, especially men who have sex with men (MSM) of color, are at a disproportionately higher risk for HIV (MSM is used to describe all men who have sex with men, including those who may not identify as gay). Among adolescent males 13 to 19 years old, 91 percent of HIV infections were due to male-to-male sexual contact. The rate of new infections for adolescent MSM increased 48 percent from 2006 to 2009; this cohort represented 27 percent of all new infections and 69 percent of new infections for young persons (ages 13 to 29). African American (14 percent) and Latino (6.9 percent) males are four and two times more likely than white males to be infected (CDC, 2012), accounting for 63 percent of all HIV infections for 13- to 24-year-olds.

These disparities continue in spite of aggressive outreach efforts to increase testing in these populations. Research to address these disparities has focused on a number of potential causes: lack of condom use and/or decreased condom knowledge, differences in social/partner networks, number of partners, and sociocultural barriers such as racism, homophobia, poverty, and homelessness (Millett et al., 2012). Sadly, despite being a well-known high-risk group for the acquisition of HIV, there has been very limited attention paid to intervention development in this area targeting YMSM.

One promising intervention to prevent HIV transmission in young persons is pre-exposure prophylaxis (PrEP). PrEP, if taken daily, has been shown to reduce the risk of HIV acquisition by over 92 percent (CDC, 2018). As of May 2018, the FDA expanded the indication for PrEP to include adolescents ages 15–17, which creates legal (e.g., consent for treatment), behavioral (e.g., ability to take a daily pill), and financial (e.g., ability to afford medications with and without insurance coverage) challenges for dissemination to adolescents. In spite of the clinical promise of PrEP, uptake in adolescents and young adults, particularly black and Latino MSM, has not matched the disproportionate incidence of HIV in these two groups.

Eating Disorders and Weight Management

There has been significant attention on childhood obesity rates overall, given the increasing prevalence of obesity nationwide, but little specific data on obesity on LGBT youth. Austin et al. utilized the Growing Up Today Study (1998–2005) to show that heterosexual adolescent males had a steeper increase in BMI from early to late adolescence than their nonheterosexual peers. The same study, though, found that LGBT female adolescents had elevated BMI compared to their peers (Austin et al., 2009).

There are a limited number of studies examining eating disorders in this demographic group. These studies, often done with large data sets, have shown that LGBT adolescents have higher rates of body dissatisfaction, dieting, and binge eating. The above-mentioned Growing Up Today Study (1998–2005) found that self-described LGBT adolescents demonstrate higher rates of binge eating than their heterosexual peers, and all subgroups with the exception of lesbians had higher rates of purging (vomiting and/or using laxatives to control weight) throughout adolescence (Austin et al., 2009; IOM, 2012). Limited data suggests that transgender youth face increased body dissatisfaction and eating disorders. A recent study at the Washington State University found that 40 of 65 respondents were dissatisfied with their bodies and 17 percent had reported previously having an eating disorder.

Homelessness

LGBT youth often experience homelessness, most commonly as a result of familial conflict and lack of social support after coming out. This is compounded by a national shortage of youth housing programs and shelter policies requiring separation by birth sex (Durso & Gates, 2012). As early as 1999, data showed a disproportionately high percentage of LGBT youth as homeless. According to the National Coalition for the Homeless, between 20 and 40 percent of the 1.6 million homeless youth in the United States are LGBT. Homeless LGBT adolescents are at increased risk of victimization, substance abuse, unsafe sexual practices, and mental illness in comparison to heterosexual homeless youth. Additionally, they are over 7 times more likely to be sexually assaulted and to commit suicide (62 percent) than het-erosexual homeless youth (National Coalition for the Homeless, 2009).

Mental Illness

Limited studies have revealed a possible relationship between sexual identity and onset of mood and anxiety disorders, including major depression, generalized anxiety disorder, and conduct disorder (Fergusson, Horwood, & Beautrias, 1999). It is important to note, however, that these studies have not been based on formal diagnoses but instead on symptom and distress scales (Mustanski, Garofalo, & Emerson, 2010; IOM, 2011).

A collection of recent studies in this area have consistently shown an increased risk for suicidal ideation and attempts, even when controlling for depression and substance use (Almeida, Johnson, Corliss, Molnar, & Azrael, 2009; Birkett, Espelage, & Koenig, 2009; Bontempo & D'Augelli, 2002; Garofalo, Wolf, Wissow, Woods, & Goodman, 1999; IOM, 2011; Jiang, Perry, & Hesser, 2010; Russell & Joyner, 2001; Saewyc et al., 2007). The overall data was consistent across race, age, gender, and sexual identity (IOM, 2011). Several generic risk factors have been identified as possible explanations for this increased risk among LGBT youth, including inadequate social support, substance use, depression, not feeling safe at school, early initiation of sexual activity (D'Augelli et al., 2005), and cigarette smoking (IOM, 2011). LGBT youth are also at increased risk of victimization and homophobia, both of which have been linked to suicidal behavior.

Family response to sexual orientation and parental support have also been found to play a significant role in suicidality. Research has shown a negative correlation between parental response and mental and physical health of LGBT adolescents, regardless of the level of severity. Ryan et al. found significantly higher rates of mental and physical health problems among LGBT young adults who experienced high levels of rejection from their parents while they were adolescents. LGBT youth who experienced higher levels of rejection compared to those who experienced very were nearly six times as likely to have high levels of depression, more than eight times as likely to have attempted suicide, more than three times as likely to use illegal drugs, and more than three times as likely to engage in unprotected sexual behaviors that put them at increased risk for HIV and other sexually transmitted infections (2009).

Less data has been collected to reflect the mental health risks of transgendered youth. Several small convenience studies have suggested that transgender youth are at increased risk for depression and suicide. A study of 515 transgender youth conducted by Clements-Nolle et al. found that 47 percent of respondents had previously attempted suicide. These findings were similar to another study by Grossman and D'Augelli (2007) in which 45 percent of adolescents in sample had considered suicide and 26 percent reported an attempt. Nuttbrock and colleagues (2010) also found stronger associations of depression and suicidality with younger participants in their sample.

PROVIDER RELATIONSHIP

Creating an environment that LGBT adolescents deem to be user-friendly and welcoming is the first step in overcoming barriers to care. In 2009, Philadelphia ninth graders were asked about what qualities they most desired in their health care provider (Hoffman, Freeman, & Swann, 2009). They found that providers' interpersonal skills were the most important quality; additionally, they listed qualities such as provider comfort, experience, and knowledge and attitude about LGBT youth. Provider gender and sexual orientation were rated lowest in importance (Ginsburg et al., 2002). Consistent with this previous research by Ginsburg, LGBT youth shared concerns with non-LGBT youth, such as about insurance, accessibility in making appointments, and provider experience. LGBT youth ranked their highest health concerns as depression, risky sexual behavior, and harassment as well as general health prevention and nutrition. Young LGBT women ranked mental health services as more important than did their male counterparts. African American students rated youth-only centers and ability to discuss sexual behavior, family problems, and career goals as most important.

One of the most intriguing aspects of treating adolescent patients is the balance of autonomy and confidentiality. Adequate measures must be taken to establish rapport with patients and to establish an open communicative environment. This is vital for addressing potential patient concerns about disclosure of sexual identity or reporting concerns about home life and fear of parental or guardian retribution. It is imperative to conduct a thorough examination and history without parents in the room, although a provider may start off the clinical encounter with both the patient and parent present to go over things like history of medical allergies or pertinent past medical history. Additionally, youth may take other cues about openness and comfort by witnessing LGBT-friendly literature or resources for patients to read.

Communication is also crucial with this population. Providers must establish an open, confident environment that extends to all staff in the clinical setting. Similar to working with other adolescent demographic groups, providers must avoid medical jargon and use whenever possible culturally appropriate language when addressing patients as well as when explaining medical procedures, as patients may then have more autonomy in making their own treatment decisions. Culturally competent communication extends to understanding the impact of emerging social media (e.g., Facebook, Twitter) on patients and how they respond to treatment decisions. The Internet can serve as a powerful social networking tool among youth, especially those who have little familial and environmental support. The Internet can provide a vehicle to connect to communities that have been traditionally difficult to engage and provide public-health-related information (Garofalo, 2007). Conversely, the Internet provides opportunities to facilitate anonymous and high-risk sexual encounters.

While there are specific areas of care and health concerns for LGBT youth as noted above, providers must also provide basic primary care, such as immunizations and nutrition, dental, vision, and family planning, plus general health education. A significant portion of the adolescent clinic visit should be dedicated to completing a home, education, activities, drugs, sex, suicidality, and safety (HEADS) exam that investigates the patient's home and school life and identify potential risks in behavior such as smoking, sexual activity, and victimization. Table 5.2 contains a list of sample questions that providers may use during an adolescent patient encounter.

Table 5.2   Sample Questions for Adolescent Patient Interview

I. Sexual Activity

- Do you have sex with men (boys), women (girls), or both?
- Some of my patients your age begin to find themselves attracted to other people. Have you ever been romantically or sexually attracted to men (boys), women (girls), or both?
- Have you ever dated or gone out with someone? Are you currently dating or in a relationship with a boy or a girl?
- There are many ways of being sexual or intimate with another person: kissing, hugging, or touching; or having oral sex, anal sex, or vaginal sex. Have you ever had any of these experiences? Which ones? Were they with boys, girls, or both?
- How do you protect yourself against sexually transmitted diseases and pregnancy?
- When you use condoms for anal (or vaginal) sex, do you use them 5%, 50%, 75%, or 100% of the time? Are there times that you don't use condoms when you are having sex?
- Do you have sex (oral, anal, or vaginal) with anyone other than your boyfriend or girlfriend? If so, how often are you using condoms in those situations?
- Has anyone ever pressured you or forced you into doing something sexually that you didn't want to do?

II. Sexual Identity and Disclosure

- What term (if any) do you prefer that I use to best describe your sexual orientation? For example, do you consider yourself gay, lesbian, bisexual, heterosexual (straight), or are you not sure?
- Have you ever talked to your parents, brothers or sisters, or any other adult besides me about this? Any of your friends? What did they say?
- Have you thought about disclosing your sexuality to your parents or friends? Are you concerned at all about their response or your safety?

(continued)

Table 5.2 (continued)

- Was "coming out" stressful? Or, do you get stressed out thinking about "coming out?"
- It is normal for young people to sometimes be confused about their feelings and experiences. Do you have any questions you'd like to ask me or things you would like to talk about?

III. Mental Health and Depression

- Over the past few weeks, have you ever felt down or depressed? Have you had less interest in doing things that you normally enjoy?
- Have you ever thought about hurting yourself? Have you ever actually tried to hurt yourself? What did you do? Tell me what happened.
- Have you ever been treated for depression or other psychological issues? Have you ever been in the hospital for these issues or for trying to hurt yourself?
- Who do you turn to when you are down, lonely, or need someone to talk to?
- Do you have a close friend or family member who is a good source of support?
- Have you ever thought about seeing a counselor or therapist? Do you think that might be helpful?

IV. Tobacco, Alcohol, and Other Substance Use

- Do you currently smoke cigarettes? How much and for how long? Have you ever tried quitting? Do you need or want help quitting?
- Do you drink alcohol? How often? Where do you get it, and whom do you drink with? How many drinks do you typically have? Do you ever get drunk?
- Have you ever used any other drugs, such as marijuana, cocaine, ecstasy, GHB, crystal meth, etc.? Which drugs do you currently use? How often?
- Do you think your alcohol or drug use is a problem? Would you like help in trying to quit?
- Do you have any questions about any drugs or drug use that I might be able to answer?
- Do you ever have sex while drunk or high? Have you ever done something sexually while high or drunk that you regretted or didn't really want to?
- Have you ever driven a car or motor vehicle while high or drunk? Have you ever gotten a ride from someone else who was high or drunk?

V. Safety and Violence

- How are things going at home or at school? Do you feel safe when you are at home? Do you feel safe in your neighborhood and at school?
- Has anyone ever picked on you? Can you tell me about it? Was this because you are LGBTQ?
- Who can you turn to for advice, support, or protection?

(Adapted from Garofalo & Church, 2007)

POLICY ISSUES AFFECTING LGBT ADOLESCENTS

LGBT adolescents are affected by number of policy and legal issues. Specific examples of issues unique to adolescents include constructing anti-bullying and victimization policies, school support for LGBT students, and gender identification. The challenge in constructing policies for youth is that they are not able to vote or to represent themselves independently and are reliant on others for financial support.

Anti-Bullying Policy

Given the increasing publicity about bullying, state and local lawmakers have enacted a series of laws to offer protection for victims of bullying. As it currently stands, every state has some form of anti-bullying policy or law, with 41 states having both a law and policy in place to curtail bullying. The range of provisions varies significantly from state to state. It is important to note that not all provide specific protections for sexual identity and gender orientation. There is currently no anti-bullying legislation at the federal level; however, if bullying is connected to sex, race, ethnicity, religious status, and disability status, Title IX and Title IV provisions may provide protection. These provisions do not prohibit discrimination based solely on sexual orientation (U.S. Department of Health and Human Services, 2012).

As previously stated, schools are the most common site of bullying targeting LGBTQ youth. Research has shown though that LGBTQ students report not getting support they need after reporting a bullying episode; in fact, four out of five LGBTQ adolescents do not know of a supportive adult in their school. This underscores the need for school systems to be involved in any anti-bullying efforts targeting youth.

Transgender Identity Policy

More children are expressing transgender identity and at earlier ages. As a result, families encounter a number of decisions, such as whether to proceed with hormone therapy to help with their child's transition and subsequently navigating an insurance system that has not fully addressed how to fund transgender health, and the legal process of identity reassignment. While there are currently no universal protocols for applying hormone therapies such as pubertal-delaying treatments and administration of exogenous hormones, a number of research centers, including the Children's Hospital of Los Angeles, Boston Children's Hospital, and the Ann & Robert H. Lurie Children's Hospital of Chicago, are developing multidisciplinary approaches to treating transgender children. These programs utilize teams of physicians from endocrinology, adolescent medicine, surgery, and urology as well as social workers and psychologists to provide support for families and refine clinical techniques to improve patient outcomes.

There are currently 18 states, the District of Columbia, and 160 municipalities that have laws prohibiting discrimination based on gender identity. The policies regarding identification change vary tremendously by state. All states require a letter of documentation from the individual's physician, including a physical and mental assessment. Additionally, a number of states require individuals to have successfully undergone gender reassignment surgery before identification change can be completed (Tobin, 2011).

SUMMARY

Many advances have been made socially, politically, and clinically to improve health care delivery to LGBT adolescents, as evidenced by the increasing number of youth who express their sexual and gender identities at earlier ages. It is important for providers to remember that LGBT adolescents face many of the same health issues and concerns that all adolescents face. However, providers must pay careful attention to this population given their increased risk of mental illness, substance use, bullying and victimization, and HIV. More research is needed on health behaviors and must be more inclusive of racial minorities and transgender youth. Improved research will allow for health interventions better tailored to the health needs of this population that will ultimately improve health outcomes of LGBT adolescents.

REFERENCES

Almeida, J. R., Johnson, M., Corliss, H. L., Molnar, B. E., & Azrael, D. (2009). Emotional distress among LGBT youth: The influence of perceived discrimination based on sexual orientation. *Journal of Youth and Adolescence, 38*(7), 1001–1014.

Austin, S. B., Ziyadeh, N., Corliss, H. L., Haines, J., Rockett, H. R., Wypij, D., & Field, A. E. (2009). Sexual orientation disparities in weight status in adolescence: Findings from a prospective study. *Obesity, 17*(9), 1776–1782.

Bird, J. D., Kuhns, L., & Garofalo, R. (2012). The impact of role models on health outcomes of lesbian, gay, bisexual, and transgender youth. *Journal of Adolescent Medicine, 50*(4), 353–357.

Birkett, M., Espelage, D. L., & Koenig, B. (2009). LGB and questioning students in schools: The moderating effects of homophobic bullying and school climate on negative outcomes. *Journal of Youth and Adolescence, 38*(7), 989–1000.

Bontempo, D. E., & D'Augelli, A. R. (2002). Effects of at-school victimization and sexual orientation on lesbian, gay, or bisexual youths' health risk behavior. *Journal of Adolescent Health, 30*(5), 364–374.

Brill, S., & Pepper, R. (2008). *The transgender child: A handbook for families and professionals.* San Francisco: Cleiss Press.

Brown, L. K., DiClemente, R., Crosby, R., Fernandez, M. I., Pugatch, D., Cohn, S., . . . Schlenger, W. E. (2008). Condom use among high-risk adolescents: Anticipation of partner disapproval and less pleasure associated with not using condoms. *Public Health Reports, 123*(5), 601–607.

Cass, V. (1979). Homosexual identity formation: A theoretical model. *Journal of Homosexuality, 4*(3), 219–235.

Centers for Disease Control and Prevention (CDC). (2015). *Youth risk behavior survey.* Retrieved from http://www.cdc.gov/HealthyYouth/yrbs/index.htm

Centers for Disease Control and Prevention (CDC). (2016a). *Adolescent and School Health.* Retrieved from http://www.cdc.gov/healthyyouth/

Centers for Disease Control and Prevention (CDC). (2016b). *Healthy people 2020.* Retrieved from http://www.cdc.gov/nchs/healthy_people.htm

Clements-Nolle, K., Marx, R., & Katz, M. (2006). Attempted suicide among transgender persons: The influence of gender-based discrimination and victimization. *Journal of Homosexuality, 51*(3), 53–69.

Coker, T., Austin, S. B., & Schuster, M. A. (2010). The health and health care of lesbian, gay, and bisexual adolescents. *Annual Review of Public Health, 31*(1), 457–477.

D'Augelli, A. R. (2002). Mental health problems among lesbian, gay, and bisexual youths ages 14 to 21. *Clinical Child Psychology and Psychiatry, 7*(3), 439–462.

D'Augelli, A. R., Grossman, A. H., Salter, N. P., Vasey, J. J., Starks, M. T., & Sinclair, K. O. (2005). Predicting the suicide attempts of lesbian, gay, and bisexual youth. *Suicide and Life-Threatening Behavior, 35*(6), 646–660.

Durso, L. E., & Gates, G. J. (2012). *Serving our youth: Findings from a national survey of service providers working with lesbian, gay, bisexual, and transgender youth who are homeless or at risk of becoming homeless.* Los Angeles: The Williams Institute with True Colors Fund and the Palette Fund.

Espelage, D. L., & Swearer, S. M. (2008). Current perspectives on linking school bullying research to effective prevention strategies. In T. W. Miller (Ed.), *School violence and primary prevention* (pp. 335–353). Secaucus, NJ: Springer Press.

Fergusson, D. M., Horwood, L. J., & Beautrais, A. L. (1999). Is sexual orientation related to mental health problems and suicidality in young people? *Archives of General Psychiatry, 56*(10), 876–880. doi:10.1001/archpsyc.56.10.876

Garofalo, R., & Church, S. (2007). Addressing LGBT youth in the clinical setting. In H. J. Makadon, K. H. Mayer, J. Potter, & H. Goldhammer (Eds.), *The Fenway Guide to LGBT Health* (pp. 75–99). Boston: American College of Physicians.

Garofalo, R., Herrick, A., Mustanski, B. S., & Donenberg, G. R. (2007). Tip of the iceberg: Young men who have sex with men, the internet, and HIV risk. *American Journal of Public Health, 97*(6), 1113–1117.

Garofalo, R., Wolf, R. C., Kessel, S., & Palfrey, J. (1998). The association between health risk behaviors and sexual orientation among a school-based sample of adolescents. *Pediatrics, 101*(5), 895–902.

Garofalo, R., Wolf, R. C., Wissow, L. S., Woods, E. R., & Goodman, E. (1999). Sexual orientation and risk of suicide attempts among a representative sample of youth. *Archives of Pediatrics and Adolescent Medicine, 153*(5), 487–493.

Gay, Lesbian, and Straight Education Network (GLSEN). (2012). *2011 National school climate survey.* Retrieved from http://www.glsen.org/cgi-bin/iowa /all/library/record/2897.html?state=research&type=research

Ginsburg, K. R., Winn, R. J., Rudy, B. J., Crawford, J., Zhao, H., & Schwarz, D. F. (2002). How to reach sexual minority youth in the health care setting: The teens offer guidance. *Journal of Adolescent Health, 31*(5), 407–416.

Grossman, A. H., & D'Augelli, A. R. (2007). Transgender youth and life-threatening behaviors. *Suicide and Life Threatening Behavior, 37*(5), 527–537.

Herdt, G. H., & Boxer, A. M. (1993). *Children of horizons: How gay and lesbian teens are leading a new way out of the closet.* Boston: Beacon Press.

Hoffman, N. D., Freeman, K., & Swann, S. (2009). Healthcare preferences for lesbian, gay, bisexual, transgender and questioning youth. *Journal of Adolescent Health, 45*(3), 222–229.

Human Rights Campaign (HRC). (2012). *Growing up LGBT in America.* Retrieved from http://www.hrc.org/files/assets/resources/Growing-Up-LGBT-in-America _Report.pdf

Institute of Medicine (IOM). (2011). *Lesbian, gay, bisexual and transgender health issues and research gaps and opportunities.* Washington, DC: IOM.

Jiang, Y. D., Perry, K., & Hesser, J. E. (2010). Adolescent suicide and health risk behaviors: Rhode Island's 2007 youth risk behavior survey. *American Journal of Preventative Medicine, 38*(5), 551–555.

Kaufman, J., & Johnson, C. (2004). Stigmatized individuals and the process of identity. *The Sociological Quarterly, 45*(4), 807–833.

Levine, S. B. (2009). Adolescent consent and confidentiality. *Pediatrics in Review, 30*(11), 457–458.

Marshall, M. P., Friedman, M. S., Stall, R., King, K. M., Miles, J., Gold, M. A., . . . Morse, J. Q. (2008). Sexual orientation and adolescent substance use: A meta-analysis and methodological review. *Addiction, 103*(4), 546–556.

Millett, G. (2012). Comparisons of disparities and risks of HIV infection in black and other men who have sex with men in Canada, UK, and USA: A meta-analysis. *The Lancet, 380*(9839), 341–348. doi:10.1016/S0140-6736(12)60899-X

Mulye, T. P., Park, M. J., Nelson, C. D., Adams, S. H., Irwin, C. E., & Brindis, C. (2009). Trends in adolescent and young adult health in the United States. *Journal of Adolescent Health, 45*(1), 8–24.

Mustanski, B. S., Garofalo, R., & Emerson, E. M. (2010). Mental health disorders, psychological distress, and suicidality in a diverse sample of lesbian, gay, bisexual, and transgender youths. *American Journal of Public Health, 100*(12), 2426–2432.

National Coalition for the Homeless. (2009). Retrieved from http://www.national homeless.org/factsheets/lgbtq.html

Nuttbrock, L., Hwahng, S., Bockting, W., Rosenblum, A., Mason, M., Macri, M., & Becker, J. (2010). Psychiatric impact of gender-related abuse across the life course of male-to-female transgender persons. *Journal of Sex Research, 47*(1), 12–23.

Pilkington, N. W., & D'Augelli, A. R. (2006). Victimization of lesbian, gay, and bisexual youth in community settings. *Journal of Community Psychology, 23*(1), 34–56.

Reis, B., & Saewyc, E. (1999). *Eighty-three thousand youth: Selected findings of eight population-based studies as they pertain to anti-gay harassment and the safety and well-being of sexual minority students.* Seattle: Safe Schools Coalition of Washington.

Russell, S. T., & Joyner, K. (2001). Adolescent sexual orientation and suicide risk: Evidence from a national study. *American Journal of Public Health, 91*(8), 1276–1281.

Ryan, C., Heubner, D., Diaz, R. M., & Sanchez, J. (2009). Family rejection as a predictor of negative health outcomes in white and latino lesbian, gay, and bisexual young adults. *Pediatrics, 123*(1), 346–352.

Saewyc, E. M., Bearinger, L. H., Heinz, P. A., Blum, R. W., & Resnick, M. (1998). Gender differences in health and risk behaviors among bisexual and homosexual adolescents. *Journal of Adolescent Health, 23*(2), 181–188.

Saewyc, E. M., Skay, C. L., Hynds, P., Pettingell, S., Bearinger, L. H., Resnick, M. D., & Reis, E. (2007). Suicidal ideation and attempts in North American school-based surveys: Are bisexual youth at increased risk? *Journal of LGBT Health Research, 3*(2), 25–36.

Tobin, H. J. (2011). Fair and accurate identification of transgender people. *LGBTQ Policy Journal at the Harvard Kennedy School.* Retrieved from http://isites.harvard.edu/icb/icb.do?keyword=k78405&pageid=icb.page414493

U.S. Department of Health and Human Services (HHS). (2012). *Stopbullying.gov.* Retrieved from http://www.stopbullying.gov/

Wilchins, R., Lombardi, E., Priesing, D., & Malouf, D. (1997) *The first national survey on transviolence.* New York: Gender Public Advocacy Coalition.

6

The Health of LGBT Elders

W. Christopher Skidmore, Mark J. Simone, Manuel A. Eskildsen,
David O. Staats, and Jonathan S. Appelbaum

Older adults who are lesbian, gay, bisexual, or transgender (LGBT) belong to vulnerable communities with specific health care needs. However, health care professionals often lack training in how to respond to those needs. This is partly due to lack of recognition by the health care professions, and society in general, of the growing numbers of LGBT older adults. Many of them have concealed their sexual orientation or variation in gender identity due to a lifetime of widespread exposure to stigma and discrimination, which makes them less visible in studies of older adults. Attitudes in the United States toward LGBT people are improving; however, LGBT older adults continue to be affected by a long history of stigma and mistreatment, which may have particular significance for their health status and health care needs.

Unfortunately, little research or education has focused on their health care needs or how they differ from their aging non-LGBT peers (Graham et al., 2011). In addition to typical aging-related concerns, they face unique and significant health and psychosocial issues. For example, LGBT people in general experience a variety of health disparities compared to non-LGBT peers, including higher rates of common and life-threatening physical and mental health conditions, and the effects of these conditions can persist as people age (American Geriatrics Society Ethics Committee, 2015; Daniel & Butkus, 2015; Fredriksen-Goldsen et al., 2011; Graham et al., 2011; U.S. Department of Health and Human Services, 2010). LGBT older adults are also more at risk of disconnection from family and discrimination by the services and facilities that are supposed to serve them, leaving them less able to rely on family and social services for support as their health declines.

This chapter describes the medical and psychosocial care needs of LGBT older adults, broadly those older than 65 years of age, to help readers better understand and support them. Next, we explore some unique challenges faced by LGBT older adults, including the coming-out experience, social and housing problems, and the specific health impacts of a lifetime of minority stress. Finally, we explore how discriminatory policies have affected their financial security, interactions with health care systems, and overall well-being. Of note is that we discuss lesbian, gay, bisexual, and transgender older adults together in many places to highlight their shared disparities and needs; however, each group also has distinct challenges and needs. We also remind readers that each individual is diverse on a variety of intersecting variables such as race and ethnicity, and health and resilience are the norm in LGBT people rather than the exception.

BACKGROUND

Demographics and Socioeconomic Status

Estimating the number of LGBT older adults is challenging due to differing labels and estimation methods and also underidentification and undercounting due to stigma. However, some sources estimate that there are between 1 and 3 million LGBT older adults in the United States, and by 2030, there will be an estimated 2 to 6 million (Cahill, South, & Spade, 2000; Services and Advocacy for Gay, Lesbian, Bisexual and Transgender Elders [SAGE], 2010). Analyses of U.S. Census data from 2000 found same-sex–headed households in 93 percent of all counties, with more than 1 in 10 same-sex couples including a partner over the age of 65 (Bradford & Mayer, 2008). Unfortunately, even fewer sources of reliable data exist for estimates of the number of transgender older adults.

Regarding other demographic variables, LGBT people in general appear to be as racially and economically diverse as the general population, though they may be more likely than non-LGBT peers to live in urban areas and be a part of an interracial couple if partnered (Gates, 2012). They are also more likely than non-LGBT peers to live alone, less likely to be living with a partner, and less likely to have children (American Society on Aging & MetLife Mature Market Institute, 2010; Rosenfeld, 1999). They may have strained relationships with family members and children due to a lack of acceptance or due to their attempts to conceal their sexual orientation or gender identity. The resulting lack of support can be especially problematic as they age, and they may need to rely more on informal or nonfamilial support networks, such as extensive groups of friends (Hash, 2006; Kean, 2006). These networks may be particularly crucial for LGBT older adults but can deteriorate as friends age or die, putting LGBT older adults at further risk.

Minority Stress, Sexual Stigma and Prejudice, and Their Effects

LGBT people exist in a world that has historically discriminated against them, often in violent ways. Minority stress theory (Meyer, 2003) argues that this creates a special kind of stress for LGBT people. Herek's (2009b) conceptual framework of sexual stigma and prejudice offers another lens through which to view these experiences. Minority stress and prejudice may be associated with a variety of physical and mental health concerns, including depression, suicide, substance abuse, unhealthy or risky coping behavior, lower life satisfaction, and lower self-esteem (D'Augelli & Grossman, 2001; Herek, 2009b; Meyer, 2003; Simone, Meyer, Eskildsen, & Appelbaum, 2015). Despite the risks, there are social and psychological benefits to being open about one's identity and key relationships, while concealment can damage emotional, psychological, and physical wellbeing. This may be particularly relevant for LGBT older adults for several reasons.

While all LGBT older adults in the United States have lived knowing about extreme stigma and prejudice, they may have had somewhat different experiences depending on whether they came of age before or after the Stonewall riots in 1969. These were demonstrations of protest against a police raid that targeted the Stonewall Inn in New York City. Many consider the demonstrators to have sparked the gay civil rights movement in the United States and the event as a watershed moment of history for many LGBT people. As a result, people began to confront societal views of homosexuality and variation in gender identity on a more public and broad scale beginning in the 1970s.

The pre-Stonewall generation lived most of their adult lives exposed to widespread discrimination against LGBT persons and without any organized supports or social movements. Their existence and behavior were criminalized by the government and pathologized by the medical community. For instance, it was not until 1962 that the first state decriminalized private, consensual homosexual acts, and it was not until 1973 that the American Psychiatric Association ceased designating homosexuality as a mental disorder. Until then, LGBT people could have been involuntarily hospitalized or "treated" against their will. This generation likely witnessed or experienced discrimination and abuse even in health care settings, with understandable long-term consequences for their trust in the medical profession and willingness to seek care (Simone et al., 2015).

In contrast, the post-Stonewall generation came of age during the 1960s, a time of social unrest and emerging social acceptance of LGBT people. It also participated in or benefited from the activism and advocacy of the gay civil rights movement and were likely impacted by the HIV/AIDS epidemic and activism in the 1980s. Thus, LGBT baby boomers may be more open, at least to some degree, about their sexual orientation or gender identity (Appelbaum, 2008; Fredriksen-Goldsen et al., 2011). These cohort differences should be considered when working with LGBT older adults of different ages, along with the general effects of minority stress and sexual stigma.

CHALLENGES FOR LGBT ELDERS

Concealment Versus "Coming Out"

For LGBT older adults of different ages, their year of birth in relation to the Stonewall Riots may define somewhat different coming-out trajectories and levels of comfort (see Figure 6.1).

The more that individuals experienced minority stress and negative treatment as younger adults, the less likely they are to be out of the closet. Thus, the greater institutionalized discrimination faced by the pre-Stonewall generation prevented many from coming out. In contrast, the post-Stonewall generation has lived in a time influenced by the gay civil rights movement and may be more likely to be out (Rawls, 2004; Simone et al., 2015), though they also may have personally experienced more discrimination and abuse due to being more out and visible (D'Augelli & Grossman, 2001). They also may rightly fear having to go back into the closet if they ever need long-term care in an assisted living facility or nursing home.

These cohort effects can impact patients' disclosure of sexual orientation or variation in gender identity to their health care providers, which in

					1969: Stonewall Riots				
Decade of Birth									
20	30	40	50	60	70	80	90	00	10
Age in 2020									
100	90	80	70	60	50	40	30	20	10

Figure 6.1 Decade of Birth and Respective Age in the Year 2020

turn can affect their health (SAGE, 2010). For example, concealing identity and behavior from a provider may prevent a patient from receiving appropriate targeted health care and may be associated with health disparities. Despite this, surviving and living as part of a stigmatized minority group necessitates many resiliencies in LGBT people (Meyer, 2003). As such, all LGBT older adults should also be viewed as hearty survivors.

Medical schools have lagged behind in preparing providers to understand unique issues for LGBT older adults. In fact, most medical schools provide little to no education on LGBT issues, with the quality and content being highly variable in those that do (Makadon, 2006; Obedin-Maliver et al., 2011). However, some educators, administrators, and health care systems are leading the way in curriculum and policy development to teach and empower providers to better care for LGBT older adults. The American Medical Student Association, the Association of American Medical Colleges' MedEd Portal, the Department of Veterans Affairs, and the Human Rights Campaign's Healthcare Equality Index all work to advance or track these achievements.

Social Support and Family Structure

Social supports and family structure are key areas in which LGBT older adults may face struggles. Many LGBT persons are caregivers for friends, parents, partners/spouses, children, and sometimes grandchildren. For example, more gay men may be more likely to be caregivers than heterosexual men (MetLife Mature Market Institute, Lesbian and Gay Aging Issues Network of the American Society on Aging, & Zogby International, 2006). However, when LGBT older adults need their own care, many of them will lack adequate support. Partners, spouses, or children who are accepting may provide support for some, but LGBT older adults who are not partnered must look to a network of close friends or "families of choice" for support. For example, the lack of traditional marriage benefits for LGBT people created a grassroots movement in some areas to develop communal housing among groups of friends, especially among lesbians (King, 2007). Not all LGBT older adults have access to the support they need, however, and they also may be at risk for neglect or physical, verbal, emotional, and financial abuse by caregivers. Thus, health care providers should place special emphasis on assessing LGBT older adults' access to appropriate support and vulnerability to abuse.

Housing, Home Care, and Long-Term Care

LGBT older adults have unique and justified concerns about housing and long-term care. As a general rule, antidiscrimination laws in housing do not extend to LGBT people. In addition, assisted living facilities may discriminate against or lack protections for LGBT older adults. By 2030, there will be an estimated 120,000 to 300,000 LGBT older adults living in nursing homes (Cohen, Curry, Jenkins, Walker, & Hogstel, 2008). For them and others, entering a long-term care facility is a vulnerable and potentially dangerous time. They rightly may anticipate discrimination and abuse from staff and other residents or at least lack confidence that they will be treated with dignity and respect, allowed to be out, or allowed to dress according to their gender identity (Cohen et al., 2008; Henning-Smith, Gonzales, & Shippee, 2015; Porter et al., 2016). One study found that 73 percent of lesbian and gay adults expected discrimination in retirement settings, 60 percent believed they would not have equal access to social and health services, and 34 percent believed they would have to hide their orientation upon entry into a retirement facility (Johnson, Jackson, Arnette, & Koffman, 2005).

Home care agencies and long-term care facilities are making much-needed strides along with other health care facilities in becoming more inclusive and respectful of LGBT people. Groups such as the LGBT Aging Project and the Fenway Institute in Massachusetts and the Center of Excellence for Transgender Health offer training and guidance in these areas. Institutional discrimination and negative attitudes also are increasingly recognized by regulatory and accrediting bodies as harmful, and they can and should be cited as such. In addition, large urban areas offer naturally occurring retirement centers in LGBT communities, which can be infused with supports and resources for LGBT older adults.

Provider-Related Barriers to Care

Due to the social and historical factors described above, LGBT older adults face barriers to accessing health care and social services, including those created by providers and health care systems. Actual or perceived negative attitudes among care providers can be a significant concern, which may be part of the reason that many LGBT patients do not feel comfortable coming out to their health care providers (Lambda Legal, 2014; Simone et al., 2015). Their often-well-founded fears about prejudice in providers and instructions, combined with actual deficits in providers' cultural competence, add to barriers to care (Lambda Legal, 2014; Makadon, 2006; Portz et al., 2014). This can then lead to delays in care, inappropriate care, and worsening mental health concerns (Brotman, Ryan, & Cormier, 2003; Simone et al., 2015).

Medical education has not kept pace with the need to teach specialized assessment and communication strategies in either geriatric medicine or the care of LGBT patients, so many health care providers are still not comfortable with treating younger or older LGBT patients (Henry J. Kaiser Family Foundation, 2002; Honigberg et al., 2017). They may also communicate inadvertently or intentionally that they are unaware of, or even hostile toward, the needs of LGBT older adults. LGBT older adults need culturally competent health care providers who can help them to feel comfortable. Providers should ask older patients about their sexual health, including their sexual behavior and orientation and their gender identity. However, they should also recognize that many LGBT older adults are still unwilling or unable to disclose, even if asked directly (Simone et al., 2015). Regardless, providers' ability to show awareness of and sensitivity to these topics can lead to improved care relationships and better access to targeted health care and information for patients.

Efforts to create a welcoming environment both within and outside of the exam room also help. These include simple but powerful changes to communicate respect and inclusion such as gender- or LGBT-inclusive intake forms, LGBT-affirming health literature in exam and waiting rooms, or unisex bathrooms (Gay and Lesbian Medical Association, 2018a). Social service organizations for older people are among those that have taken the lead in this area. The Gay and Lesbian Medical Association (GLMA) also works tirelessly to advance equality and competency in LGBT health care nationally and has resources for both patients and providers on its Web site. These include comprehensive guidelines for the care of LGBT patients and lists of top ten health care issues for LGBT patients to discuss with providers (GLMA, 2018b, 2018c). Many other organizations and professionals have also published training- and care-related guidelines that should be reviewed (Boroughs, Bedoya, O'Cleirigh, & Safren, 2015; Deutsch, 2016; Hollenbach, Eckstrand, & Dreger, 2014; Kauth & Shipherd, 2018; Wylie, et al., 2016).

Health Disparities

Health disparities are increasingly recognized as significant challenges for LGBT people (Daniel & Butkus, 2015; Graham et al., 2011). In 2010, the U.S. Department of Health and Human Services designated LGBT people as one of six groups affected by health disparities and included sexual orientation in 29 of its objectives related to eliminating disparities (Sell & Becker, 2001; U.S. Department of Health & Human Services, 2000). Its plan for 2020 continues to prioritize LGBT health disparities associated with high rates of psychiatric disorders, substance abuse, and suicide, which may be linked to widespread societal stigma, discrimination, and minority stress (Fredriksen-Goldsen et al., 2011; Haas et al., 2010; Herek,

2009b; Hoy-Ellis & Fredriksen-Goldsen, 2016; Simone & Appelbaum, 2011; Zelle & Arms, 2015). LGBT people also suffer from disparities in rates of impoverishment and access to health care (Fredriksen-Goldsen et al., 2011; Zelle & Arms, 2015). Finally, there are long-lasting effects from direct and indirect experiences of violence and victimization and struggles with personal, familial, and social acceptance.

Much less attention has been devoted to these disparities in LGBT older adults specifically, and this is especially true for transgender older adults (Graham et al., 2011). In addition to stigma and lack of attention to the health status of LGBT people in general, differences in how people self-identify make data collection and analysis more challenging. However, some evidence suggests that older gay and bisexual men experience more depression than heterosexual peers, while older lesbian and bisexual women may struggle more with increased physical disability and functional limitations (Gonzales & Henning-Smith, 2015).

Some investigators and groups are slowly reducing deficits in data about LGBT older adults with focused research and advocacy. For older transgender people in particular, the Transgender Aging Network (TAN) at FORGE has encouraged efforts to collect data about their health care needs. Notably, the number one health care–related disparity is exposure to violence, which will be discussed in a later section of this chapter. The TAN Web site includes a self-help guide and resource for accessing treatment for transgender people and tips for their caregivers (http://forge -forward.org/aging/). These efforts and others like them will hopefully lead to reductions in LGBT health disparities, improved health, and greater inclusion in health care settings.

SPECIFIC HEALTH CARE NEEDS FOR LGBT OLDER ADULTS

Most LGBT older adults report good health and health-related behaviors, an important reminder about their health and resilience (Fredriksen-Goldsen et al., 2011). As they age, they can suffer from the usual geriatric syndromes, including incontinence, falls, and cognitive impairment, and they need the same health promotion and maintenance in these areas as non-LGBT people. LGBT older adults also face unique health challenges that require special attention. For example, they may be more susceptible to some physical health problems due to long-term concealment of their identity and a lifetime of exposure to minority stress (e.g., Fredriksen-Goldsen et al., 2011; Graham et al., 2011). People also tend to assume incorrectly that older adults do not have sex or use substances simply because they are elderly or may avoid asking about these areas due to their own discomfort. However, taking a history of sexual practices, identity, and substance use, and providing risk reduction counseling when indicated, remains a critical aspect of good health care for LGBT older adults (Simone & Appelbaum, 2011). The following sections describe specific issues for lesbian and bisexual women, gay and bisexual men, and transgender women and men separately to highlight each group's unique needs.

Health Care Needs for Older Lesbian and Bisexual Women

Lesbian and bisexual women appear to receive less preventive care and screening, access health care services less often, and enter the health care system later than heterosexual women (Appelbaum, 2008; Valanis et al., 2000). This appears to be associated with stigma-related concerns and may result in poorer physical health status (Fredriksen-Goldsen, Kim, Shui, & Bryan, 2017; Valanis et al., 2000).

Women of childbearing age tend to be asked about contraception and counseled about the use of male barrier protection without consideration for their actual sexual practices. In contrast, older women may not be asked or counseled at all due to assumptions that they are both heterosexual and sexually inactive. This can result in failures to inquire about sexual orientation and behavior, to screen for issues such as cervical cancer, domestic abuse, and sexually transmitted infections (STIs), or to provide the preventive care necessary for optimal health (Valanis et al., 2000). Health care providers can thus promote better care in all of their female patients by:

- Understanding that women, including older women, may be sexually active with men or women or both, regardless of sexual orientation;

- Remembering that sexual identity and behavior can and do change over time. A woman who currently has sex exclusively with women may have had sex with men in the past or may do so in the future, and;

- Realizing that many lesbian and bisexual women have children and grandchildren or desire or plan to in the future.

There are also other key needs providers should monitor to optimize the health of older lesbian and bisexual women:

- *Cardiovascular health and risk factors* should be a key focus of assessment and treatment (Fredriksen-Goldsen et al., 2011). Heart disease is the leading cause of death in older women in general, and lesbian and bisexual women may be at greater risk than heterosexual women due to higher rates of risk factors for cardiovascular disease such as cigarette smoking, obesity, or other effects of minority stress and stigma (Appelbaum, 2008; Fredriksen-Goldsen et al., 2011; Simone et al., 2015; Valanis et al., 2000).

- *Obesity* remains a major concern for many older women, particularly as a risk factor for cardiovascular disease (Fredriksen-Goldsen et al., 2011; Simone et al., 2015). Lesbian and bisexual women on average have a higher body mass index (BMI) than their straight counterparts, again likely due to risk factors, stigma, and stress (Valanis et al., 2000). With patients' permission, providers should offer nutritional and general health counseling in a manner that enhances motivation while respecting patient autonomy.

- *Cancers of certain types* appear to affect LGBT people at disproportionate rates, with breast cancer being the most commonly reported cancer affecting lesbian and bisexual women (Fredriksen-Goldsen et al., 2011; Quinn et al., 2015; Valanis et al., 2000). Lesbian and bisexual women who do not have regular mammograms may struggle with barriers to care, so this remains an important area for screening and intervention (Appelbaum, 2008; Simone et al., 2015; Lauver et al., 1999; Valanis et al., 2000). Cervical cancer screening is also important (Appelbaum, 2008).

- *Osteoporosis* is more common in older women than older men and appears to affect a substantial minority of lesbian and bisexual women (Fredriksen-Goldsen et al., 2011). General risk factors include age, estrogen deficiency, smoking, family background, sedentary lifestyle, and inadequate calcium and vitamin D intake. Some risk factors such as smoking may be more prevalent in lesbian and bisexual women. Screening, performing bone mineral density testing when indicated, offering nutritional counseling, and providing treatment to women who fit treatment criteria are crucial (Appelbaum, 2008).

- *Safer sex* is a concern given that lesbian and bisexual older women can develop the same STIs as heterosexual women. In addition, they have a higher incidence of bacterial vaginosis and can transmit this to their partners. Woman-to-woman transmission of HIV, however, is very rare. The preventative use of barriers (dental dams) is recommended for oral-vaginal and oral-anal contact (Appelbaum, 2008).

- *Mental health concerns and exposure to violence* put many lesbian and bisexual women at significant risk for a variety of health concerns. See a following section devoted to this topic for details.

Health Care Needs for Older Gay and Bisexual Men

In large part, gay and bisexual older men require the same screening and preventative care as their heterosexual peers (Appelbaum, 2008). Providers should also monitor the following specific issues when providing care to older gay and bisexual men:

- *STIs* are of concern for men of all ages, including older gay and bisexual men, and regular screening is recommended for at least some STIs (Appelbaum, 2008; GLMA, 2018c; Simone et al., 2015). Both patients and providers often avoid discussing sexual health issues including STIs, but it remains vital to assess and discuss sexual identity, function, and behavior.

  Gonorrhea, chlamydia, syphilis, hepatitis, herpes, human papillomavirus (HPV), and HIV can be sexually transmitted at any age, and many of these can also be transmitted through oral-anal sex. While the Centers for Disease Control and Prevention (CDC) currently recommend that HIV testing be a routine part of primary care for men younger than 65, it is important for sexually active men at any age to consider this test (Appelbaum, 2008; Branson et al., 2006). Depending on sexual practices, samples for gonorrhea and chlamydia screening may be obtained from anal, urethral, and pharyngeal sites; however, a nucleic-acid amplification test (NAAT) using a urine sample for both urethral gonorrhea and chlamydia may be considered (CDC, 2017a, 2017b). Because of a recent rise in incidence, testing for syphilis is also important (CDC, 2017c). Routine blood testing for antibodies to herpes is not advised, but culture of a suspected outbreak is (Appelbaum, 2008). Routine anal Pap smears every two to three years may be indicated, especially in men who have unprotected receptive anal intercourse or who have HIV, to screen for HPV and early signs of precancerous cells caused by certain strains (Appelbaum, 2008). Some specialists recommend the use of high-resolution anoscopy as superior for screening for anal HPV infection (Benson, Kaplan, Masur, Pau, & Holmes, 2004; Park & Palefsky, 2010). Transmission of anal cancer–producing HPV can be prevented by one of several HPV vaccinations, though this is typically recommended for young men. Older gay and bisexual men should also be vaccinated against hepatitis B. In terms of preventative care, condoms should be used for oral-anal, oral-genital, and genital-anal sex.

- *Erectile dysfunction and/or low sexual desire* typically increase in frequency as men age, and there is some evidence of decreases in blood levels of testosterone and decreased sexual desire in older men. Testosterone replacement may sometimes be a treatment option, as are PDE5 inhibitors, although there are medical risks associated with both. PDE5 inhibitors can interact with other medications such as alpha-blockers used for hypertension and prostate enlargement, nitrates used for heart disease, or protease inhibitors used to treat HIV (Appelbaum, 2008). A full medical evaluation should be completed, including screens for diabetes, thyroid disease, and vascular disease, as well as anxiety and depressive disorders. A prostate exam and PSA level should also be part of an evaluation before testosterone replacement therapy, and regular monitoring should be done during testosterone replacement treatment due to risks of cardiovascular disease (Appelbaum, 2008).

- *Cardiovascular health and risk factors* are also important to monitor (Fredriksen-Goldsen et al., 2011). Heart disease remains the leading cause of death in older men in general, and gay and bisexual men are more likely to smoke cigarettes, a major risk factor for cardiovascular disease including stroke and heart attacks (Appelbaum, 2008; Simone et al., 2015). Smoking cessation should be a major treatment goal, and there are many options—such as smoking cessation programs, nicotine replacement therapies, nicotine-containing vapors, medications such as bupropion (Zyban) and varenicline (Chantix), psychotherapy, and alternative approaches using acupuncture (Appelbaum, 2008). Besides smoking, other cardiovascular risk factors such as control of blood pressure, cholesterol, and diabetes should be addressed. Encouraging a healthy body weight, a healthy amount of aerobic exercise, and a daily aspirin dose if indicated may be helpful (Appelbaum, 2008).

- *Cancer* is the second leading cause of death in older men, and certain types may affect gay and bisexual men at disproportionate rates compared to heterosexual peers. These include: anal cancer associated with HPV infection; lung cancer; colorectal cancer; endometrial and lung cancers; liver cancer associated with increased risks of hepatitis B and C infections; and prostate cancer (Appelbaum, 2008; Quinn et al., 2015; Simone et al., 2015). This should be a priority for screening and treatment among older gay and bisexual men.

- *Prostate health* is a key concern for older men, and gay and bisexual men are no exception (Quinn et al., 2015; Simone et al., 2015). Discussions concerning the merits of prostate cancer screening should begin at age 50, and earlier in those at higher risk—such as African Americans and those with a family history of prostate cancer (Appelbaum, 2008; Simone et al., 2015). When considering treatment for prostate cancer, since the prostate gland can be involved in the sexual response during receptive anal intercourse, the effects of treatment options on sexual health should be discussed thoroughly (Appelbaum, 2008; Drescher & Perlman, 2005; Simone et al., 2015).

- *Other aspects of anal health* are important to discuss with men who engage in receptive anal intercourse. For gay and bisexual men who do, the anus is also a sexual organ, and dysfunction or injury to it can cause pain and distress. Proctitis, which is an inflammation of the lower rectum, is more commonly associated with STIs such as chlamydia and gonorrhea; anal fissures and hemorrhoids are also common and are treated per usual recommendations, such as stool softeners, astringents, hydrocortisone creams, and suppositories (Appelbaum, 2008). Occasionally, these conditions require surgery.

• *Mental health concerns and exposure to violence* exacerbate health issues for many gay and bisexual men and are described in more detail in a following section.

Health Care Needs for Older Transgender Women and Men

Transgender people are often marginalized by society and may have particularly significant barriers to care that impact their health. As they age, they may encounter diseases or conditions associated either with assigned birth sex or with gender-affirming treatments (Appelbaum, 2008; Gooren, 2011). They may have additional stress as they must cope with reminders of an assigned birth sex that did not fit their gender identity, or they may have inadequate or absent care if they have not come out to their providers (Appelbaum, 2008). Health screenings corresponding to assigned birth sex are thus important preventive care, but they must be conducted with substantial sensitivity (Brown & Jones, 2015; Simone & Appelbaum, 2011). Transgender women and men also may lack health insurance altogether or have insurance that does not cover transgender-specific health care needs such as gender-affirming treatments (Appelbaum, 2008; Deutsch, 2016; Torke & Carnahan, 2017). Thus, many transgender people must find ways to take hormones without a prescription and may lack access to preventive health care (Appelbaum, 2008; den Heijer, Bakker, & Gooren, 2017).

As an important reminder, transgender women and men also have distinct health needs from each other. In addition, even something as relatively straightforward (to providers) as a physical exam may be fraught with anxiety and stress for patients. There are several specific and distinct considerations and knowledge needs for physical exams of which providers should be aware (Deutsch, 2016).

Providers should also monitor several key health issues when providing care to transgender older adults:

• *Improper gender-affirming hormone use* may be a concern for some transgender women and men (Appelbaum, 2008). Either due to use of nonprescription hormones or due to insufficient provider training, many transgender people do not receive safe or proper doses. For example, they may be forced to buy gender-affirming hormones from unsafe sources without a prescription due to poverty, lack of health insurance that covers these medications, or lack of access to appropriate health care. Inquire about past or current improper dosing and consider appropriate dosing if medically indicated, a normal standard of care within the scope of practice of many providers (Deutsch, 2016). There are published articles and guidelines on appropriate dosing and gender-affirming surgeries that can guide clinical decision making (Asscheman, Giltay, Megens, van Trotsenburg, & Gooren, 2011; den Heijer et al., 2017; Deutsch, 2016).

- *Adverse effects from use of gender-affirming hormones and other medications* are a concern for many transgender women and men, though relative risks for specific conditions vary based on assigned birth sex and type, source, and extent of hormones used (Deutsch, 2016; Mahan, Bailey, Bibb, Fenney, & Williams, 2016; Wierckx et al., 2012). These include higher risks for factors related to cardiovascular disease with hormone use, venous thromboembolism in particular with estrogen, and liver toxicity and mood and libido changes in particular with testosterone (Appelbaum, 2008; den Heijer et al., 2017; Deutsch, 2016; Mahan et al., 2016; Simone et al., 2015; Wierckx et al., 2012). These may be even more problematic for transgender older adults, so providers should be aware of and actively monitor for a host of possible adverse effects.

- *Screening for osteoporosis* should be considered in transgender older adults because of potential adverse effects of estrogen and testosterone treatment in addition to normal age-related changes. The risk of osteoporosis with hormonal treatment varies depending on factors such as timing and specific regimens used (Deutsch, 2016; Mahan et al., 2016; Wierckx et al., 2012). Risk appears to be greater for transgender women than for transgender men; however, providers should encourage calcium and vitamin D supplementation and consider bone mineral density screening regardless of gender identity, potentially at earlier ages for people with other known risk factors and longer durations of gender-affirming treatments (Deutsch, 2016; Mahan et al., 2016).

- *Risk factors for cardiovascular disease such as smoking and obesity* should also be targeted (Appelbaum, 2008; Deutsch, 2016; Fredriksen-Goldsen et al., 2011; Simone et al., 2015). Evidence is mixed as to whether their risks for cardiovascular problems are higher than average for transgender women and men (Deutsch, 2016). However, for those at risk, primary prevention strategies are important, including encouragement of regular aerobic exercise, proper diet, and smoking cessation. Again, providers should offer counseling with patients' permission in a manner that enhances motivation while respecting their autonomy.

- *Cancer* risks should also be closely monitored, although relative risks for transgender women and men compared to birth-sex controls are not yet well documented (Deutsch, 2016; Fredriksen-Goldsen et al., 2011; Quinn et al., 2015). Cancers from use of gender-affirming hormones are rare, so screening should be conducted for cancers related to assigned birth sex and any organ that typically meets criteria for screening, regardless of hormone use (Deutsch, 2016). These include prostate exams and monitoring for breast and testicular cancer risks in older transgender women and breast and pelvic exams and Pap smears for transgender men, particularly those who have not completed gender-affirming surgeries (Appelbaum, 2008; Deutsch, 2016; Gooren, 2011; Mahan et al., 2016).

- *Sexual health and functioning* are important to the health and well-being of transgender older adults as they are for other people (Daskalakis, Radix, & Mayer, 2015; Sheffield & Keuroghlian, 2017). Effective assessment and discussion of their needs in this area requires substantial knowledge, sensitivity, and openness among providers, and providers should be the ones to invite discussions about these issues in appropriate clinical encounters (Sheffield & Keuroghlian, 2017).

- *HIV and other STIs* affect disproportionate numbers of transgender people due in part to behavioral risk factors and barriers to care (Appelbaum, 2008; Fredriksen-Goldsen et al., 2011). Transgender people who are also racial or ethnic minority group members may be at even higher risk (Appelbaum, 2008; Deutsch, 2016). Regular testing and monitoring of risk factors for infection are recommended, though providers should also take accurate sexual histories that include discussion of anatomy-specific sexual behavior (Deutsch, 2016). The next section discusses HIV screening and treatment in older adults in more detail.

- *Hepatitis* also affects transgender women and men. Increased prevalence of sharing needles (e.g., for "black market" hormones or silicone) due to poverty, decreased access to health care, and stigma plays a role, though the actual prevalence of this risk factor is still relatively low (Appelbaum, 2008; Deutsch, 2016). Regular screening and treatment are recommended in affected transgender older adults (Appelbaum, 2008).

- *Mental health concerns and exposure to violence* disproportionately affect transgender women and men and are discussed in more detail in a following section.

HIV in Older Adults

HIV is an often overlooked but significant health issue in older adults (Simone & Appelbaum, 2008). For example, about one-quarter of all those infected with HIV in the United States are over the age of 55, and more than half are over 50 (Bhavan, Kampalath, & Overton, 2008). The management and prognosis of HIV/AIDS has changed dramatically since the introduction of antiretroviral therapy (ART) in 1996, but unfortunately, many new infections continue to occur. In fact, over 18 percent of new HIV infections occur in people over the age of 50, with most of these occurring in adults between the ages of 50 and 54 (CDC, 2018). HIV screening and prevention are thus important in the care of LGBT older adults, particularly given then additional risk factors for infection described earlier.

The unexpectedly high numbers of older adults living with HIV result from several factors. Besides new infections, individuals living with HIV are living longer and aging into this demographic due to treatment advances (Bhavan et al., 2008; Simone & Appelbaum, 2008). In addition, older adults are often ignored or forgotten in prevention efforts, and many older people do not consider themselves at risk for infection (Simone & Appelbaum, 2008; Simone et al., 2015). Older adults in general use condoms or other safer-sex practices less frequently (Simone et al., 2015; Stall & Catania, 1994). Finally, health care providers often do not think of older adults as sexually active or otherwise at risk and therefore do not perform adequate HIV risk assessments or counseling with them. When appropriate to the clinical encounter, providers for LGBT older adults thus should take sensitive and thorough sexual histories and explain safer-sex practices (Simone et al., 2015).

Despite advances in detection and treatment, HIV infection still poses significant health risks for older adults (Simone & Appelbaum, 2008; Simone et al., 2015). HIV may be diagnosed later in older adults, who also may show a faster decline in immune functioning, more comorbid conditions, and increased mortality than younger people (Luther & Wilkin, 2007; Simone et al., 2015; Smith, Delpech, Brown, & Rice, 2010). HIV infection also may accentuate several aging-related comorbidities in older adults, including abnormal cholesterol (dyslipidemia), diabetes, reduced bone density (osteoporosis), kidney and liver diseases, psychiatric illness, neurocognitive impairment, and coronary artery disease (Bhavan et al., 2008; CDC, 2018). Finally, about one-third of AIDS-related deaths occur in older adults, and racial and ethnic minorities may be at even greater risk, particularly older black and Hispanic people (CDC, 2018). The additional health disparities and barriers to care faced by LGBT older adults likely increase risks and morbidity further.

Specific treatment issues for older adults living with HIV should also be considered. They have a higher risk of adverse events, more comorbidities, and a greater risk of toxicity and drug-drug interactions due to normal aging, other illnesses, and other medications; despite these concerns, they still appear to maintain better adherence to ART (Simone & Appelbaum, 2008).

Thus, age and the presence of other illnesses should not deter the use of ART. Several published treatment strategies or guidelines describe the optimal care of older adults living with HIV.

Mental Health and Exposure to Violence

Mental health concerns and exposure to violence affect many LGBT people and deserve special attention. Of note, studies of LGBT people in general find similar rates of most mental health disorders as in the general population, suggesting that they are as mentally healthy overall as non-LGBT people. Mental health concerns thus should not be assumed a priori to be associated with sexual orientation or gender identity (Deutsch, 2016). However, LGBT people may have higher rates of suicidality and depressive and anxiety disorders, which can persist as they age (D'Augelli, Grossman, Hershberger, & O'Connell, 2001; Dean et al., 2000; Fredriksen-Goldsen et al., 2013; Graham et al., 2011; Simone et al., 2015). The psychological burdens of exposure to discrimination and minority stress likely contribute to this (Dean et al., 2000; Graham et al., 2011). LGBT older adults, who have lived with minority stress and sexual stigma much longer, may be at even greater risk. In addition, mental health concerns such as adjustment disorders, depressive and anxiety disorders, and post-traumatic stress disorder may not be addressed effectively, particularly as they age (Dean et al., 2000; Simone et al., 2015).

LGBT people in general experience abuse, violence, and trauma at higher rates than non-LGBT people, with bisexual and transgender people possibly at greatest risk (D'Augelli & Grossman, 2001; Walters, Chen, & Breiding, 2013). Older adults in general also may be at relatively high risk for violence and abuse (Acierno et al., 2010). Thus, LGBT older adults are dually at risk. Violence and abuse can impact physical and mental health in significant ways and also affect patient-provider relationships and dynamics in the exam room. A review is beyond the scope of this chapter, but the Substance Abuse and Mental Health Services Administration (SAMHSA) guide to trauma-informed care provides an excellent foundation and approach for all providers and patients (SAMHSA, 2014).

Minority-specific hate crimes can severely affect physical and mental health, and many survivors choose not to report them due to fears of indifference or mistreatment by law enforcement and legal systems (Dean et al., 2000; Dunbar, 2006; Fredriksen-Goldsen et al., 2013; Herek, 2009a; Langenderfer-Magruder, Walls, Kattari, Whitfield, & Ramos, 2016). Perpetrators also target LGBT people at disproportionate rates for physical and sexual assault and abuse, beginning in childhood, which can result in lifelong struggles with recovery (Dean et al., 2000; Dunbar, 2006; Gold, Feinstein, Skidmore, & Marx, 2011; Langenderfer-Magruder et al., 2016;

Rothman, Exner, & Baughman, 2011; Schneeberger, Dietl, Muenzenmaier, Huber, & Lang, 2014). Transgender people in particular are at startlingly high risk for exposure to potentially traumatic events and violence (Shipherd, Maguen, Skidmore, & Abramovitz, 2011; Stotzer, 2009). LGBT people also experience greater lifetime rates of intimate partner violence (IPV) than non-LGBT people (Edwards, Sylaska, & Neal, 2015; Landers & Gilsanz, 2009). Factors that further heighten risk include racial/ethnic minority status and substance use (Edwards et al., 2015). Caregivers can also target LGBT older adults for harm, abuse, and neglect (Grossman et al., 2014). Screening and intervention for impacts of violence and abuse should thus be high priorities in the care of LGBT older adults, who have lived a lifetime facing these risks.

Some older LGBT women and men engage in risky coping behaviors such as substance use or unprotected or risky sex, which in turn can worsen their health (Dean et al., 2000; Fredriksen-Goldsen et al., 2011; Simone et al., 2015; Valanis et al., 2000). For example, lesbian and bisexual women may use alcohol and tobacco at higher rates than heterosexual peers, which affects cardiovascular health (Simone et al., 2015; Valanis et al., 2000). Gay and bisexual men who use methamphetamine or "crystal meth" or other "club drugs" are at increased risk for depression, mania, and psychosis, in addition to risky sex that can lead to STIs (Brennan-Ing, Porter, Seidel, & Karpiak, 2014; Dean et al., 2000; Fredriksen-Goldsen et al., 2011; Halkitis, Green, & Mourgues, 2005). HIV-positive men with substance use problems may be at risk for nonadherence with antiretroviral therapy (ART) protocols and transmission of HIV to their partners. Women and men living with HIV who use tobacco or other substances may be less likely to have an undetectable viral load and more likely to have opportunistic infections (Ompad et al., 2014). These issues are even more complex and deserving of attention in LGBT older adults.

LGBT older adults may view the aging process in unique ways that also impact their mental health and well-being. For example, many LGBT persons may be better able to cope with aging than their non-LGBT counterparts due to resiliencies, adaptive skills, and increased social support from other LGBT people (Fredriksen-Goldsen et al., 2011; Quam & Whitford, 1992). However, in addition to the usual concerns of aging adults, they identify unique needs such as inclusive senior housing, transportation, or help accessing LGBT-oriented social services and events, as well as legal services and protections (Czaja et al., 2016; Fredriksen-Goldsen et al., 2011). They also rightly worry about rejection by children, grandchildren, or other family members, decreased social support, and discrimination in health care, employment, housing, and long-term care (Czaja et al., 2016; D'Augelli & Grossman, 2001; Simone et al., 2015; Stein, Beckerman, & Sherman, 2010). LGBT older adults also may worry more than non-LGBT people about loneliness and isolation (Simone et al., 2015). Finally, some evidence suggests that lesbian and bisexual women may view aging more positively, while ageism may be greater in communities of gay and bisexual men (Grossman, 2008; Schope, 2005; Simone et al., 2015). Providers should explore the extent to which these concerns do or do not apply for each individual patient and consider how they should be addressed in treatment and case management plans.

POLICY ISSUES AFFECTING LGBT OLDER ADULTS

Unequal Treatment Under Laws, Programs, and Services

LGBT older adults face many policy and systemic challenges that impact their well-being and financial security. Some of these derive from their need to rely on nontraditional family structures, but many exist because of institutionalized discrimination and hostility present in laws and regulations. For example, the federal government did not recognize same-sex marriage or domestic partnerships until landmark rulings by the Supreme Court in 2013 and extension of marriage equality to same-sex couples in all 50 U.S. states in 2015. Prior to this, more than 1,100 benefits and protections were denied to same-sex couples. For example:

- Survivor or retirement benefits were denied to partners and children in LGBT families, at an estimated cost to elderly LGBT persons of $124 million a year in unaccessed benefits (Cahill et al., 2000).

- Federal employees could not provide health insurance for their same-sex partners or receive paid sick leave to care for a partner (29 U.S.C. § 2601). The federal government also taxed such benefits if offered by a private employer.

- Tax laws and regulations on joint assets, 401(k) plans, and pensions also discriminated against same-sex partners (Cahill et al., 2000).

- Job stability, and the health insurance that comes with it, remain threatened for LGBT adults in the many states that do not have laws prohibiting employment discrimination based on sexual orientation or gender identity (Hash, 2006).

Despite positive developments in recent years, law and policy changes may have come too late for many LGBT older adults. For example, many older couples did not have the opportunity to legally marry, even if they did feel comfortable disclosing their relationships to others. Without proactive legal protections established through wills and trusts, the lack of marital recognition for inheritance, social security benefits, federal benefits, and pensions will have gravely impacted the financial security of countless older LGBT couples.

Medical Decision Making and Visitation

The Defense of Marriage Act and other measures of institutionalized discrimination toward LGBT people (1 U.S.C. § 7; 28 U.S.C. § 1738C) also have had significant consequences for LGBT older adults in health care settings. Prior to the legal recognition of LGBT couples by most states and the federal government, long-term partners could be viewed by health care providers and officials as legal strangers in situations of illness and disease. This in turn could lead to unfortunate medical situations for many LGBT older adults.

In the absence of legal documentation of marriage or advance health directives, providers often give priority in medical decision making to bio-logical relatives or former opposite-sex spouses, which can be disempow-ering and tragic for LGBT patients and their partners (Cahill et al., 2000). It may even be dangerous if those individuals are unaware of patients' wishes, unaccepting of them, or even hostile or abusive. Visitation policies also have prioritized biological family and ignored same-sex partners or chosen family, particularly when same-sex relationships were not legally recognized in that state (Cahill et al., 2000; Lambda Legal, 2014). A 2011 executive order signed by President Obama attempted to remedy this by mandating that hospitals extend visitation rights to the partners of LGBT women and men (75 Fed. Reg. 20511). The significance of this cannot be overstated, though it lacked the force of congressional legislation and may be overturned or ignored by unsupportive or prejudiced staff. Recognition of marriage equality further protected this right. However, some older couples still may not benefit from these changes if they are unable to get married due to difficulties with being open about their relationship or if they are too ill, frail, or poor to get married.

Advance Care Planning

Even with the protections afforded by marriage equality, many LGBT older adults may be ill prepared to navigate the legal and medical chal-lenges associated with aging (Porter et al., 2016). As such, they should be advised to complete medical powers of attorney or advance health direc-tives, one of the most important things they can do to protect themselves in health care settings (Cahill et al., 2000; Lambda Legal, 2014; Simone et al., 2015). These legal documents generally fall into two categories. One is a living will, which declares individuals' preferences for end-of-life care, such as choices regarding artificial feeding and breathing tubes. The main dis-advantage of relying solely on a living will is that it does not designate a sur-rogate decision maker. As a result, LGBT older adults should also be encouraged to obtain legal documentation that clearly designates a surrogate decision maker in the case of incapacitation (Cahill et al., 2000). These documents are named differently in different states (e.g., "health care proxy" or "durable power of attorney for health care") and can help LGBT older adults to legally safeguard their choice of decision makers and honor treatment preferences (Simone et al., 2015).

Future Policy Issues and New Resources for LGBT Older Adults

Several new developments and resources can continue to improve the care and health of LGBT older adults. More funding and research on their demographics and health concerns, and more positive and holistic conceptual models of their health and aging, will lead to improved health promotion and equity (Fredriksen-Goldsen et al., 2014). In addition, their health care needs should be addressed at future White House Conferences on Aging. National organizations such as the American Geriatrics Society continue to raise awareness and create educational opportunities for improving health care and services for LGBT older adults. GLMA and other organizations also offer models for others in advocacy, education, and efforts to improve services.

Services and Advocacy for GLBT Elders (SAGE) is another key resource for providers and patients. In partnership with 10 leading national organizations, SAGE obtained a federal grant from the Department of Health and Human Services in 2010 to develop the National Resource Center on LGBT Aging (SAGE, 2018). This is the first digital national resource to assist communities across the country in their efforts to provide services and supports for LGBT older adults by centralizing access to the necessary culturally appropriate supports and services they need to successfully age. The Center includes a clearinghouse of LGBT resources by state to help LGBT older adults and their supporters find appropriate care and support.

SUMMARY

LGBT older adults have survived a lifetime of discrimination and disparities. While they struggle with many of the same issues as the general elderly population, LGBT older adults also face unique health challenges. Health care providers need awareness of and training in LGBT-specific competencies. They will not always know the sexual orientation or gender identity of their patients, so cultural competence in these areas may be important in a variety of settings and situations. Providers should seek further education about the needs and disparities of LGBT patients, advocate for improved laws and policies, and fight discrimination when it is witnessed (Lambda Legal, 2014; Simone et al., 2015). They should also work to ensure their health care systems have fair and inclusive policies that recognize LGBT partners and family members; systems should also create pathways for reporting and resolution of discrimination, require LGBT-specific cultural competency training for trainees and staff, and develop laws and accreditation standards that ensure equitable care (Lambda Legal, 2014).

Importantly, the negative experiences and disparities described here are not true for every LGBT older adult; there are many happy, healthy, and inspiring LGBT people of all ages, and they are all the more remarkable for what they have lived through and overcome (Monin, Mota, Levy, Pachankis, & Pietrzak, 2017; Simone et al., 2015). These women and men deserve to be cared for by sensitive and knowledgeable providers who provide appropriate services that address their needs.

REFERENCES

1 U.S.C. § 7 (1996).

28 U.S.C. § 1738C (1997).

29 U.S.C. § 2601 (1993).

75 Fed. Reg. 20,511 (2010).

Acierno, R., Hernandez, M. A., Amstadter, A. B., Resnick, H. S., Steve, K., Muzzy, W., & Kilpatrick, D. G. (2010). Prevalence and correlates of emotional, physical, sexual, and financial abuse and potential neglect in the United States: The National Elder Mistreatment Study. *American Journal of Public Health, 100*(2), 292–297. https://doi.org/10.2105/AJPH.2009.163089

American Geriatrics Society Ethics Committee. (2015). American Geriatrics Society care of lesbian, gay, bisexual, and transgender older adults position statement: American Geriatrics Society Ethics Committee. *Journal of the American Geriatrics Society, 63*(3), 423–436. https://doi.org/10.1111/jgs.13297

American Society on Aging & MetLife Mature Market Institute. (2010). *Still out, still aging: The MetLife study of lesbian, gay, bisexual, and transgender baby boomers.* San Francisco: American Society on Aging & MetLife Mature Market Institute. Retrieved from https://www.giaging.org/documents/mmi-still-out-still-aging.pdf

Appelbaum, J. S. (2008). Late adulthood and aging: Clinical approaches. In H. J. Makadon, K. H. Mayer, J. Potter, & H. Goldhammer (Eds.), *The Fenway guide to lesbian, gay, bisexual, and transgender health* (pp. 135–154). Philadelphia: American College of Physicians.

Asscheman, H., Giltay, E. J., Megens, J. A., van Trotsenburg, M. A., & Gooren, L. J. (2011). A long-term follow-up study of mortality in transsexuals receiving treatment with cross-sex hormones. *European Journal of Endocrinology, 164*(4), 635–642. https://doi.org/10.1530/EJE-10-1038

Benson, C. A., Kaplan, J. E., Masur, H., Pau, A., & Holmes, K. K. (2004). Treating opportunistic infections among HIV-infected adults and adolescents;

recommendations from CDC, the National Institutes of Health, and the HIV Medicine Association/Infectious Diseases Society of America. *Morbidity & Mortality Weekly Report: Recommendations & Reports, 53*(RR15), 1–112. Retrieved from https://www.cdc.gov/mmwr/preview/mmwrhtml/rr5315a1.htm

Bhavan, K. P., Kampalath, V. N., & Overton, E. T. (2008). The aging of the HIV epidemic. *Current HIV/AIDS Reports, 5*(3), 150–158. http://dx.doi.org/10.1007/s11904-008-0023-3

Boroughs, M. S., Bedoya, C. A., O'Cleirigh, C., & Safren, S. A. (2015). Toward defining, measuring, and evaluating LGBT cultural competence for psychologists. *Clinical Psychology: Science & Practice, 22*(2), 151–171. https://doi.org/10.1111/cpsp.12098

Bradford, J. B., & Mayer, K. (2008). Demography and the LGBT population: What we know, don't know, and how the information helps to inform clinical practice. In H. J. Makadon, K. H. Mayer, J. Potter, & H. Goldhammer (Eds.), *The Fenway guide to lesbian, gay, bisexual, and transgender health* (pp. 25–41). Philadelphia: American College of Physicians.

Branson, B. M., Handsfield, H. H., Lampe, M. A., Janssen, R. S., Taylor, A. W., Lyss, S. B., & Clark, J. E. (2006). Revised recommendations for HIV testing of adults, adolescents, and pregnant women in health-care settings. *Morbidity & Mortality Weekly Report: Recommendations & Reports, 55*(RR14), 1–17. Retrieved from https://www.cdc.gov/mmwr/preview/mmwrhtml/rr5514a1.htm

Brennan-Ing, M., Porter, K. E., Seidel, L., & Karpiak, S. E. (2014). Substance use and sexual risk differences among older bisexual and gay men with HIV. *Behavioral Medicine, 40*(3), 108–115. http://dx.doi.org/10.1080/08964289.2014.889069

Brotman, S., Ryan, B., & Cormier, R. (2003). The health and social service needs of gay and lesbian elders and their families in Canada. *The Gerontologist, 43*(2), 192–202. http://dx.doi.org/10.1093/geront/43.2.192

Brown, G. R., & Jones, K. T. (2015). Incidence of breast cancer in a cohort of 5,135 transgender veterans. *Breast Cancer Research & Treatment, 149*(1), 191–198. http://dx.doi.org/10.1007/s10549-014-3213-2

Cahill, S., South, K., & Spade, J. (2000). *Outing age: Public policy issues affecting gay, lesbian, bisexual and transgender elders.* New York: Policy Institute of the National Gay and Lesbian Taskforce. Retrieved from https://static1.squarespace.com/static/566c7f0c2399a3bdabb57553/t/566cc1ea4bf118e6b4487654/1449968106637/2000-NGLTF-Outing-Age2.pdf

Centers for Disease Control and Prevention. (2017a). *Gonorrhea—CDC Fact Sheet (Detailed).* Retrieved from https://www.cdc.gov/std/gonorrhea/stdfact-gonorrhea-detailed.htm

Centers for Disease Control and Prevention. (2017b). *Chlamydia—CDC Fact Sheet (Detailed).* Retrieved from https://www.cdc.gov/std/chlamydia/stdfact-chlamydia-detailed.htm

Centers for Disease Control and Prevention. (2017c). *Syphilis—CDC Fact Sheet (Detailed).* Retrieved from https://www.cdc.gov/std/syphilis/stdfact-syphilis-detailed.htm

Centers for Disease Control and Prevention. (2018). *HIV among people aged 50 and over.* Retrieved from https://www.cdc.gov/hiv/group/age/olderamericans/index.html

Cohen, H. L., Curry, L. C., Jenkins, D., Walker, C. A., & Hogstel, M. O. (2008). Older lesbians and gay men: Long-term care issues. *Annals of Long Term Care, 16*(2), 33–38.

Czaja, S. J., Sabbag, S., Lee, C. C., Schulz, R., Lang, S., Vlahovic, T., . . . Thurston, C. (2016). Concerns about aging and caregiving among middle-aged and older lesbian and gay adults. *Aging & Mental Health, 20*(11), 1107–1118. http://dx.doi.org/10.1080/13607863.2015.1072795

Daniel, H., & Butkus, R. (2015). Lesbian, gay, bisexual, and transgender health disparities: Executive summary of a policy position paper from the American College of Physicians. *Annals of Internal Medicine, 163*(2), 135–137. http://dx.doi.org/10.7326/M14-2482

Daskalakis, D. C., Radix, A., & Mayer, G. (2015). Sexual health of LGBTQ people. In H. J. Makadon, K. H. Mayer, J. Potter, & H. Goldhammer (Eds.), *The Fenway guide to lesbian, gay, bisexual, and transgender health, second edition* (pp. 289–324). Philadelphia: American College of Physicians.

D'Augelli, A. R., & Grossman, A. H. (2001). Disclosure of sexual orientation, victimization, and mental health among lesbian, gay, and bisexual older adults. *Journal of Interpersonal Violence, 16*(10), 1008–1027. http://dx.doi.org/10.1177/088626001016010003

D'Augelli, A. R., Grossman, A. H., Hershberger, S. L., & O'Connell, T. S. (2001). Aspects of mental health among older lesbian, gay, and bisexual adults. *Aging & Mental Health, 5*(2), 149–158. http://dx.doi.org/10.1080/13607860120038366

Dean, L., Meyer, I. H., Robinson, K., Sell, R. L., Sember, R., Silenzio, V. M., . . . Dunn, P. (2000). Lesbian, gay, bisexual, and transgender health: Findings and concerns. *Journal of the Gay and Lesbian Medical Association, 4*(3), 102–151. http://dx.doi.org/10.1023/A:1009573800168

den Heijer, M., Bakker, A., & Gooren, L. (2017). Long term hormonal treatment for transgender people. *BMJ, 359*, j5027. http://dx.doi.org/10.1136/bmj.j5027

Deutsch, M. B. (Ed.). (2016). *Guidelines for the primary and gender-affirming care of transgender and gender nonbinary people.* San Francisco: Center for Excellence in Transgender Health, University of California. Retrieved from http://transhealth.ucsf.edu/pdf/Transgender-PGACG-6-17-16.pdf

Dunbar, E. (2006). Race, gender, and sexual orientation in hate crime victimization: Identity politics or identity risk? *Violence & Victims, 21*(3), 323–337. http://dx.doi.org/10.1891/vivi.21.3.323

Edwards, K. M., Sylaska, K. M., & Neal, A. M. (2015). Intimate partner violence among sexual minority populations: A critical review of the literature and agenda for future research. *Psychology of Violence, 5*(2), 112–121. http://dx.doi.org/10.1037%2Fa0038656

Fredriksen-Goldsen, K. I., Cook-Daniels, L., Kim, H. J., Erosheva, E. A., Emlet, C. A., Hoy-Ellis, C. P., . . . Muraco, A. (2013). Physical and mental health of transgender older adults: An at-risk and underserved population. *The Gerontologist, 54*(3), 488–500. https://doi.org/10.1093/geront/gnt021

Fredriksen-Goldsen, K. I., Kim, H.-J., Emlet, C. A., Muraco, A., Erosheva, E. A., Hoy-Ellis, C. P., . . . Petry, H. (2011). *The aging and health report: Disparities and resilience among lesbian, gay, bisexual, and transgender older adults.* Seattle: Institute for Multigenerational Health. Retrieved from https://www.homophobie.org/wp-content/uploads/2016/02/Full-Report -FINAL-11-16-11.pdf

Fredriksen-Goldsen, K. I., Kim, H. J., Shui, C., & Bryan, A. E. (2017). Chronic health conditions and key health indicators among lesbian, gay, and bisexual older US adults, 2013–2014. *American Journal of Public Health, 107*(8), 1332–1338. http://dx.doi.org/10.2105/AJPH.2017.303922

Fredriksen-Goldsen, K. I., Simoni, J. M., Kim, H. J., Lehavot, K., Walters, K. L., Yang, J., . . . Muraco, A. (2014). The health equity promotion model: Reconceptualization of lesbian, gay, bisexual, and transgender (LGBT) health disparities. *American Journal of Orthopsychiatry, 84*(6), 653–663. http://dx.doi.org/10.1037/ort0000030

Gates, G. J. (2012). *Same-sex couples in census 2010: Race and ethnicity.* Los Angeles: Williams Institute. Retrieved from https://williamsinstitute.law.ucla. edu/research/census-lgbt-demographics-studies/same-sex-couples-census -2010-race-ethnicity/

Gay and Lesbian Medical Association. (2018a). *Creating a welcoming clinical environment for lesbian, gay, bisexual, and transgender (LGBT) patients.* Washington, DC: Gay and Lesbian Medical Association. Retrieved from http://www.rainbowwelcome.org/uploads/pdfs/Creating%20a%20Welcome %20Clinical%20Environment%20for%20LGBT%20Patients.pdf

Gay and Lesbian Medical Association. (2018b). *Guidelines for the care of lesbian, gay, bisexual, and transgender patients.* Washington, DC: Gay and Lesbian Medical Association. Retrieved from http://glma.org/_data/n_0001/resources /live/GLMA%20guidelines%202006%20FINAL.pdf

Gay and Lesbian Medical Association. (2018c). *Top ten issues to discuss with your healthcare provider.* Washington, DC: Gay and Lesbian Medical Association. Retrieved from http://www.glma.org/index.cfm?fuseaction=Page.vie wPage&pageId=947&grandparentID=534&parentID=938&nodeID=1

Gold, S. D., Feinstein, B. A., Skidmore, W. C., & Marx, B. P. (2011). Childhood physical abuse, internalized homophobia, and experiential avoidance among lesbians and gay men. *Psychological Trauma: Theory, Research, Practice, & Policy, 3*(1), 50–60. http://dx.doi.org/10.1037/a0020487

Goldstone, S. E. (2005). The ups and downs of gay sex after prostate cancer treatment. In J. Drescher & G. Perlman (Eds.), *A gay man's guide to prostate cancer.* Binghampton, NY: Haworth Medical Press.

Gonzales, G., & Henning-Smith, C. (2015). Disparities in health and disability among older adults in same-sex cohabiting relationships. *Journal of Aging and Health, 27*(3), 432–453. http://dx.doi.org/10.1177/0898264314551332

Gooren, L. J. (2011). Care of transsexual persons. *New England Journal of Medicine, 364*(13), 1251–1257. http://dx.doi.org/10.1056/NEJMcp1008161

Graham, R., Berkowitz, B., Blum, R., Bockting, W., Bradford, J., de Vries, B., . . . Makadon, H. (2011). *The health of lesbian, gay, bisexual, and transgender people: Building a foundation for better understanding.* Washington, DC: Institute of Medicine. Retrieved from https://www.ncbi.nlm.nih.gov /books/NBK64806/pdf/Bookshelf_NBK64806.pdf

Grossman, A. H. (2008). The unique experiences of older gay and bisexual men: Associations with health and well-being. In R. J. Wolitski, R. Stall, & R. O. Valdiserri (Eds.), *Unequal opportunity: Health disparities affecting gay and bisexual men in the United States* (pp. 303–326). New York: Oxford UniversityPress.http://dx.doi.org/10.1093/acprof:oso/9780195301533.003.0011

Grossman, A. H., Frank, J. A., Graziano, M. J., Narozniak, D. R., Mendelson, G., El Hassan, D., & Patouhas, E. S. (2014). Domestic harm and neglect among lesbian, gay, and bisexual older adults. *Journal of Homosexuality, 61*(12), 1649–1666. http://dx.doi.org/10.1080/00918369.2014.951216

Haas, A. P., Eliason, M., Mays, V. M., Mathy, R. M., Cochran, S. D., D'Augelli, A. R., . . . Russell, S. T. (2010). Suicide and suicide risk in lesbian, gay, bisexual, and transgender populations: Review and recommendations. *Journal of Homosexuality, 58*(1), 10–51. http://dx.doi.org/10.1080/00918369.2011.534038

Halkitis, P. N., Green, K. A., & Mourgues, P. (2005). Longitudinal investigation of methamphetamine use among gay and bisexual men in New York City: Findings from Project BUMPS. *Journal of Urban Health, 82*(1), i18–i25. http://dx.doi.org/10.1093/jurban/jti020

Hash, K. (2006). Caregiving and post-caregiving experiences of midlife and older gay men and lesbians. *Journal of Gerontological Social Work, 47*(3–4), 121–138. http://dx.doi.org/10.1300/J083v47n03_08

Henning-Smith, C., Gonzales, G., & Shippee, T. P. (2015). Differences by sexual orientation in expectations about future long-term care needs among adults 40 to 65 years old. *American Journal of Public Health, 105*(11), 2359–2365. http://dx.doi.org/10.2105/AJPH.2015.302781

Henry J. Kaiser Family Foundation. (2002). *National Survey of Physicians, part 1: Doctors on disparities in medical care.* Menlo Park, CA: Henry J. Kaiser Family Foundation. Retrieved from https://www.kff.org/uninsured /national-survey-of-physicians-part-i-doctors/

Herek, G. M. (2009a). Hate crimes and stigma-related experiences among sexual minority adults in the United States: Prevalence estimates from a national probability sample. *Journal of Interpersonal Violence, 24*(1), 54–74. http:// dx.doi.org/10.1177/0886260508316477

Herek, G. M. (2009b). Sexual stigma and sexual prejudice in the United States: A conceptual framework. In D. Hope (Ed.), *Contemporary perspectives on lesbian, gay, and bisexual identities* (pp. 65–111). New York: Springer. http://dx.doi.org/10.1007/978-0-387-09556-1

Hollenbach, A. D., Eckstrand, K. L., & Dreger, A. D. (Eds.). (2014). *Implementing curricular and institutional climate changes to improve health care for individuals who are LGBT, gender nonconforming, or born with DSD: A resource for medical educators.* Washington, DC: Association of American Medical Colleges.

Honigberg, M. C., Eshel, N., Luskin, M. R., Shaykevich, S., Lipsitz, S. R., & Katz, J. T. (2017). Curricular time, patient exposure, and comfort caring for lesbian, gay, bisexual, and transgender patients among recent medical graduates. *LGBT Health*, *4*(3), 237–239. http://dx.doi.org/10.1089/lgbt .2017.0029

Hoy-Ellis, C. P., & Fredriksen-Goldsen, K. I. (2016). Lesbian, gay, & bisexual older adults: linking internal minority stressors, chronic health conditions, and depression. *Aging & Mental Health*, *20*(11), 1119–1130. http://dx.doi.org /10.1080/13607863.2016.1168362

Johnson, M. J., Jackson, N. C., Arnette, J. K., & Koffman, S. D. (2005). Gay and lesbian perceptions of discrimination in retirement care facilities. *Journal of Homosexuality*, *49*(2), 83–102. http://dx.doi.org/10.1300/J082v49n02_05

Kauth, M. R., & Shipherd, J. C. (Eds.). (2018). *Adult transgender care: An interdisciplinary approach for training mental health professionals*. New York: Routledge.

Kean, R. (2006). Understanding the lives of older gay people. *Nursing Older People*, *18*(8), 31–36. http://dx.doi.org/10.7748/nop.18.8.31.s18

King, M. (2007, June 17). Elder co-housing project is aimed at gay women. *The Seattle Times*. Retrieved from https://www.seattletimes.com/seattle-news /elder-co-housing-project-is-aimed-at-gay-women/

Lambda Legal. (2014). *When health care isn't caring: Lambda Legal's survey of discrimination against LGBT people and people with HIV*. New York: Lambda Legal. Retrieved from https://www.lambdalegal.org/sites/ default/files/publications/downloads/whcic-report_when-health-care -isnt-caring.pdf

Landers, S. J., & Gilsanz, P. (2009). *The health of lesbian, gay, bisexual and transgender (LGBT) persons in Massachusetts: A survey of health issues comparing LGBT persons with their heterosexual and non-transgender counterparts*. Commonwealth of Massachusetts, Department of Public Health. Retrieved from http://masslib-dspace.longsight.com/bitstream /handle/2452/112258/ocn728179770.pdf?sequence=1&isAllowed=y

Langenderfer-Magruder, L., Walls, N. E., Kattari, S. K., Whitfield, D. L., & Ramos, D. (2016). Sexual victimization and subsequent police reporting by gender identity among lesbian, gay, bisexual, transgender, and queer adults. *Violence & Victims*, *31*(2), 320–331. https://doi.org/10.1891/0886-6708 .VV-D-14-00082

Lauver, D. R., Karon, S. L., Egan, J., Jacobson, M., Nugent, J., Settersten, L., & Shaw, V. (1999). Understanding lesbians' mammography utilization. *Women's Health Issues*, *9*(5), 264–274. http://dx.doi.org/10.1016/S1049-3867(99)00024-9

Luther, V. P., & Wilkin, A. M. (2007). HIV infection in older adults. *Clinics in Geriatric Medicine*, *23*(3), 567–583. http://dx.doi.org/10.1016/j.cger.2007.02.004

Mahan, R. J., Bailey, T. A., Bibb, T. J., Fenney, M., & Williams, T. (2016). Drug therapy for gender transitions and health screenings in transgender older adults. *Journal of the American Geriatrics Society*, *64*(12), 2554–2559. https://doi.org/10.1111/jgs.14350

Makadon, H. J. (2006). Improving health care for the lesbian and gay communities. *New England Journal of Medicine*, *354*(9), 895–897. http://dx.doi .org/10.1056/NEJMp058259

MetLife Mature Market Institute, Lesbian and Gay Aging Issues Network of the American Society on Aging, & Zogby International. (2006). *Out and aging: The MetLife study of lesbian and gay baby boomers*. Westport, CT: MetLife

Mature Market Institute, Lesbian & Gay Aging Issues Network of the American Society on Aging, & Zogby International. Retrieved from https://lgbtagingcenter.org/resources/pdfs/OutandAging.pdf

Meyer, I. H. (2003). Prejudice, social stress, and mental health in lesbian, gay, and bisexual populations: Conceptual issues and research evidence. *Psychological Bulletin*, *129*(5), 674–697. http://dx.doi.org/10.1037/0033-2909.129.5.674

Monin, J. K., Mota, N., Levy, B., Pachankis, J., & Pietrzak, R. H. (2017). Older age associated with mental health resiliency in sexual minority US veterans. *The American Journal of Geriatric Psychiatry*, *25*(1), 81–90. http://dx.doi.org/10.1016/j.jagp.2016.09.006

Obedin-Maliver, J., Goldsmith, E. S., Stewart, L., White, W., Tran, E., Brenman, S., . . . Lunn, M. R. (2011). Lesbian, gay, bisexual, and transgender–related content in undergraduate medical education. *JAMA*, *306*(9), 971–977. http://dx.doi.org/10.1001/jama.2011.1255

Ompad, D. C., Kingdon, M., Kupprat, S., Halkitis, S. N., Storholm, E. D., & Halkitis, P. N. (2014). Smoking and HIV-related health issues among older HIV-positive gay, bisexual, and other men who have sex with men. *Behavioral Medicine*, *40*(3), 99–107. http://dx.doi.org/10.1080/08964289.2014.889067

Park, I. U., & Palefsky, J. M. (2010). Evaluation and management of anal intraepithelial neoplasia in HIV-negative and HIV-positive men who have sex with men. *Current Infectious Disease Reports*, *12*(2), 126–133. http://dx.doi.org/10.1007/s11908-010-0090-7

Porter, K. E., Brennan-Ing, M., Chang, S. C., Dickey, L. M., Singh, A. A., Bower, K. L., & Witten, T. M. (2016). Providing competent and affirming services for transgender and gender nonconforming older adults. *Clinical Gerontologist*, *39*(5), 366–388. http://dx.doi.org/10.1080/07317115.2016.1203383

Portz, J. D., Retrum, J. H., Wright, L. A., Boggs, J. M., Wilkins, S., Grimm, C., . . . Gozansky, W. S. (2014). Assessing capacity for providing culturally competent services to LGBT older adults. *Journal of Gerontological Social Work*, *57*(2–4), 305–321. http://dx.doi.org/10.1080/01634372.2013.857378

Quam, J. K., & Whitford, G. S. (1992). Adaptation and age-related expectations of older gay and lesbian adults. *The Gerontologist*, *32*(3), 367–374. http://dx.doi.org/10.1093/geront/32.3.367

Quinn, G. P., Sanchez, J. A., Sutton, S. K., Vadaparampil, S. T., Nguyen, G. T., Green, B. L., . . . Schabath, M. B. (2015). Cancer and lesbian, gay, bisexual, transgender/transsexual, and queer/questioning (LGBTQ) populations. *CA: A Cancer Journal for Clinicians*, *65*(5), 384–400. http://dx.doi.org/10.3322/caac.21288

Rawls, T. W. (2004). Disclosure and depression among older gay and homosexual men: Findings from the Urban Men's Health Study. In G. Herdt & B. De Vries (Eds.), *Gay and lesbian aging: Research and future directions* (pp. 117–141). New York: Springer.

Rosenfeld, D. (1999). Identity work among lesbian and gay elderly. *Journal of Aging Studies*, *13*(2), 121–144. http://dx.doi.org/10.1016/S0890-4065(99)80047-4

Rothman, E. F., Exner, D., & Baughman, A. L. (2011). The prevalence of sexual assault against people who identify as gay, lesbian, or bisexual in the United

States: A systematic review. *Trauma, Violence, & Abuse, 12*(2), 55–66. http://dx.doi.org/10.1177/1524838010390707

Schneeberger, A. R., Dietl, M. F., Muenzenmaier, K. H., Huber, C. G., & Lang, U. E. (2014). Stressful childhood experiences and health outcomes in sexual minority populations: A systematic review. *Social Psychiatry and Psychiatric Epidemiology, 49*(9), 1427–1445. http://dx.doi.org/10.1007/s00127-014-0854-8

Schope, R. D. (2005). Who's afraid of growing old? Gay and lesbian perceptions of aging. *Journal of Gerontological Social Work, 45*(4), 23–39. https://doi .org/10.1300/J083v45n04_03

Sell, R. L., & Becker, J. B. (2001). Sexual orientation data collection and progress toward Healthy People 2010. *American Journal of Public Health, 91*(6), 876–882. https://doi.org/10.2105/AJPH.91.6.876

Services and Advocacy for Gay, Lesbian, Bisexual and Transgender Elders. (2010). *Improving the lives of LGBT older adults.* New York: Services & Advocacy for Gay, Lesbian, Bisexual & Transgender Elders, 2010. Retrieved from https://sageusa.org/files/Improving%20the%20Lives%20of%20LGBT%20 Older%20Adults%20-%20full%20report.pdf

Services and Advocacy for Gay, Lesbian, Bisexual and Transgender Elders. (2018). *National resource on LGBT aging.* Retrieved from https://www.lgbtaging center.org/

Sheffield, L., & Keuroghlian, A. S. (2017). Sexual health among transgender people. In M. R. Kauth & J. C. Shipherd (Eds.), *Adult transgender care: An interdisciplinary approach for training mental health professionals* (pp. 194–207). New York: Routledge.

Shipherd, J. C., Maguen, S., Skidmore, W. C., & Abramovitz, S. M. (2011). Potentially traumatic events in a transgender sample: Frequency and associated symptoms. *Traumatology, 17*(2), 56–67. http://dx.doi.org/10.1177/153476 5610395614

Simone, M. J., & Appelbaum, J. S. (2008). HIV in older adults. *Geriatrics, 63*(12), 6–12.

Simone, M. J., & Appelbaum, J. S. (2011). Addressing the needs of older lesbian, gay, bisexual, and transgender adults. *Clinical Geriatrics, 19*(2), 38–45. Retrieved from https://www.consultant360.com/articles/addressing-needs -older-lesbian-gay-bisexual-and-transgender-adults

Simone, M. J., Meyer, H., Eskildsen, M. A., & Appelbaum, J. S. (2015). LGBT late adulthood and aging: Clinical approaches. In H. J. Makadon, K. H. Mayer, J. Potter, & H. Goldhammer (Eds.), *The Fenway guide to lesbian, gay, bisexual, and transgender health,* 2nd ed. (pp. 133–156). Philadelphia: American College of Physicians.

Smith, R. D., Delpech, V. C., Brown, A. E., & Rice, B. D. (2010). HIV transmission and high rates of late diagnoses among adults aged 50 years and over. *AIDS, 24*(13), 2109–2115. http://dx.doi.org/10.1097/QAD.0b013e32833c7b9c

Stall, R., & Catania, J. (1994). AIDS risk behaviors among late middle-aged and elderly Americans. *Archives of Internal Medicine, 154*(1), 57–63. http://dx .doi.org/10.1001/archinte.1994.00420010085010

Stein, G. L., Beckerman, N. L., & Sherman, P. A. (2010). Lesbian and gay elders and long-term care: Identifying the unique psychosocial perspectives and challenges. *Journal of Gerontological Social Work, 53*(5), 421–435. http://dx.doi.org/10.1080/01634372.2010.496478

Stotzer, R. L. (2009). Violence against transgender people: A review of United States data. *Aggression & Violent Behavior, 14*(3), 170–179. http://dx.doi.org/10.1016/j.avb.2009.01.006

Substance Abuse and Mental Health Services Administration. (2014). *Trauma-informed care in behavioral health services.* Treatment Improvement Protocol (TIP) Series 57. HHS Publication No. (SMA) 13-4801. Rockville, MD: Substance Abuse & Mental Health Services Administration.

Torke, A. M., & Carnahan, J. L. (2017). Optimizing the clinical care of lesbian, gay, bisexual, and transgender older adults. *JAMA Internal Medicine, 177*(12), 1715–1716. http://dx.doi.org/10.1001/jamainternmed.2017.5324

U.S. Department of Health and Human Services. (2000). *Healthy People 2010: Understanding and improving health.* Washington, DC: U.S. Government Printing Office.

Valanis, B. G., Bowen, D. J., Bassford, T., Whitlock, E., Charney, P., & Carter, R. A. (2000). Sexual orientation and health: Comparisons in the Women's Health Initiative sample. *Archives of Family Medicine, 9*(9), 843–853. http://dx.doi.org/10.1001/archfami.9.9.843

Walters, M. L., Chen, J., & Breiding, M. J. (2013). *The National Intimate Partner and Sexual Violence Survey (NISVS): 2010 findings on victimization by sexual orientation.* Atlanta: National Center for Injury Prevention & Control, Centers for Disease Control & Prevention. Retrieved from https://www.cdc.gov/ViolencePrevention/pdf/NISVS_SOfindings.pdf

Wierckx, K., Mueller, S., Weyers, S., Van Caenegem, E., Roef, G., Heylens, G., & T'Sjoen, G. (2012). Long-term evaluation of cross-sex hormone treatment in transsexual persons. *The Journal of Sexual Medicine, 9*(10), 2641–2651. https://doi.org/10.1111/j.1743-6109.2012.02876.x

Wylie, K., Knudson, G., Khan, S. I., Bonierbale, M., Watanyusakul, S., & Baral, S. (2016). Serving transgender people: Clinical care considerations and service delivery models in transgender health. *The Lancet, 388*(10042), 401–411. https://doi.org/10.1016/S0140-6736(16)00682-6

Zelle, A., & Arms, T. (2015). Psychosocial effects of health disparities of lesbian, gay, bisexual, and transgender older adults. *Journal of Psychosocial Nursing and Mental Health services, 53*(7), 25–30. http://dx.doi.org/10.3928/02793695-20150623-04

7

Lesbian, Gay, Bisexual, and Transgender Parents

Megan C. Lytle

Literature about children with lesbian, gay, bisexual, and transgender (LGBT) parents tends to take a defensive approach; more often it has been used to justify the suitability of LGBT parents and to demonstrate the psychological well-being of their children (Patterson, 2005). Organizations such as Children of Lesbians and Gays Everywhere (COLAGE, n.d.a.) and researchers have suggested that scholars move away from investigating the impact of stigma and to start exploring resiliency. By disseminating empirical research and sharing the beneficial aspects of having a LGBT parent, researchers can help break down stereotypes, reduce legalized discrimination, and help practitioners provide better care to LGBT families.

Therefore, this chapter will begin with a description of family relationships and parent-child bonds; next, the unique experiences of gay fathers, lesbian mothers, bisexual parents, and transgender parents will be addressed; the influence of culture on LGBT families will be examined; and then the current policies that impact LGBT families will be explored. Recommendations and resources are also provided.

FAMILY RELATIONSHIPS

The idea of a nuclear family with two parents and children is no longer the norm, and what constitutes as a family differs based on a number of factors such as culture and institutions (Human Rights Campaign, 2013b). The notion of what defines a family has continuously evolved since the 1970s, and the postmodern conceptualization of a family varies significantly (Kelley & Sequeira, 1997). A postmodern family may consist of one or more individuals who may or may not choose to have children in the context of a heterosexual, same-sex, or gender-diverse relationship. Family relationships are often measured by the self-reported behaviors and emotions or the family function of each family member (Epstein, Baldwin, & Bishop, 1983). However, the family constellation must be understood in order to assess family relationships.

Aside from cultural and societal assumptions of what it means to be a family, the health care system has a different definition of family. According to the Human Rights Campaign (HRC) (2013b), some hospitals and health care organizations tend to view family members as "any person(s) who plays a significant role in an individual's life." Therefore, families are not always limited to biological relatives but may include step family members and legal guardians, among others. Yet, some health care systems limit visitation and health care decision making to immediate family members (i.e., legal spouses, parents, and children), and depending on state laws, some coparents would not be considered immediate family (Movement Advancement Project, Family Equality Council, & Center for American Progress, 2012b).

Regardless of how the term "family" is defined, a common experience among LGBT individuals is the concept of creating a family of choice, especially when their families of origin are not accepting (Riggle, Whitman, Olson, Rostosky, & Strong, 2008). As a result, many individuals will seek out support from the broader LGBT community (Riggle et al., 2008; Riggle, Rostosky, McCants, & Pascale-Hague, 2011; Rostosky, Riggle, Pascale-Hague, & McCants, 2010). Yet, some ethnically diverse LGBT individuals report that their culture impedes disclosing their sexual orientation to family members, whereas white gay or lesbian individuals may not feel as inhibited by their culture in coming out to their families (Merighi & Grimes, 2000). Therefore, some LGBT individuals may consider the homonegativity and transnegativity from ethnic communities in addition to racism with the LGBT community before coming out or creating their own families of choice.

Indeed, many LGBT individuals consider familial reactions before choosing to come out. For example, when LGBT individuals have had children in the context of a heterosexual relationship, their disclosure impacts the whole family (Armesto, 2002; Beeler & DiProva, 1999; Bozett, 1980; Van Voorhis & McClain, 1997). Therefore, LGBT parents may delay their disclosure and/or choose to stay distant from their families to avoid rejection (Armesto, 2002). Just as LGBT parents must learn how, when, and to whom they want to come out, their children also need to negotiate their own coming-out process. For instance, Beeler and DiProva (1999) found that family members not only have a "finding out story," but they also have their own coming-out process as the relative of a LGBT individual. Additionally, adult children tend to be protective of their LGB parents due to the awareness that their parents' suitability is constantly being scrutinized due to societal homonegativity, heterosexism (Goldberg, 2007), and cisgenderism. They are not only aware of how their families are misrepresented in the media, but they report wanting to break down these stereotypes.

Literature on LGBT families used to focus on divorce and comparing divorced lesbian mothers to divorced heterosexual mothers without separating the influence of sexual orientation (Patterson, 2005) and gender identity from the impact of divorce. However, Lytle, Foley, and Aster (2013) as well as Goldberg (2007) found that adult children of LGBT parents often report that watching their families divide due to a divorce caused more distress than having a LGBT parent. In the book *Families Like Mine*, 50 children of LGBT parents were interviewed about their unique experiences. One noted concern was that children born to a LGBT parent and a heterosexual, cisgender parent often receive homonegative and transnegative messages from the heterosexual parent during the divorce process and/or through the legal system during custody battles. Although young adults may experience distress over their parents' divorce as well as not having a closer relationship with their fathers, the levels of depression and anxiety did not differ between individuals whose parents had divorced or remain married (Laumann-Billings & Emery, 2000).

PARENT-CHILD BONDS

There is no empirical support to suggest that LGBT parents are any less suitable than heterosexual parents (Armesto, 2002; Bigner, 1996; Tasker & Golombok, 1995); however, Armesto suggested that the strain of deciding whether or not to come out to their children may impact the parental bond of LGBT parents. For instance, gay fathers believe that their children may experience stigma and discrimination if they disclose their sexual orientation; however, the consequences of not coming out may lead to detachment in the father-child relationship. Indeed, gay men may decide to distances themselves both psychologically and emotionally from their children to evade rejection (Armesto, 2002), but the bond between parent and child is impacted by a number of factors, including: security, proximity, personality, and values (Mortimer, 1984; Weiss, 1991). According to Patterson (2006), a "warm and affectionate" parent-child bond was the most influential factor on development, whereas the child's development was not impacted by the parent's sexual orientation.

Not to mention, the dynamics of parent-child bonds evolve over time. Although adult children may have affection and concern for their parents, their sense of security is no longer enhanced by their parent-child bond. Specifically, children often view their parents as "wiser and stronger," whereas in a bond between adult children and their parents, whether the person is viewed as wise and strong often fluctuates (Weiss, 1991). Hence, the parent-child bond may change, depending on the age when children learn about their parents' sexual orientation or gender identity and how the disclosure is made, as well as bias among family and friends, among other factors (Lytle et al., 2013).

Children of Gay Men

Aside from gay men who have had children while in heterosexual relationships (Armesto, 2002; Bigner, 1996; Patterson, 2000), few studies have focused on gay fathers. In fact, due to social barriers, many gay men used to believe that their sexual orientation was mutually exclusive with fatherhood. However, gay men have used a number of methods to become fathers, such as adoption, marriage, and alternative forms of surrogacy and insemination (Berkowitz & Marsiglio, 2007; Bigner, 1996). Therefore, over the years, more and more gay men are actively choosing fatherhood.

Even though the mental health field has worked toward depathologizing LGB individuals, some gay men are choosing to remain in heterosexual relationships (i.e., mixed-orientation relationships) out of their desires for both acceptance and to have children. Tornello and Patterson (2012) used the Gay Dads Study to further examine the experiences of gay men who had children in mixed-orientation relationships and explored how their current relationship status (e.g., female partner, male partner, or single) is associated with relationship satisfaction, outness, and parenting stress. Gay men who remained married to female partners had less relationship satisfaction and were less out about their sexual orientation than men who were partnered with men (Tornello & Patterson, 2012). Unfortunately, this study only examined the parents' perspective and did not investigate the child's perspective or the strength of the parent-child bonds.

Researchers have also started to examine the experiences of men who are choosing parenthood through such means as adoption and surrogacy. As culture has shifted, there may be a cohort effect in the pathways that gay men choose for becoming fathers, with younger gay men choosing adoption and foster care among other means to become parents while older gay fathers were more likely to enter parenthood through heterosexual marriages (Patterson & Tornello, 2010). To learn more about the experiences of gay men who became parents through surrogacy, Bergman, Rubio, Green, and Padrón (2010) interviewed 40 gay fathers and found that work transitions allowed fathers to spend more time with their families (e.g., becoming a stay-at-home parent or working part time), financial shifts (i.e., less income, more expenses) were common, they identified sources of support (e.g., improved relationships with families of origin and socializing more with other parents), and their well-being improved (i.e., fathers reported increase in self-esteem but less self-care). While this study focused on gay parenthood through surrogacy, many of these themes may apply to LGBT parents in general.

Overall, gay fathers do not differ from heterosexual fathers in their parenting ability, but they do differ in their parenting styles (Bigner, 1996). Specifically, gay fathers may not adhere to male gender roles when parenting and tend to be more emotionally expressive and nurturing. Both gay and heterosexual fathers are equally involved with their children (Armesto, 2002), and while gay fathers are often stern, they explain the reasons for their discipline and are more approachable. Unfortunately, assumptions about the relationship between sexual orientation and parenting has been the main focus for researchers rather than exploring how the desire for fatherhood impacts parent-child relationships.

Children of Lesbian Women

Similar to research about children with gay fathers, the majority of literature on lesbian parenting used to focus on the psychological impact of children who were conceived into a heterosexual relationship (Tasker & Golombok, 1995). However, some scholars have started to investigate the lesbian baby boom that resulted from women choosing to adopt or have a child born into a same-sex relationship (Patterson, 2001). For instance, improved access to donor insemination in the Netherlands has facilitated the process for lesbians to choose motherhood, and planned lesbian parenthood has become increasingly common in Western countries as well (Bos, 2013; Bos, van Balen, & van den Boom, 2003).

In a 15-year longitudinal study, Tasker and Golombok (1995) found that children raised by lesbian mothers did not differ from those with heterosexual mothers regarding their parent-child relationships; however, children with lesbian parents reported better relationships with their mother's partner than the relationship participants who had heterosexual mothers had with their mother's male partner. In addition, children with lesbian mothers tend to be proud of their mother's sexual orientation and therefore often became social advocates for LGBT rights (Tasker & Golombok, 1995). Similarly, Bos (2013) compared parenting and child well-being between planned lesbian families with heterosexual families in a review and found that although planned lesbian mothers often consider their reasons for having children for a longer duration than heterosexual parents, their motives do not differ from those of heterosexual couples. Additionally, planned lesbian mothers do not differ from heterosexual parents in their levels of parental stress, but their style of parenting differs, especially in comparison to heterosexual fathers (Bos, 2013). Specifically, planned lesbian mothers tend to have more emotional involvement, are less likely to spank their children as a means of discipline, and make more time for caregiving; thus, their children did not report any significant differences in terms of psychological well-being, let alone other developmental concerns. When comparing lesbian mothers, single mothers, and heterosexual mothers, data from a longitudinal study suggests that lesbian parents had less separation anxiety and more emotional involvement (Golombok & Badger, 2010). In terms of their children, most comparisons were insignificant, but children of lesbian parents reported fewer psychological concerns, greater self-worth, and better academic capabilities (Golombok & Badger, 2010). Perhaps future researchers will also examine whether these positive differences apply to children of gay men, bisexual parents, and transgender parents.

Children of Bisexual Men and Bisexual Women

More often than not, scholars have focused on the parenting styles and child outcomes of gay and lesbian parents, and when bisexual parents are included, they are often grouped together with LGBT parents. On occasion, researchers have focused on the gender of the parent and have grouped bisexual mothers with lesbian parents and bisexual fathers with gay parents, but very few studies have examined the unique experiences of bisexual parents and their children. According to Ross and Dobinson (2013), children of bisexual parents are believed to have similar experiences as children of gay and lesbian parents in that their parents may have concealed their sexual orientation from them, they may experience stigma, and their sexual orientation was not related to their parent's sexual orientation. Specifically, Murray and McClintock (2005) reported that the age of children during their parent's disclosure was similar when comparing gay and lesbian parents with bisexual parents; however, mothers tend to come out when their children are younger when compared to fathers. Although children of bisexual parents were grouped with children of gays and lesbians, these children did not differ from children of heterosexual parents in terms of social desirability, anxiety, or self-esteem. Similar to the progression of research on children of gays and lesbians, research focused on children of a bisexual parent's ability to parent and the well-being of their children rather than considering the potential strengths of having a bisexual parent.

Despite the similarities to gay and lesbian parents, bisexual parents face unique experiences. For instance, the amount of stigma that bisexual couples and their children face may be associated with the parent's partner status. If a bisexual parent is partnered with an other-sex partner, she or he may experience less stigma than when parented with a same-sex partner (Fassinger & Arseneau, 2007), and this privilege may also limit the stigma experienced by their children. However, Ross and Dobinson (2013) suggested that the privilege associated with a perceived heterosexual orientation may influence the level of support received from the LGBT community. In addition, there is an assumption that bisexual individuals cannot commit to a monogamous relationship and that exposing their children to polyamory will have negative consequences (Ross & Dobinson, 2013). Yet, research suggests that these assumptions are not true, as many bisexual individuals have monogamous relationships; and, although they are attracted to both sexes, bisexuals may consistently partner with one gender over time (Weinberg, Williams, & Pryor, 2001). Moreover, Pallotta-Chiarolli, Haydon, and Hunter (2013) described some of the benefits that children of polyamorous families may experience, such as a being raised in a nonsexist environment, access to collective resources, and more parenting time; however, additional research is needed.

Children of Transgender Individuals

The literature on transgender parenting is extremely scant. One of the few studies presented on the parenting experiences of three transgender individuals in the form of case studies (Hines, 2006). One commonality was that all of three of the transgender parents explored how important it was for them to be open and honest with their children. Being open gave the families time to work through this transition together by negotiating how the children would refer to their parents, working with the schools to prevent bullying, and being transparent about the process (Hines, 2006). As a result, the transgender parents were able to maintain the parent-child bonds, and as with LGB parents, the disclosure appears to have improved some of these relationships.

Downing (2013) took a different approach and explored some of the experiences that transgender parents may go through. For instance, the preconceived and often heteronormative (and cisgendernormative) beliefs about what constitutes as a family do not apply to transgender households.

The binary assumptions about being a mother or father may not be true for transgender parents, not to mention the gender roles and norms have started to diversify among postmodern parents in general. According to Downing (2013), children of transgender parents may share similar experiences as children of LGB parents in that they may feel pressure to take on traditional gender roles to prove the aptness of their parents, they too have a coming-out process, and they may experience stigma. As with LGB individuals, the psychological well-being of transgender parents is related to their family relationships.

Due to the paucity of literature about transgender parents and their children, additional research is needed. To begin with, qualitative studies addressing how families negotiate and work through the transition process are especially important. Rather than focusing on how children of transgender parents differ from children of heterosexual parents, it will be more important to understand how these families can succeed. In addition, since transgender is an umbrella term that groups individuals with diverse gender identities and expressions together, it will be important to learn about the heterogeneity among transgender families as well as their unique needs. For instance, children of a transitioning parent will have different experiences and needs compared to children of genderqueer parents.

INFLUENCE OF CULTURE ON LGBT FAMILIES

Strategies for managing stigma, parenting, the family's adjustment, culture, and religion are among some of the issues that LGBT families face. Indeed, many families, regardless of sexual orientation and gender identity, face these same issues—but researchers have started to investigate the influence of heterosexism and homonegativity in society on LGBT individuals as well as their families. And more recently, scholars have started to examine how race, ethnicity, and religion impact not only LGBT individuals (Buchanan, Dzelme, & Hecker, 2001; Greene, 1997; Lease, Horse, & Noffsinger-Frazier, 2005) but also the parent-child relationships of children with LGBT parent(s) (Lytle et al., 2013).

Lease and Shulman (2005), offer a foundation for further exploration of this topic by providing insight as to how family members of gay and lesbian individuals use religion to either assist or obstruct their relationships with their gay or lesbian relatives. Later on, Lytle and colleagues (2013) explored the influence of religion on the parent-child relationships adult children with a gay or lesbian parent as well as a heterosexual parent and found that although some individuals may need to reevaluate their religiosity as they accept or reject their gay or lesbian parents, some individuals are able to negotiate having an affirming relationship with their gay or lesbian parent and a religious identity. Indeed, the adult children interviewed for this study described how family breakups were more difficult than the parents' coming out, how they discovered that parent was gay or lesbian, the initial shame they felt over having a gay or lesbian parent, positive aspects of having a gay or lesbian parent, how they redefined a relationship with religion, and the impact of culture on how gay and lesbian individuals are viewed.

In order to understand the cultural context that may impact the parent-child relationships of adult children with LGBT parents, it is necessary to consider how religious and ethnic groups perceive LGBT individuals. For instance, individuals from Christian, Jewish, Muslim, and Hindu denominations all report prejudice toward LGBT individuals, especially among fundamental and conservative sects (Hunsberger, 1996). However, adherents to various Christian and Jewish denominations varied in how they viewed LGBT individuals (Pew Forum on Religion, 2007). Hence, both religious identity and religiosity may influence the parent-child relationships of children with an LGBT parent. Moreover, family support, religious morals, connectedness to ethnic community, and acculturation are all factors that not only impact the disclosure or LGBT individuals but could also affect how children bond with their gay or lesbian parent. Lastly, the homonegative messages in society supported by religiously-based prejudice and legal discrimination must be considered when researching these parent-child relationships.

POLICIES THAT IMPACT LGBT FAMILIES

Heterosexism and cisgenderism have impacted the family relationships of LGBT individuals. For example, judicial decisions regarding children of LGBT parents used to be based on the stereotypes that LGBT parents were unfit (Patterson, 2000). However, research has demonstrated that LGBT parents are as suitable as heterosexual parents and that children with LGBT parents do not differ from children of heterosexual parents in regard to self-esteem, gender identity, sexual orientation, intelligence, behavioral problems, psychological development, developing peer relationships, or developing romantic relationships (COLAGE, n.d.; Patterson, 2005). Since there is no empirical support for these legal decisions, a number of professional organizations have fought against this legalized discrimination toward LGBT families. For example, the American Psychological Association offered an amicus curiae brief in 2008 for *Varnum v. Brien* (Docket No. 07-1499) that stated the advantages of marriage equality for children of LGBT parents included custodial stability, providing family resources (e.g., health care), and their stigma would be reduced through recognition of their families.

However, LGBT individuals continue to have limited rights in regard to protection against discrimination, adoption, custody, hospital visitation, marriage, and housing, among other areas (HRC, 2013c). Although the Supreme Court ruled that the Defense of Marriage Act (DOMA), a law that used to deny federal benefits to individuals in same-sex marriages, was unconstitutional, LGBT individuals were not guaranteed marriage equality until *Obergefell v. Hodges* made bans on same-sex marriage unconstitutional (Supreme Court, 2015). Further, some states have used a parent's sexual orientation to deny or limit custody and visitations, and many have restricted custody or visitation if a parent's sexual orientation is a perceived as harmful to the children (Maxwell & Donner, 2006). Currently, nondiscrimination laws for transgender and same-sex parents (e.g., both parents simultaneously adopt a child and are recognized as legal parents) is only allowed in nine states as well as the District of Columbia, with four more states protecting the adoption rights for same-sex couples (HRC, 2016). According to Maxwell and Donner (2006), until 2000 it was not uncommon for courts to assume that LGBT parents were unfit and made such rulings as allowing visitation only on the condition that children would not find out about their parent's sexual orientation, prohibiting visitation while the same-sex partner was present, restricting such activities as attending a gay-affirming church, and using supervised visitation to further limit children's involvement in the LGBT community. However, as previously noted, restrictions such as forcing a parent to hide their sexual orientation tend to have negative consequences on the parent-child relationship (Armesto, 2002), and the same may be true when transgender parents attempt to hide their gender identity.

LGBT parents' ability to provide a stable home may be impacted by housing discrimination and other forms of discrimination (e.g., employment). According to the HRC (2016), only 20 states as well as the District of Columbia protect LGBT individuals from housing discrimination, and two more states protect LGB individuals from housing discrimination. In addition, only 16 states as well as the District of Columbia protect LGBT individuals from hate crimes (HRC, 2016), and another 14 states protect LGB individuals from bias crimes. While the Equal Employment Opportunity Commission recently amended its regulations to protect gender identity from discrimination in employment, LGB individuals can be fired based on their sexual orientation in more than half of all states. While the DOMA and *Obergefell v. Hodges* rulings are a step toward providing LGBT families more rights, a lot more work needs to be done to end legalized discrimination.

IMPLICATIONS FOR PRACTICE

LGBT individuals and their families face a number of health disparities. Although the DOMA and *Obergefell v. Hodges* rulings may alleviate barriers in some states, the fact is that most LGBT families do not have equal access to health care due to exclusions in insurance plans; because coparents may not have legal rights to make health care decisions; and because of bias in the health care system and health disparities that are exacerbated by cultural factors (Movement Advancement Project, Family Equality Council, & Center for American Progress, 2012b). For instance, LGBT families of color may experience additional health disparities associated with their ethnic backgrounds. According to Movement Advancement Project (MAP), Family Equality Council (FEC), and Center for American Progress (CAP) (2012a), higher proportions of ethnically diverse LGBT individuals reported that they were parents, regardless of the pathway to parenthood. However, LGBT families of color tend to live in poverty in higher proportions compared to both white LGBT families and families with heterosexual, cisgender parents (MAP, FEC, & CAP, 2012a). And just as LGBT individuals are at risk of stigma based on multiple minority statuses, LGBT families of color may experience homonegativity and/or transnegativity in addition to racism. Therefore, it is important for providers to recognize the potential barriers that their LGBT patients may face. If appropriate, it may be helpful to connect these families with a social worker who may be able to help them navigate the health care system and, when necessary, connect them to services. However, these families will benefit the most from an LGBT-affirming social worker who is aware of the aforementioned legal barriers these families may face.

In addition to the obvious barriers to health, MAP, FEC, and CAP (2011) provide a list of safety net programs that do not provide the same level of support to LGBT families. Now that DOMA and state-level bans on same-sex marriage have been deemed unconstitutional, many of the following programs will change, but the disproportionate levels of support will continue in most states due to the state-by-state definitions of family. Therefore, aside from TANF and FMLA, Medicaid, children's health insurance programs, supplemental security income, child care, and early-education assistance programs, among other services, do not provide equal assistance to LGBT families since they only consider legal parents as family members. Hence, LGBT families may not receive such safety net programs such as health care, income, and prevention programs. What practitioners can do is stay informed about how the laws and policies in their states impact LGBT families and advocate for change. Moreover, providers can make recommendations based on the programs available to LGBT families rather than making the assumption that LGBT families are eligible for services.

As previously mentioned, most states do not protect LGBT parents from discrimination in terms of second-parent and joint adoptions. When coparents are not allowed to become legal parents, they may not have hospital visitation rights or the right to make health care decisions for their partners or children (MAP, FEC, & CAP, 2011). In 2010, the Obama administration took an important step toward giving LGBT families equal treatment and requested that hospitals allow patients to designate visitors and decision makers. Although hospitals are expected to follow these guidelines, they may expect to receive these designations in writing, and they usually do not apply to medical decisions for children since minors do not have the right to legally designate a decision maker (MAP, FEC, & CAP, 2011). Therefore, providers can help LGBT families navigate the system by making these designations in advance.

Aside from overcoming the negative impact of legalized discrimination, providers should be aware of how their own biases may impact LGBT families. Chapman, Wardrop, Freeman, Zappia, Watkins, and Shields (2011) used qualitative methods to learn about how the health care decisions that LGBT parents make for their children are based on their own personal experiences with stigma and discrimination. For example, providers may not receive training in how to respectfully inquire about which individuals are the biological parents of the children, let alone how to interact with the parents in a culturally competent manner (Chapman et al., 2011). One way that practitioners could address this concern is to revise the intake forms to inquire about parents rather than mothers and fathers; the form could also be used to determine which individuals are the biological parents and, if applicable, ask about how to address each parent (e.g., preferred names and pronouns). In addition, providers can not only show their willingness to become agents of change by making their offices more inclusive, but they can also show their support by attending local LGBT meetings and trainings.

CONCLUSIONS

Families are becoming increasingly diverse and have unique needs depending on social and cultural factors. Over the years, more LGBT individuals are choosing parenthood, and just like any other parents, they want the best for their children. Although additional research is needed to better understand the needs of LGBT families, there are many things providers can do to offer optimal health care. To begin with, it is important that health care professionals learn about LGBT families, recognize their own biases, and identify local resources to support LGBT families. Although there are a number of laws and policies that exacerbate the health disparities these families often face, there are a number organizations that can help LGBT individuals overcome these obstacles.

RESOURCES

Adopt US Kids
    ◆ http://www.adoptuskids.org/for-families/who-can-foster-and-adopt /adoption-laws-and-resources-for-lgbt-families
American Psychological Association
    ◆ http://www.apa.org/pi/lgbt/resources/marriage-and-family.aspx

Centers for Disease Control and Prevention
- ◆ http://www.cdc.gov/lgbthealth/youth-resources.htm

Children of Lesbians and Gays Everywhere (COLAGE)
- ◆ http://www.colage.org/resources/

Family Equality Council
- ◆ http://www.familyequality.org

Fenway Health: LGBT Family and Parenting Services
- ◆ https://fenwayhealth.org/care/wellness-resources/lgbt-family-services/

GLAAD
- ◆ http://www.glaad.org/resources

Human Rights Campaign
- ◆ https://www.hrc.org/explore/topic/all-children-all-families
- ◆ http://www.hrc.org/resources/category/marriage
- ◆ http://www.hrc.org/resources/category/parenting
- ◆ https://www.hrc.org/hei/lgbtq-inclusive-definitions-of-family
- ◆ http://www.hrc.org/resources/entry/maps-of-state-laws-policies

Parents, Families, and Friends of Lesbians and Gays (PFLAG)
- ◆ www.pflag.org

REFERENCES

Adopt US Kids. (2013). Adoption laws and resources for lesbian, gay, bisexual, and transgender (LGBT) families. Retrieved from http://www.adoptuskids.org /for-families/who-can-foster-and-adopt/adoption-laws-and-resources -for-lgbt-families

American Fertility Association. (2013). LGBT family building. Retrieved from http://www.theafa.org/family-building/lgbt-family-building/

American Psychological Association. (2013). Marriage and family issues for LGBT people: Resources. Retrieved from http://www.apa.org/pi/lgbt/resources /marriage-and-family.aspx

Armesto, J. C. (2002). Developmental and contextual factors that influence gay fathers' parental competence: A review of the literature. *Psychology of Men and Masculinity, 3*(2), 67–78.

Barrett, H., & Tasker, F. (2001) Growing up with a gay parent: Views of 101 gay fathers on their sons' and daughters experiences. *Educational and Child Psychology, 18*, 62–77.

Beeler, J., & DiProva, V. (1999). Family adjustment following disclosure of homosexuality by a member: Themes discerned in narrative accounts. *Journal of Marriage and Family Therapy, 25*(4), 443–459.

Bergman, K., Rubio, R. J., Green, R. J., & Padrón, E. (2010). Gay men who become fathers via surrogacy: The transition to parenthood. *Journal of GLBT Family Studies, 6*(2), 111–141.

Berkowitz, D., & Marsiglio, W. (2007). Gay men: Negotiating procreative, father, and family identities. *Journal of Marriage and Family, 69*(2), 366–381.

Bigner, J. J. (1996). Working with gay fathers: Developmental, postdivorce parenting and therapeutic issues. In J. Laird & R. J. Green (Eds.), *Lesbians and gays in couples and families: A handbook for therapists* (pp. 370–403). San Francisco: Jossey-Bass.

Bigner, J. J., & Jacobsen, R. B. (1989). Parenting behaviors of homosexual and heterosexual fathers. In F. W. Bozett (Ed.), *Homosexuality and the family* (pp. 173–186). Binghamton, NY: Haworth Press.

Bos, H. (2013). Lesbian-mother families formed through donor insemination. In A. E. Goldberg & K. R. Allen (Eds.), *LGBT-parent families: Innovations in research and implications for practice* (pp. 21–37). New York: Springer.

Bos, H. M. W., van Balen, F., & van den Boom, D. C. (2003). Planned lesbian families: Their desire and motivation to have children. *Human Reproduction, 18*(10), 2216–2224.

Bozett, F. W. (1980). Gay fathers: How and why they disclose their homosexuality to their children. *Family Relations, 29*(2), 173–179.

Buchanan, M., Dzelme, K., & Hecker, L. (2001). Challenges of being simultaneously gay or lesbian and spiritual and/or religious: A narrative perspective. *The American Journal of Family Therapy, 29*, 435–449.

Centers for Disease Control and Prevention. (2013). Lesbian, gay, bisexual, and transgender health. Retrieved from http://www.cdc.gov/lgbthealth/youth-resources.htm

Chapman, R., Wardrop, J., Freeman, P., Zappia, T., Watkins, R., & Shields, L. (2012). A descriptive study of the experiences of lesbian, gay and transgender parents accessing health services for their children. *Journal of Clinical Nursing, 21*(7–8), 1128–1135.

Children of Lesbians and Gays Everywhere. (n.d.a). *Facts about kids with LGBT parents.* Retrieved from http://www.colage.org/resources/facts.htm

Children of Lesbians and Gays Everywhere. (n.d.b.). Resources. Retrieved from http://www.colage.org/resources/

Downing, J. B. (2013). Transgender-parent families. In A.E. Goldberg & K. R. Allen (Eds.), *LGBT-parent families: Innovations in research and implications for practice* (pp. 105–115). New York: Springer.

Epstein, N. B., Baldwin, L. M., & Bishop, D. S. (1983). The McMaster family assessment device. *Journal of Marital and Family Therapy, 9*, 171–180.

Family Equality Council. (2013a). Family equality. Retrieved from http://www.familyequality.org

Family Equality Council. (2013b). Parent resources. Retrieved from http://www.familyequality.org/get_informed/parent_resources/

Fassinger, R. E., & Arseneau, J. R. (2007). "I'd rather get wet than be under that umbrella": Differentiating the experiences and identities of lesbian, gay, bisexual, and transgender people. In K. J. Bieschke, R. M. Perez, & K. A. Debord (Eds.), *Handbook of counseling and psychotherapy with lesbian, gay, bisexual, and transgender clients* (pp. 19–49). Washington, DC: American Psychological Association.

Fenway Health. (n.d.). Fenway health: LGBT family and parenting services. Retrieved August 7, 2013, from http://www.fenwayhealth.org/site/PageServer?pagename=FCHC_srv_services_LGBT

Garner, A. (2004). *Families like mine: Children of gay parents tell it like it is.* New York: Harper Collins.

GLADD. (n.d.). Resources and programs. Retrieved August 7, 2013, from http://www.glaad.org/resources

Goldberg, A. E. (2007). (How) does it make a difference? Perspectives of adults with lesbian, gay, and bisexual parents. *American Journal of Orthopsychiatry, 77*(4), 550–562.

Goldberg, A. E., Kashy, D. A., & Smith, J. Z. (2012). Gender-typed play behavior in early childhood: Adopted children with lesbian, gay, and heterosexual parents. *Sex roles, 67*(9–10), 503–515.

Golombok, S., & Badger, S. (2010). Children raised in mother-headed families from infancy: A follow-up of children of lesbian and single heterosexual mothers, at early adulthood. *Human Reproduction, 25*(1), 150–157.

Greene, B. (1997). Ethnic minority lesbians and gay men: Mental health and treatment issues. In B. Greene (Ed.), *Psychological perspectives on lesbian and gay issues: Vol. 3. Ethnic and cultural diversity among lesbians and gay men* (pp. 216–239). Thousand Oaks, CA: Sage.

Hines, S. (2006). Intimate transitions: Transgender practices of partnering and parenting. *Sociology, 40*(2), 353–371.

Human Rights Campaign. (2013a). All children—all families: About the initiative. Retrieved from http://www.hrc.org/resources/entry/all-children-all-families -about-the-initiative

Human Rights Campaign. (2013b). LGBT—inclusive definitions of family. Retrieved from http://www.hrc.org/resources/entry/lgbt-inclusive-definitions-of -family

Human Rights Campaign. (2013c). Maps of state laws and policies. Retrieved from http://www.hrc.org/resources/entry/maps-of-state-laws-policies

Human Rights Campaign. (2013d). Resources: DOMA: Get the facts. Retrieved from http://www.hrc.org/resources/entry/doma-get-the-facts

Human Rights Campaign. (2013e). Resources: Marriage. Retrieved from http:// www.hrc.org/resources/category/marriage

Human Rights Campaign. (2013f). Resources: Parenting. Retrieved from http:// www.hrc.org/resources/category/parenting

Human Rights Campaign. (2016). Maps of state laws and policies. Retrieved from http://www.hrc.org/state_maps

Hunsberger, B. (1996). Religious fundamentalism, right-wing authoritarianism, and hostility toward homosexuals in non-Christian religious groups. *The International Journal for the Psychology of Religion, 6*(1), 39–49.

Kelley, D. L., & Sequeira, D. L. (1997). Understanding family functioning in a changing America. *Communication Studies, 48,* 93–108.

Laumann-Billings, L., & Emery, R. (2000). Distress among young adults from divorced families. *Journal of Family Psychology, 14*(4), 671–687.

Lease, S. H., Horse, S. G., & Noffsinger-Frazier, N. (2005). Affirming faith experiences and psychological health for Caucasian lesbian, gay, and bisexual individual. *Journal of Counseling Psychology, 52*(3), 378–388.

Lease, S. H., & Shulman, J. L. (2003). A preliminary investigation of the role of religion for family members of lesbian, gay male, and bisexual male and female individuals. *Counseling and Values, 47*(3), 195–209.

Lytle, M. C., Foley, P. F., & Aster, A. M. (2013). Adult children of gay and lesbian parents Religion and the parent-child relationship. *The Counseling Psychologist, 41*(4), 530–567.

Maxwell, N. G., & Donner, R. (2006). Psychological consequences of judicially imposed closets in child custody and visitation disputes involving gay and lesbian parents. *William & Mary Journal of Women and the Law, 13*(1), 305–348.

Merighi, J. R., & Grimes, M. D. (2000). Coming out to families in a multicultural context. *Families in Society, 81*(1), 32–41.

Mortimer, J. T. (1984). Commentary: Psychological and sociological perspectives on parent-child relations. In M. Perlmutter (Ed.), *Parent-child interaction and parent-child relations in child development* (pp. 150–166). Hillside, NJ: Lawrence Erlbaum Associates.

Movement Advancement Project, Family Equality Council, & Center for American Progress. (2011). All children matter: How legal and social inequalities hurt LGBT families. Retrieved from http://www.lgbtmap.org/file/all-children -matter-full-report.pdf

Movement Advancement Project, Family Equality Council, & Center for American Progress. (2012a). LGBT families of color: Facts at a glance. Retrieved from http://www.lgbtmap.org/policy-and-issue-analysis/lgbt-families-of -color-facts-at-a-glance

Movement Advancement Project, Family Equality Council, & Center for American Progress. (2012b). Obstacles and opportunities: ensuring health and wellness for LGBT families. Retrieved from http://action.familyequality.org /site/DocServer/LGBTFamiliesHealthandWellnessBriefFinal03222012.pdf

Murray, P., & McClintock, K. (2005). Children of the closet: A measurement of the anxiety and self-esteem of children raised by a non-disclosed homosexual or bisexual parent. *Journal of Homosexuality, 49*(1), 77–95. doi:10.1300 /J082v49n01

Obama, B. (2010). Presidential memorandum—Hospital visitation. Retrieved from http://www.whitehouse.gov/the-press-office/presidential-memorandum -hospital-visitation

Pallotta-Chiarolli, M., Haydon, P., & Hunter, A. (2013). "These are our children": Polyamorous parenting. In A. E. Goldberg & K. R. Allen (Eds.), *LGBT-parent families: Innovations in research and implications for practice* (pp. 117–131). New York: Springer.

Parker, G., & Gladstone, G. L. (1996). Parental characteristics as influences on adjustment in adulthood. In G. R. Pierce, B. R. Sarason, & I. G. Sarason (Eds.), *Handbook of social support and the family* (pp. 195–218). New York: Plenum Press.

Patterson, C. J. (2000). Family relationships of lesbians and gay men. *Journal of Marriage and the Family, 64*(4), 1052–1069.

Patterson, C. J. (2001). Families of the lesbian baby boom. *Journal of Gay & Lesbian Psychotherapy, 4*, 91–107.

Patterson. C. J. (2005). *APA public interest directorate: Lesbian & gay parenting.* American Psychological Association. Retrieved November 30, 2007, from http://www.apa.org/pi/parent.html.

Patterson, C. J. (2006). Children of lesbian and gay parents. *Current Directions in Psychological Science, 15*(5), 241–244.

Patterson, C. J., & Tornello, S. L. (2010). Gay fathers' pathways to parenthood: International perspectives. *Zeitschrift für Familienforschung—Journal of Family Research—Sonderheft, 5,* 103–116.

Pew Forum on Religion. (2007). Views about homosexuality by religious tradition. Retrieved from http://religions.pewforum.org/pdf/table-views-about-homo sexuality-by-religious-tradition.pdf

Riggle, E. D., Rostosky, S. S., McCants, L. E., & Pascale-Hague, D. (2011). The positive aspects of a transgender self-identification. *Psychology & Sexuality, 2*(2), 147–158.

Riggle, E. D., Whitman, J. S., Olson, A., Rostosky, S. S., & Strong, S. (2008). The positive aspects of being a lesbian or gay man. *Professional Psychology: Research and Practice, 39*(2), 210.

Ross, L. E., & Dobinson, C. (2013). Where is the "B" in LGBT parenting? A call for research on bisexual parenting. In A. E. Goldberg & K. R. Allen (Eds.), *LGBT-parent families: Innovations in research and implications for practice* (pp. 87–103). New York: Springer.

Rostosky, S. S., Riggle, E. D., Pascale-Hague, D., & McCants, L. E. (2010). The positive aspects of a bisexual self-identification. *Psychology & Sexuality, 1*(2), 131–144.

Supreme Court of the United States. (2015). Obergefell et al. v. Hodges, director, Ohio Department of Health, et al. Retrieved from http://www.supremecourt .gov/opinions/14pdf/14-556_3204.pdf

Tasker, F. (2010). Same-sex parenting and child development: Reviewing the contribution of parental gender. *Journal of Marriage and Family, 72*(1), 35–40.

Tasker, F. L., & Golombok, S. (1995). Adults raised as children in lesbian families. *The American Journal of Orthopsychiatry, 65,* 203–215.

Tornello, S. L., & Patterson, C. J. (2012). Gay fathers in mixed-orientation relationships: Experiences of those who stay in their marriages and of those who leave. *Journal of GLBT Family Studies, 8*(1), 85–98.

van Gelderen, L., Bos, H. M., Gartrell, N., Hermanns, J., & Perrin, E. C. (2012). Quality of life of adolescents raised from birth by lesbian mothers: The US National Longitudinal Family Study. *Journal of Developmental & Behavioral Pediatrics, 33*(1), 17–23.

Van Voorhis, R., & McClain, L. (1997). Accepting a lesbian mother. *Families in Society, 78*(6), 642–650.

Varnum v. Brien, No. 07-1499 (S.C. Iowa April 3, 2009).

Weinberg, M. S., Williams, C. J., & Pryor, D. W. (2001). Bisexuals at midlife: Commitment, salience, and identity. *Journal of Contemporary Ethnography, 30*(2), 180–208.

Weiss, R. S. (1991). The attachment bond in childhood and adulthood. In C. M. Parkes, J. Stevenson-Hinde, & P. Marris (Eds.), *Attachment across the life cycle* (pp. 66–76). New York: Routledge.

Wyers, N. L. (1987). Homosexuality in the family: Lesbian and gay spouses. *Journal of the National Association of Social Workers, 32*(2), 143–148.

8

Preventive Health for Gay, Bisexual, and Queer Men

Russell G. Buhr and Tri D. Do

The field of preventive medicine focuses on disease prevention and harm reduction. Prevention is often split into categories: *primary prevention* focuses on health practices to improve health and reduce risk of contracting a disease; *secondary prevention* focuses on early detection of a disease, or *screening*, and aims to catch disease before complications arise to allow for early intervention; while *tertiary prevention* focuses on reducing harm from an already-manifested disease. Some of these efforts fall within the sphere of public health and address environmental, community, and systemic factors that may influence health outcomes. Much of preventive medicine, however, focuses on disease prevention and early detection of disease on an individual level, which is the primary focus of this chapter.

Recommendations for preventive medicine come from a number of sources. The United States Preventive Services Taskforce (USPSTF) is a government body that convenes groups of experts to produce *evidence-based guidelines*, or sets of recommendations for health care practitioners based on the available data from medical trials and consensus opinions from experts in particular fields (Agency for Healthcare Research and Quality, 2014; Office of Disease Prevention and Health Promotion, 2014). The USPSTF produces guidelines on many topics, from cancer and cardiovascular screening to immunization for different populations. Men who have sex with men (MSM)* are a special population, and as such, there are often not thorough studies about this population available to formulate a rigorous guideline on particular topics. As a result, the USPSTF may not have specific recommendations, and other bodies, such as an academic medical society in a particular field, or in this case, the Gay and Lesbian Medical Association (GLMA), help guide best practices with a combination of medical science and expert opinions on a topic.

This chapter will focus on preventive medicine practices for MSM, focusing on those assigned male at birth. A separate chapter in this book specifically addresses the health care needs of transgender people. We should state that we will also discuss some topics pertinent to men in general, regardless of their sexual practices, but will focus on how MSM may be faced with special circumstances that alter their risk. The main objectives are to introduce the concept of MSM as a population with special preventive health needs, provide an overview of topics that MSM and those who provide care to them should be aware of, and go into more depth in areas not otherwise covered elsewhere in this book.

GAY AND BISEXUAL MEN: A POPULATION OF SPECIAL NEEDS AND RISKS

The differences in health needs and outcomes in MSM have been widely studied and occur as a function of many factors (Cochran & Mays, 2015; Conron, Mimiaga, & Landers, 2010; Fredriksen-Goldsen et al., 2013). One major factor is *structural homophobia*, defined as a tacit undercurrent of discrimination against the LGBT community, including MSM, that influences the way these men experience social institutions. The AIDS crisis in the 1980s provides an example of structural homophobia in that the Reagan administration failed to recognize and act on the growing number of cases of newly discovered HIV. Dismissed largely as a disease of gay men and a result of promiscuity, several years of inaction passed before Surgeon General C. Everett Koop directed the National Public Health Service to send information about AIDS and its prevention to every household in the United States. In the last decade, efforts toward inclusion and health promotion for the LGBT community have increased multifold, but there are still many areas where this community experiences health disparities on a

---

* We will use "men who have sex with men" (MSM) throughout the chapter, which is a preferred medical designation. This is intended to include gay, bisexual, questioning, and heterosexual-identified men who engage in sexual behavior with other men.

regular basis (Altman et al., 2012). Everyday occurrences of discrimination are called "micro trauma" and can affect self-care and health care–seeking behaviors. Discriminatory environments can impose stress and lead to both physical and mental manifestations of stress, which will be discussed in greater detail later in this chapter (Hatzenbuehler, Slopen, & McLaughlin, 2014; Mays & Cochran, 2001; Meyer, 2003).

The Affordable Care and Patient Protection Act of 2010, known colloquially as "Obamacare," set minimum standards for basic health insurance coverage and out-of-pocket spending limits on preventive health care services and screening and will hopefully lead to improved health outcomes through increased prevention. *Obergefell v. Hodges*, the 2015 landmark Supreme Court case that effectively legalized same-sex marriage across all 50 states, is expected to reduce some of the disparity in obtaining health insurance and access to care. While circumstances are improving, LGBT persons remain at higher risk of not having health insurance or access to affordable and reliable healthcare (Knight & Jarrett, 2015).

Men who have sex with men also have unique health risks as a result of *health behaviors*, individual practices that influence health. The sexual practices of MSM may expose them to different patterns of infectious diseases than heterosexuals. Disparate rates of noninfectious diseases such as cardiovascular disease and certain types of cancers have also been documented. Lack of a relationship with a primary care provider can amplify this through lower rates of screening and other preventive services like vaccinations that would normally be offered during primary care visits. The influence of discrimination and fear of victimization has been shown to both increase risky health behaviors and reduce protective behaviors like seeking preventive services (Garofalo et al., 1998). Often, a type of prevention called "harm reduction" can be used when it is not possible to entirely remove the risks a person faces. For example, people who use recreational drugs may not be able to quit but can take steps such as using clean needles, setting limits on their use, or using a buddy system to reduce the harm that might happen during drug use.

In addition, there are influences called social ecological factors that change the occurrence of diseases among subgroups of MSM, even when health behaviors are similar. For example, among African American MSM, the rate of HIV is much higher than other racial groups even though rates of unprotected sex are relatively low. This is due to the high background rate of HIV within black men's sexual networks. It is also well-established that the norms and values of one's social networks affect one's sense of health (Millett et al., 2006).

This leads to an important third factor in outcomes: a differential in the quality of care received as a result of *cultural competence*. While training of medical school graduates has more recently included dedicated instruction on LGBT cultural issues, disparities, and risk factors, many practicing physicians have not either received or retained this type of training (Obedin-Maliver et al., 2011). Similarly, nursing and physician assistant training programs generally have little LGBT health content (Lim, Brown, & Jones, 2013; Seaborne, Prince, & Kushner, 2015). Professional societies such as GLMA, the American Medical Student Association (AMSA), and the American Public Health Association (APHA), among others, have helped craft guidelines to train and provide a framework for practitioners working with LGBT populations (Dean et al., 2000; Gay and Lesbian Medical Association, 2006). Establishing care with a primary care provider who is aware of the unique issues that MSM face is important and allows for frank discussions on sensitive topics such as health behaviors. In general, young men are less likely to have a usual source of primary care than others, and this likely is even more the case for MSM, who may defer seeking care due to difficulty finding a provider with whom they are comfortable. GLMA has published a guide developed by LGBT health experts and available online that outlines the top 10 things that men who have sex with other men should discuss with their primary care provider (Silenzio, 2002).

SEXUAL HEALTH: SCREENING AND PREVENTING SEXUALLY TRANSMITTED INFECTIONS AND HIV

Perhaps the most obvious way that the health needs of MSM differ from the general population is related to their sexual practices. Sexual health involves more than just sexually transmitted infections (STIs), and other chapters in this text will cover these elements in more detail than this overview. With regard to STIs, this chapter will focus on the primary methods of preventing sexually transmitted illnesses. Knowledge of one's own health issues—including HIV/STI status and having frank conversations with sexual partners—is a crucial component of managing sexual health.

Primary Prevention: Reducing Risk of Disease Transmission

While the landscape of HIV prevention in particular is changing with the advent of *pre-exposure prophylaxis* (PrEP), barrier precautions, such as condoms, remain the primary method of preventing its transmission. Consistent condom use with every sexual encounter and partner has been shown to be highly effective at reducing the risk of transmission of STIs including HIV (Centers for Disease Control and Prevention, 2016b). Regular condom use among MSM has been shown on average to be less than that of heterosexual couples, with increased rates of HIV transmission among those who use them inconsistently (Smith et al., 2015).

Condoms should be put on before penetration occurs and remain in use for the duration of intercourse for the most effective protection. Doubling up condoms provides no extra protection and can actually increase risk of rupture due to excess friction. A condom of appropriate size should be selected, and it should fit snugly. Condoms should be inspected for damage, holes, packaging defects, and expiration date for best results. Use of a water- or silicone-based personal lubricant is important both for comfort and to prevent excess friction from damaging the condom. Some personal lubricants are oil based, and these are not safe for use with latex condoms, as the oils can weaken the latex and increase the risk of leaks or tears. After ejaculation, the condom should be removed promptly and discarded to prevent any leaking as the penis becomes soft again. Use of condoms on any shared sex toys and changing them between sharing with others is also important for reducing the transmission of infections related to bodily fluids that may remain on the toys after use.

While condoms provide excellent protection from infections transmitted through semen, including HIV, gonorrhea, chlamydia, and syphilis, they do not cover the entire genital area, and so diseases that can be spread from skin-to-skin contact alone, including pubic lice (also called "crabs"), genital warts, and herpes may be contracted even while wearing condoms. One should pay careful attention to any new rashes, sores, or symptoms such as burning, itching, or discharge and seek prompt medical attention in these cases. Grooming practices undertaken by MSM such as pubic hair removal ("manscaping") have been associated with small cuts and scrapes that may increase risk of contracting STIs (Gaither et al., 2015).

Oral sex is considered to be exceedingly low-to-no risk for transmission of HIV, but syphilis, herpes, HPV, gonorrhea, and chlamydia can all be transmitted this way. Sexually transmitted infections in the throat can also be transmitted to another partner during subsequent oral sex. In addition, oral-anal contact, or *analingus* ("rimming"), can transmit these infections as well as viral hepatitis A, and bacterial and parasitic infections that can cause gastrointestinal distress. Risk can be reduced using barrier precautions (condoms for oral-penile contact and dental dams for rimming), as well as avoiding oral sexual contact if any oral sores or recent dental work has been done and avoiding swallowing bodily fluids, including semen (Saini, Saini, & Sharma, 2010).

Occasionally, condoms may fail, and in these cases, medical attention should be considered, especially when engaging in anal intercourse with a partner whose HIV status is unknown. It is estimated that the transmission rate of HIV infection from unprotected anal sex is less than 1 percent. This risk varies some depending on the exposure, the prevalence rates of

HIV in a given area, the presence of an STI, and whether the exposure is to the insertive ("top") or receptive ("bottom") partner. In cases where exposure to HIV may have occurred due to unprotected sex or condom failure, *post-exposure prophylaxis* (PEP) with anti-HIV medications can reduce the risk of contracting HIV if administered promptly, i.e., within 36 to 72 hours (Landovitz & Currier, 2009). Local LGBT centers and public health clinics are generally well versed in the appropriate post-exposure care and are an excellent resource.

Pre-exposure prophylaxis for HIV has advanced rapidly in the last several years. In 2010, the *New England Journal of Medicine* published the iPrEx trial, which investigated the use of tenofovir plus emtracitabine (TDF/FTC), currently marketed as Truvada, a daily oral medication to reduce the risk of contracting HIV. This groundbreaking study found that daily use of this medication in a study of around 1,200 cisgender men and transgender women who had sex with men resulted in a 45 percent reduction in the rate of contracting HIV across the entire group and a 92 percent reduction in those with high rates of taking the drug daily, with other subsequent studies confirming its effectiveness (Grant et al., 2010).

As a result of these studies, the Centers for Disease Control and Prevention (CDC) have recommended that PrEP be offered to high-risk MSM as one option for reducing their chances of contracting HIV. Because the state of the science around this is changing rapidly, the 2014 guidelines do not necessarily reflect the practices of every individual clinician. In general, per Centers for Disease Control and Prevention guidelines, PrEP is suggested as an option for adult, HIV-negative MSM who are:

- not in a monogamous relationship with another HIV-negative male partner and
- at high risk for HIV, defined as
  - having had any unprotected sex or an STI in the last six months,
  - or having had sexual partners who are HIV-positive (Centers for Disease Control and Prevention, 2014).

While a great advance in the fight against HIV, it should be noted that PrEP may not be the best option for all people, and the decision on when to start and stop use of PrEP should be made after consultation with a primary care provider with familiarity in its use. Daily use of the medication, rather than episodic use, has been shown to be the most effective, and while ongoing clinical trials are investigating on-demand use of PrEP before and after sexual encounters, the current clinical guidelines still recommend daily use (Molina et al., 2015; Centers for Disease Control and Prevention, 2014). Furthermore, studies that have validated the use of PrEP all encouraged routine condom use as part of their protocols, and it warrants reminding that the highest level of protection against HIV includes use of condoms with PrEP. PrEP does not protect against any other STIs besides HIV, and, in one PrEP study, the risk of acquisition of gonorrhea, chlamydia or syphilis was approximately 50 percent (Volk et al., 2015). Because the medication used for PrEP is also used to treat chronic hepatitis B, those taking PrEP who also have hepatitis B should be cautioned to not stop taking the medication. PrEP should also be used with caution in those with underlying kidney disease, as it may worsen kidney function.

Alcohol and substance use during sexual encounters can increase rates of STI transmission, and avoidance or judicious use of anything that can alter consciousness is advised. Drug use during sex (also called "chemsex," "party and play," or "PNP"), is associated with lower rates of health-protective behaviors like use of condoms and increased likelihood of intercourse with unknown or multiple partners. Use of drugs during sex is an independent risk factor for infectious diseases like HIV and viral hepatitis, especially if injected (McCall et al., 2015). The most commonly used drugs include crystallized methamphetamine, cocaine, gamma-hydroxybutyrate (GHB), ketamine ("K"), MDMA ("ecstasy" or "molly"), and amyl nitrate ("poppers") (Hatfield et al., 2009). Furthermore, some of these drugs have noninfectious health risks like stroke, heart attack, and lung damage. Men who use substances, especially during sex, should discuss these practices with their primary care providers in order to better understand the risks associated and how to best reduce them.

Secondary Prevention: Screening

In addition to reducing risk of transmission, preventing illness from sexually transmitted infections relies on *screening*. Routine evaluation and testing for STIs is essential in order to provide treatment and to inform individuals of their risk for transmitting the infections to others. The CDC publishes updates to guidelines describing the types and frequency of testing recommended, and the following are adapted from these guidelines (Centers for Disease Control and Prevention, 2015a).

It is generally recommended that those with one regular sexual partner undergo full screening for HIV and STIs, including syphilis, chlamydia, and gonorrhea, at least annually. Even those in presumed-monogamous relationships should consider annual screening, which offers the opportunity for early recognition and treatment in case assumptions about monogamy are incorrect and one's partner has contracted an infection from another partner. Those who have multiple sexual partners, who are in a *sero-discordant* relationship where one is HIV-negative while the other is HIV-positive, or who are engaging in high-risk sexual behaviors (including unprotected sex, sex work, or sex while using drugs), should undergo screening more frequently, usually every three to six months depending on the level of risk. Those in monogamous relationships may want to consider getting screened at the same time as their partners to discuss their results in order to protect each other.

Screening for syphilis, which has been on the rise among MSM, involves a blood test. Screening for gonorrhea and chlamydia can be done in multiple ways. The most common are a urethral swab or a urine test to look for urethral infection. MSM who have receptive anal intercourse (bottoming) should have a rectal swab as well, as infections can occur there without symptoms and put subsequent partners at risk. Those who engage in oral sex should also have a throat swab to look for oral infection, which, like rectal infections, may be asymptomatic but passed to others. Screening for herpes has not been found to be effective and is generally not recommended. Instead, those with symptoms, including a new rash, itching, or burning should seek medical attention and undergo examination. Providers can use tests or a physical exam to determine whether the cause of the rash is herpes, scabies, pubic lice, or something else. Genital warts are caused by the human papillomavirus (HPV), and new bumps should be evaluated by a qualified provider.

HIV screening may be done through multiple methods, including blood testing and oral swab antibody screening. HIV testing typically consists of two phases, a screening test that looks for antibodies against HIV, which appear within four to six weeks of HIV exposure, and for those with a positive antibody test, a confirmatory test that looks directly in the blood for the virus. The time it takes for the body to generate antibodies after contracting HIV is known as a "window period." During this time, an antibody test may not return positive, but an individual who carries the virus could potentially spread it to others. For this reason, those with a high-risk exposure should notify their care providers in order to inform the type of test that needs to be ordered. Newer combination antibody-antigen tests can reduce the window period to about one month. People suspected of recent exposure even within two weeks can undergo a viral test by a qualified provider to detect acute infection.

INJURY PREVENTION AND VIOLENCE

Accidents and trauma make up a large part of the causes of death and injury in young men, with twice as many men as women dying as a result of injury and violence every year (World Health Organization, 2010). A large proportion of these injuries and deaths are preventable and can be avoided through either careful behavior or use of safety equipment. One study found that gay and bisexual teenage boys were less likely than their heterosexual counterparts to use safety belts when driving (Reisner et al., 2014). The extension of this principle to bicycle and motorcycle helmets, life jackets while boating, and other safety equipment can substantially reduce the likelihood of serious disability or death from traumatic accidents.

Stabbings and shootings at gay pride events and gay nightclubs continue to be a source of physical violence against LGBT individuals. Gay men may be attacked by strangers but are also at increased risk for violence at the hands of partners or family members. Research on intimate partner and domestic violence in MSM has been limited by the difficulty in its definition and lack of large-scale studies to define its prevalence and burden. One large study analyzing over 500 smaller studies showed that rates of intimate partner violence among MSM was as high or higher than among women in heterosexual relationships (Finneran & Stephenson, 2013). Abuse can go beyond physical violence and include intimidation, stalking, financial abuse, and sexual assault. Another review of multiple studies on sexual assault of gay and bisexual men found a staggeringly high rate, where 11.8 to 54 percent had experienced some form of sexual violence during their lives (Rothman, Exner, & Baughman, 2011). Sexual and physical violence may go on without intervention due to shame or stigma by the victim and the relative power differential between the assailants and the victims (DuRant, Krowchuk, & Sinal, 1998; Lampinen et al., 2008). Unique to LGBT people, some abusers will use the threat of disclosure of their victim's sexual orientation to gain power. These issues remain a major public health concern, and expansions to violence and abuse prevention programs are needed. Men in situations of abuse or violence should seek help from their healthcare provider or another trusted source of support.

TOBACCO USE

Exposure to tobacco smoke is the top leading cause of preventable illness in the United States, and MSM have higher rates of tobacco smoking than their heterosexual counterparts (King, Dube, & Tynan, 2012; Lee, Griffin, & Melvin, 2009). Nicotine has a higher addition potential than most if not all other recreationally used drugs, and quitting smoking once one has started is often quite difficult. There is not a "safe" amount of smoking without health risks, and the benefits of quitting on health are nearly immediate. Tobacco smoke has been linked to multiple diseases, including emphysema of the lungs, multiple types of cancer, heart disease, stroke, and accelerated skin aging.

The advent of "vaping" or use of electronic cigarettes recently has been perceived by many people as less dangerous or even completely safe compared to standard cigarettes. Unfortunately, the relatively short time that e-cigarettes have been on the market has meant that long-term studies on damage from inhaling the chemicals that deliver the nicotine in these devices have not yet been carried out. It is important to know that these devices are not regulated either as medical devices (such as a nicotine inhaler for quitting smoking would be) or as tobacco products. Multiple injuries from e-cigarette device fires have been reported. In addition, flavored e-cigarette cartridges and vapor-producing heating coils have been shown to contain harmful chemicals and heavy metals associated with serious and potentially life-threatening lung disease.

ALCOHOL AND SUBSTANCE USE

While these issues will be covered in more detail elsewhere in this book, a brief overview of alcohol and substance use among MSM, which is relatively common, will be provided in this chapter. One large population study of LGB identified adults found that gay and non-gay-identified MSM were between 50 and 100 percent more likely than heterosexual-identified men to be diagnosed with alcohol dependence (Drabble, Midanik, & Trocki, 2005). While the amount of alcohol consumed before feeling drunk varies from person to person for a number of reasons, "moderate drinking" is defined for men as drinking three to four alcoholic beverages on the same occasion on five or more days in the last 30 days (Woody et al., 2001). Drinking more than 4 drinks per day or 14 drinks in one week is defined as high risk for men (National Institute on Alcohol Abuse and Alcoholism, 2016b).

Moderate alcohol use for most people has no serious health consequences, and some light use may even promote cardiovascular health. Heavy and binge drinking, however, are associated with increased risk for trauma, interpersonal and social conflict, and health risks. Alcohol-related illnesses and injuries make up the fourth leading cause of death in the United States, and alcohol is linked to nearly a third of traffic fatalities (National Institute on Alcohol Abuse and Alcoholism, 2016a). Those who are having difficulty controlling the amount of alcohol consumed, find a need to drink outside of social contexts, have feelings of anger, guilt, or anxiety about their drinking, or who have tried and failed to cut down should seek medical attention or counseling.

Drug use and abuse have been found to occur at higher rates among MSM than their heterosexual counterparts, while men in general are more likely than women to have dysfunctional or dependent drug use (Cochran et al., 2004). Men who have sex with men are more likely to use marijuana, cocaine, other sedatives and stimulants, and hallucinogens than other men (Boyd, McCabe, & d'Arcy, 2003; Fendrich et al., 2003; Woody et al., 2001). While no clearly safe levels of recreational drug use are established, some, including injection drug use and methamphetamine use, are high in risk for complications. It is well established that use of such drugs leads to higher rates of unsafe sexual practices and therefore STI and HIV infections (Hatfield et al., 2009). Frank discussions with one's primary care provider are important to best understand one's risk and to recognize problematic drug use.

INFECTION PREVENTION AND VACCINATION

Men who engage in sex with men are at higher risk of certain other communicable diseases, including some that are preventable through vaccination. Decisions about which vaccines to get and how often should be discussed with a healthcare provider, but we provide a general outline here of those recommended by the CDC's Advisory Council on Immunization Practices guidelines, as well as some special considerations for men living with HIV (Kroger et al., 2006).

Hepatitis A virus (HAV) is an infection of the liver that usually causes mild symptoms of nausea, vomiting, diarrhea, fatigue, and jaundice (yellowing of the skin and eyes). While most do recover spontaneously over the course of a few weeks, it can cause serious liver damage and even death in some cases. The virus is spread through oral contact with fecal matter from an infected person, and while worldwide, this is primarily through the handling of food and contaminated water, MSM have been found to be at increased risk, especially if they engage in oral-anal contact (rimming) or oral sex after anal sex (Kahn, 2002). Risk of sexual transmission can be reduced by using barrier precautions like dental dams or condoms. It is also recommended that MSM who engage in these practices be vaccinated for HAV (Centers for Disease Control and Prevention, 2015b).

Hepatitis B virus (HBV) can be transmitted through sexual contact, blood (e.g., transfusions or tattoos) or from mother to child during birth. MSM are at higher risk for contracting HBV sexually, mainly through contact with blood or semen during sex or contact of these fluids with broken skin or mucous membranes. While rare, there have also been cases of transmission via sharing of a toothbrush, razor, or theoretically, sharing sex toys. Hepatitis B results in an asymptomatic infection that clears spontaneously in the majority of cases, but about 5 percent will develop chronic hepatitis, which can lead to cirrhosis of the liver and liver cancer.

Universal HBV vaccination for children and young adults under age 19 began in 1999, so those who fall in this age group may have been vaccinated as children, but it is advised that all MSM consult with their physician regarding the HBV vaccine series to reduce their risk. Those who engage in intravenous drug use are at much higher risk and should both be vaccinated and avoid sharing needles to reduce risk of transmission (Mast et al., 2006). Medication regimens to treat hepatitis B are available, but studies on their effectiveness in clearing infection and who should be treated are not clear-cut, and consultation with an infectious disease or liver disease specialist in these cases is warranted. Based on consultation with GLMA experts, CDC recommends screening all MSM not vaccinated in childhood for chronic active HBV (Centers for Disease Control and Prevention, 2015b).

Post-exposure prophylaxis for HBV is available, and should a known exposure occur (e.g., having unprotected sex with an HBV-positive partner), and the exposed person is either unvaccinated or has an unknown immune status to HBV, prompt medical attention and administration of post-exposure prophylaxis should be considered. HBV-positive persons should use condoms and avoid sharing household items to reduce risk of transmission to their partners, and their partners should be vaccinated and tested to confirm immune status following vaccination.

Those born in certain regions abroad have a higher rate of carrying hepatitis B, mostly transmitted during birth and early childhood. Those from sub-Saharan Africa have the highest rates (greater than 8 percent), while those from Asia, Central and South America, and Central and Eastern Europe also have increased rates (2 to 7 percent) compared to those from North America and Western Europe (Ott et al., 2012). Immigrants from these affected regions should undergo testing and treatment. Those traveling to these regions should take this into consideration, get vaccinated, and avoid high-risk contact with bodily fluids when abroad.

Hepatitis C virus (HCV) is contracted primarily through infected blood, either during needle sharing as part of intravenous drug use or through medical treatments. Many cases have also been reported in which HCV was transmitted through unprotected anal sex, with risk increasing with multiple partners and among those with HCV-positive long-term partners, and highest risk among those already infected with HIV (Yaphe et al., 2012; Wilkin, 2015). Due to higher rate of infection, the CDC has recommended universal screening of those born between 1945 and 1965 at least once (Smith et al., 2012). In addition, those with continued high risk for contracting HCV, including those who have ongoing intravenous drug use, those with HIV, or MSM engaging in high-risk sexual practices as described above, should be screened for HCV infection. The interval to repeat screening has not been well established (Moyer, 2013; Centers for

Disease Control and Prevention, 2015b). Untreated, HCV can progress to cirrhosis, cause liver failure requiring a liver transplant, and increase risk of liver cancer. Coinfection with other viral hepatitis strains or HIV increases the risk of complications. Treatment for HCV is available and has substantially improved over the last several years. Those who have chronic HCV should seek expert consultation from an infectious disease or liver specialist for evaluation.

In the last few years, an increased rate of bacterial meningitis, a severe and life-threatening brain infection due to invasive meningococcal disease, was noted among MSM in the urban areas of New York City and Los Angeles (Wheaton et al., 2013). In general, this disease is rare and found primarily in teenagers and young adults dwelling in close quarters such as college dormitories or military barracks. Vaccination against the disease is universally recommended in children, and a booster dose is a common entry requirement for university students. The reason that MSM had an increased rate of infection is still unclear, but it has led some public health professionals to recommend that MSM, especially if planning travel to a large, urban center, in particular for events like LGBT Pride celebrations, consider vaccination (Simon, Weiss, and Gulick, 2013). There are no formal recommendations in this area, and consideration for vaccinations should be made on an individual basis in consultation with one's primary care provider.

Human papillomavirus (HPV) causes genital warts. Certain high-risk types are also implicated in increased risk for cancers of the throat, penis, and anus. Infection with HPV is very common, and one large study found that 57 percent of HIV-negative MSM had anal infections with HPV, and 26 percent of these were high-risk subtypes with higher risk for development of anal cancer (Chin-Hong et al., 2004). The biggest risk factor for developing HPV was the number of sexual partners in the previous six months. Most cases cleared spontaneously, while others required medical attention, often in the form of freezing warts with liquid nitrogen or application of topical medicines to help clear the infection. Immunization with the HPV vaccine was approved by the Food and Drug Administration for men up to age 26 in the last several years, and recent guidelines recommend its use in MSM including those with HIV (Petrosky et al., 2015). Recommendations did not include those older than 26 due to the likelihood of exposure to HPV and developing immunity through exposure by that age. Consideration for vaccination of older adults may be made on a per-case basis in consultation with one's provider. Immunization has been shown to reduce the rate of anal cancers (Palefsky et al., 2011). Not every subtype of HPV is included in the vaccine, and so it is not a complete guarantee of prevention. Appropriate barrier precautions with condoms and dental dams are still advised for maximum protection (Palefsky et al., 2011).

Additional vaccines are advised for all adults, including annual influenza vaccination (Advisory Committee for Immunization Practices, 2016). While flu deaths primarily affect the elderly and those with weakened immune systems, including those with HIV, even young and healthy adults can die from influenza infection, with about 50,000 people killed each year. The influenza vaccine varies in its effectiveness every year but is quite safe and contains no live flu virus, making it impossible to contract influenza from the vaccine. Unless a medical reason precludes it, annual flu vaccination is recommended for all adults. The tetanus, diphtheria, and pertussis (TDaP) vaccine should also be administered every 10 years as a booster (Broder et al., 2006). The pneumococcal vaccine reduces the risk of one serious type of pneumonia and should be considered in those who have HIV or other chronic medical conditions. It is also recommended for everyone above the age of 65.

CANCER PREVENTION AND SCREENING

Cancers are a leading cause of death among men over the course of a lifetime. While few studies have been directly conducted to look at differential risk for MSM compared to others for all types of cancer, differences have been observed (Boehmer, Cooley, and Clark, 2012; American Cancer Society, 2016) . Some of these differences can be explained through different rates of infections like HIV and HPV that are known to increase risk for development of cancers. We will cover both MSM-specific cancer risks as well as some recommendations for risk reduction and prevention of cancer for men in general.

The strongest evidence for a higher rate of cancer in MSM is for HPV-related anal cancers. Increased numbers of sexual partners increase the risk for acquiring HPV, while HPV vaccination reduces it (Palefsky et al., 2011). Some have recommended a specific test akin to a Pap smear in women, but there is limited information on whether this is truly beneficial and with what frequency the testing should be done. It is recommended that MSM seek medical attention if they notice any rectal symptoms, including pain, bleeding, or bumps or growths in the anus that could signal a problem. The same virus can cause penile cancer, which is overall quite rare. HPV has also been implicated in cancers of the mouth and throat, and if new trouble swallowing or hoarseness develops or progresses without resolution, medical attention is advised. Having HIV increases the risks for both penile and anal cancers.

Testicular cancer is primarily a disease of young men aged 20 to 34, with higher risk among white men and those with a family history, as well as among men with an undescended testicle. While some doctors have recommended monthly self-examinations—feeling the testicle for lumps or bumps—the studies to determine if this actually promotes early detection and therefore early treatment have been mixed. The USPSTF does not continue to recommend self-examination or routine medical examination by a provider to evaluate for testicular cancer, but those who are at potentially higher risk ought to discuss this with their physicians (Lin and Sharangpani, 2010). Any noticeable changes in the scrotum, testicle, or lower abdomen, including heaviness, pain, or a painless hard bump, should trigger concern and warrant medical evaluation.

Prostate cancer is found primarily in men over age 50 and is more prevalent in African Americans than other racial groups. Recommendations about screening have changed around prostate cancer in the last several years. There is a paucity of studies specifically on prostate cancer in MSM, and these gave mixed results as to whether MSM were at higher risk (Simon Rosser et al., 2016). In one bit of good news, one study showed that increased sexual activity, specifically the number of times per week a man ejaculated during young adulthood, was correlated with lower risk of prostate cancer, while contracting a sexually transmitted infection was correlated with higher risk (Dennis & Dawson, 2002; Giles et al., 2003; Leitzmann et al., 2004). In general, routine screening for prostate cancer, which uses a combination of a blood test (prostate surface antigen, or PSA) and a prostate examination, is not recommended for those who are not high risk, although MSM should discuss the risks and benefits of screening with their providers (American Cancer Society, 2015).

Skin cancer occurs at higher rates in MSM, who report higher rates of both indoor and outdoor tanning compared to heterosexual men (Blashill & Safren, 2014). Skin cancers are largely preventable through the use of sunscreen, protective clothing including sunglasses, and judicious exposure to the sun, and sun exposure in young adulthood can lead to long-term consequences. Those with fair skin and blond or red hair are at particularly high risk, as are those with a family history of close relatives with melanoma. Reporting changes in moles, freckles, or birthmarks, as well as a general skin examination for those at higher risk during routine annual physical examinations, can reduce the risk of serious skin cancers (Centers for Disease Control and Prevention, 2016a).

Additional cancer screenings are based primarily on an individual's risk. Colon cancer screening is recommended for all adults starting at age 50, and it can be started at a younger age for those with strong family history. Men can develop breast cancer as well, and those with family history of multiple relatives with breast or ovarian cancers may carry a genetic abnormality that increases their risk. Discussion with one's primary care provider about additional cancer risk reduction strategies and screening needs should be taken up and will vary from person to person (American Cancer Society, 2015).

CARDIOVASCULAR RISK REDUCTION AND SCREENING

Sex and gender differences in cardiovascular disease have been widely studied, and men in general are at higher risk for heart disease, including heart attacks and congestive heart failure, as well as stroke, compared to women (Mosca, Barrett-Connor, & Wenger, 2011). Difference in health status and non-HIV health concerns have also been observed among MSM, at least some of which seem to be correlated with psychological stress experienced by this community. Stress even in youth can affect likelihood of disease later in life (Cochran & Mays, 2007; Hatzenbuehler et al., 2014; Hatzenbuehler, McLaughlin, & Slopen, 2013).

Risk of heart disease, diabetes, and the associated complications increase with age. A healthy lifestyle including regular exercise, a balanced diet, and a reasonable body mass index can help mitigate future problems. At least 150 minutes of vigorous exercise weekly (which often translates to 30 minutes, five times per week) has been shown to promote both a healthy body and reduce risk of these diseases (LeFevre, 2014). As a foundation, a diet high in fruits and vegetables; with a variety of sources of protein; and limited in saturated or trans fats, added sugar, and sodium is recommended (U.S. Department of Health and Human Services & U.S. Department of Agriculture, 2015).

Men are advised to have their cholesterol checked at age 35, or at age 25 for those at increased risk for heart disease, including those with family history of heart or cholesterol disorders, and those who are obese, smoke, or are diabetic (Helfant & Carson, 2008). The interval that screening should be repeated depends on an individual's risk. Occasionally, those with higher risk may be recommended to take low-dose aspirin and/or a class of cholesterol medications called statins in order to reduce risk. Screening for diabetes is recommended at age 40 for all men who are overweight or obese, while those with a family history of diabetes and certain non-white racial and ethnic groups may have higher risk at younger ages and at lower body weights and should be considered for screening earlier (Siu, 2015). Chronic HIV infection increases the risk of diabetes and heart disease as age increases, and closer monitoring and care from a practitioner experienced in HIV management is important (Grinspoon, 2009).

Aging with chronic disease is difficult for everyone, but MSM in particular have been shown to have a harder time, which seems to be multifaceted. Many LGBT people do not have the same level of family and peer support compared to their heterosexual peers, especially in today's older generation, which did not enjoy the same openness many in the community today have. Lack of community services targeted toward LGBT elderly, compounded with societal stigma, perceived homophobia, and lack of cultural competence of health care providers in LGBT health issues can be isolating. These factors make contact with preventive health care services more infrequent and increase the chances of poor health outcomes. Special attention to aging in LGBT communities is important for addressing unique health concerns (Blank et al., 2009; Lipton, 2004).

MENTAL HEALTH BASICS

Mental health issues among LGBT communities are discussed in greater detail in other sections of this book, but we aim to provide a brief overview in this chapter. It is well established that social stigma and structural homophobia increase psychological stress and that rates of depression and anxiety are higher in MSM (Bailey, 1999; Cochran, Sullivan, and Mays, 2003). Feelings of sadness or worthlessness, lack of interest or pleasure in activities, guilt, diminished energy and change in appetite, sexual drive, and sleep can all be indicators of depression and should trigger evaluation by a qualified health care provider. Recognition is often the major barrier to treatment of depression and/or anxiety, and untreated, both can have major consequences. Suicidal thoughts and attempts are known to be higher in MSM than their heterosexual counterparts, especially among adolescents and young adults (Biernbaum and Ruscio, 2004; King et al., 2008; Russell & Joyner, 2001). Friends and loved ones should be aware of changes in mood or behavior and encourage an affected individual to seek help. Resources are available in many communities for those struggling with any of these issues.

Body image is a common problem in MSM, where ideals of a lean, muscular body portrayed in popular culture and pornography help propagate often-unrealistic expectations (Duggan & McCreary, 2004; Yelland & Tiggemann, 2003). Multiple studies have shown an increase in unhealthy eating and exercise behaviors among MSM, including anorexia, bulimia, and overexuberant exercise routines (Lakkis, Ricciardelli, & Williams, 1999; Laska et al., 2015). While maintenance of a healthy weight does help promote cardiovascular health, it is important to observe a balance. Exercises designed to increase muscle mass (weight training) can worsen heart health, whereas cardiovascular exercise reduces the risk for heart disease. In addition, an uptick in use of dietary supplements for weight loss and/or muscle gain has been reported, and it should be noted that most of these supplements are not formally evaluated for safety or effectiveness by the Food and Drug Administration, and as such, there are no guarantees as to their contents. The use of anabolic steroids for muscle mass gain is not uncommon among MSM and can cause significant heart problems. On the other end of the spectrum, those in the bear community who value gaining nonmuscle weight should consider the impact of excess caloric intake on their health. Those struggling with body image issues should seek advice from a health care provider experienced in dealing with these issues.

Sleep is important for both physical and mental health. Young adults need 8 to 10 hours of sleep per night, with the total time decreasing with age. Lack of adequate sleep has been shown to increase cardiovascular disease and is associated with weight gain and obesity (Markwald et al., 2013). *Sleep hygiene* refers to the practices known to promote good-quality sleep. Poor sleep hygiene includes watching television or using computers or other devices in bed. It is best to use the bed for nothing else but sleeping and having sex, and to restrict other activities to outside bed. Eating heavy meals, consuming alcohol, or vigorous exercise right before bed can also make sleep quality worse (UCLA Sleep Disorders Center, 2015). While alcohol helps people feel tired, it inhibits the brain's natural sleep cycle and results in poor-quality sleep (National Institute on Alcohol Abuse and Alcoholism, 1998). Those with chronic difficulty sleeping, especially after making sleep hygiene practice changes, should consult their providers and consider a referral to a sleep medicine specialist for evaluation for other underlying sleep disorders.

CONCLUSION

In this chapter, we have explored basics of prevention in MSM and how risk reduction, screening, and early treatment can decrease the burden of illness. Men who have sex with men are a population with unique health needs, and not all medical practitioners will be familiar with specific recommendations for caring for MSM, so choosing a sensitive and competent provider is important. Homophobia on a societal level continues to affect the health of MSM but is improving with time and progressive health policy. While much of health promotion for LGBT communities is focused on sexual practices and HIV, we have outlined a general overview of issues that men who have sex with men should be aware of in order to best protect their own health. If an ounce of prevention is worth a pound of cure, we at least hope that this overview has been worth the weight of the ink on the page.

REFERENCES

Advisory Committee for Immunization Practices. (2016). *ACIP vaccine recommendations.* Centers for Disease Control and Prevention. Retrieved on April 24 from http://www.cdc.gov/vaccines/hcp/acip-recs/

Agency for Healthcare Research and Quality. (2014). Implementing U.S. Preventive Services Task Force (USPSTF) recommendations. Retrieved from https://www.ahrq.gov/cpi/centers/ockt/kt/tools/impuspstf/impuspstf.html.

Altman, D., Aggleton, P., Williams, M., et al. (2012). Men who have sex with men: Stigma and discrimination. *Lancet, 380*(9839), 439–445. doi:10.1016/S0140-6736(12)60920-9

American Cancer Society. (2015). American Cancer Society guidelines for the early detection of cancer. Retrieved from http://www.cancer.org/Healthy/FindCancerEarly/CancerScreeningGuidelines/american-cancer-society-guidelines-for-the-early-detection-of-cancer

American Cancer Society. (2016). Cancer facts for gay and bisexual men. Retrieved from http://www.cancer.org/healthy/findcancerearly/menshealth/cancer-facts-for-gay-and-bisexual-men

Bailey, J. M. (1999). Homosexuality and mental illness. *Archives of General Psychiatry, 56*(10), 883–884.

Biernbaum, M. A., & Ruscio, M. (2004). Differences between matched heterosexual and non-heterosexual college students on defense mechanisms and psychopathological symptoms. *Journal of Homosexuality, 48*(1), 125–141. doi:10.1300/J082v48n01_06

Blank, T. O., Asencio, M., Descartes, L., et al. (2009). Aging, health, and GLBTQ family and community life. *Journal of GLBT Family Studies, 5*(1–2), 9–34. doi:10.1080/15504280802595238

Blashill, A. J., & Safren, S. A. (2014). Skin cancer risk behaviors among US men: The role of sexual orientation. *American Journal of Public Health, 104*(9),1640–1641. doi:10.2105/AJPH.2014.301993

Boehmer, U., Cooley, T. P., & Clark, M. A. (2012). Cancer and men who have sex with men: A systematic review. *Lancet Oncology, 13*(12), E545–E553. doi:10.1016/S1470-2045(12)70347-9

Boyd, C. J., McCabe, S. E., & D'Arcy, H. (2003). Ecstasy use among college undergraduates: Gender, race and sexual identity. *Journal of Substance Abuse Treatment, 24*(3), 209–215. doi:10.1016/S0740-5472(03)00025-4

Broder, K. R., Cortese, M. M., Iskander, J. K., et al. (2006). Preventing tetanus, diphtheria, and pertussis among adolescents: Use of tetanus toxoid, reduced diphtheria toxoid and acellular pertussis vaccines: Recommendations of the Advisory Committee on Immunization Practices (ACIP). *Morbidity and Mortality Weekly Report: Recommendations and Reports, 55*(RR-3), 1–42.

Centers for Disease Control and Prevention. (2014). *Pre-exposure prophylaxis for the prevention of HIV in the United States: A clinical practice guideline.* Atlanta, GA: Centers for Disease Control and Prevention.

Centers for Disease Control and Prevention. (2015a). Screening recommendations referenced in treatment guidelines and original recommendation sources. Retrieved from http://www.cdc.gov/std/tg2015/screening-recommendations.htm

Centers for Disease Control and Prevention. (2015b). Viral hepatitis and men who have sex with men. Retrieved from http://www.cdc.gov/hepatitis/Populations/msm.htm

Centers for Disease Control and Prevention. (2016a). Cancer and men. Retrieved from http://www.cdc.gov/cancer/dcpc/resources/features/cancerandmen/

Centers for Disease Control and Prevention. (2016b). Condom effectiveness. Retrieved from http://www.cdc.gov/condomeffectiveness/

Chin-Hong, P. V., Vittinghoff, E., Cranston, R. D., et al. (2004). Age-specific prevalence of anal human papillomavirus infection in HIV-negative sexually active men who have sex with men: The explore study. *The Journal of Infectious Diseases, 190*(12), 2070–2076.

Cochran, S. D., Ackerman, D., Mays, V. M., et al. (2004). Prevalence of non-medical drug use and dependence among homosexually active men and women in the US population. *Addiction, 99*(8), 989–998. doi:10.1111/j.1360 -0443.2004.00759.x

Cochran, S. D., & Mays, V. M. (2007). Physical health complaints among lesbians, gay men, and bisexual and homosexually experienced heterosexual individuals: Results from the California Quality of Life Survey. *American Journal of Public Health, 97*(11), 2048–2055. doi:10.2105/AJPH.2006.087254

Cochran, S. D., & Mays, V. M. (2015). Mortality risks among persons reporting same-sex sexual partners: Evidence from the 2008 General Social Survey—National Death Index Data Set. *American Journal of Public Health, 105*(2), 358–364. doi:10.2105/AJPH.2014.301974

Cochran, S. D., Sullivan, J. G., & Mays, V. M. (2003). Prevalence of mental disorders, psychological distress, and mental health services use among lesbian, gay, and bisexual adults in the United States. *Journal of Consulting and Clinical Psychology, 71*(1), 53–61. doi:10.1037/0022-006x.71.1.53

Conron, K. J., Mimiaga, M. J., & Landers, S. J. (2010). A population-based study of sexual orientation identity and gender differences in adult health. *American Journal of Public Health, 100*(10), 1953–1960. doi:10.2105/AJPH .2009.174169

Dean, L., Meyer, I. H., Robinson, K., et al. (2000). Lesbian, gay, bisexual, and transgender health: Findings and concerns. *Journal of the Gay and Lesbian Medical Association, 4*(3), 102–151. doi:10.1023/a:1009573800168

Dennis, L. K., & Dawson, D. V. (2002). Meta-analysis of measures of sexual activity and prostate cancer. *Epidemiology, 13*(1), 72–79.

Drabble, L., Midanik, L. T., & Trocki, K. (2005). Reports of alcohol consumption and alcohol-related problems among homosexual, bisexual and heterosexual respondents: Results from the 2000 National Alcohol Survey. *Journal of Studies on Alcohol, 66*(1), 111–120.

Duggan, S. J., & McCreary, D. R. (2004). Body image, eating disorders, and the drive for muscularity in gay and heterosexual men: The influence of media images. *Journal of Homosexuality, 47*(3–4), 45–58. doi: 10.1300/J082v47n03_03

DuRant, R. H., Krowchuk, D. P., & Sinal, S. H. (1998). Victimization, use of violence, and drug use at school among male adolescents who engage in same-sex sexual behavior. *Journal of Pediatrics, 133*(1), 113–118. doi:10.1016 /S0022-3476(98)70189-1

Fendrich, M., Wislar, J. S., Johnson, T. P., et al. (2003). A contextual profile of club drug use among adults in Chicago. *Addiction, 98*(12), 1693–1703. doi:10.1111/j.1360-0443.2003.00577.x

Finneran, C., & Stephenson, R. (2013). Intimate partner violence among men who have sex with men: A systematic review. *Trauma Violence Abuse, 14*(2), 168–185. doi:10.1177/1524838012470034

Fredriksen-Goldsen, K. I., Kim, H.-J., Barkan, S. E., et al. (2013). Health disparities among lesbian, gay, and bisexual older adults: Results from a population-based study. *American Journal of Public Health, 103*(10), 1802–1809. doi:10.2105/AJPH.2012.301110

Gaither, T. W., Truesdale, M., Harris, C. R., et al. (2015). The Influence of sexual orientation and sexual role on male grooming-related injuries and infections. *Journal of Sexual Medicine, 12*(3), 631–640. doi:10.1111/jsm.12780

Garofalo, R., Wolf, R. C., Kessel, S., et al. (1998). The association between health risk behaviors and sexual orientation among a school-based sample of adolescents. *Pediatrics, 101*(5), 895–902. doi:10.1542/peds.101.5.895

Gay and Lesbian Medical Association. (2006). Guidelines for care of gay, lesbian, bisexual, and transgender patients.

Giles, G. G., Severi, G., English, D. R., et al. (2003). Sexual factors and prostate cancer. *BJU International, 92*(3), 211–216. doi:10.1046/j.1464-410X.2003.04319.x

Grant, R. M., Lama, J. R., Anderson, P. L., et al. (2010). Preexposure chemoprophylaxis for HIV prevention in men who have sex with men. *New England Journal of Medicine, 363*(27), 2587–2599. doi:10.1056/NEJMoa1011205

Grinspoon, S. (2009). Diabetes mellitus, cardiovascular risk, and HIV disease. *Circulation, 119*(6), 770–772. doi:10.1161/circulationaha.108.835710

Hatfield, L. A., Horvath, K. J., Jacoby, S. M., et al. (2009). Comparison of substance use and risky sexual behavior among a diverse sample of urban, HIV-positive men who have sex with men. *Journal of Addictive Diseases, 28*(3), 208–218. doi:10.1080/10550880903014726

Hatzenbuehler, M. L., McLaughlin, K. A., & Slopen, N. (2013). Sexual orientation disparities in cardiovascular biomarkers among young adults. *American Journal of Preventive Medicine, 44*(6), 612–621. doi:10.1016/j.amepre.2013.01.027

Hatzenbuehler, M. L., Slopen, N., & McLaughlin, K. A. (2014). Stressful life events, sexual orientation, and cardiometabolic risk among young adults in the United States. *Health Psychology, 33*(10), 1185–1194. doi:10.1037/hea0000126

Helfant, M., and Carson, S. (2008). *Screening for lipid disorders in adults: Selective update of 2001 U.S. Preventive Services Task Force Review.* Evidence Synthesis No. 49. Rockville, MD: Agency for Healthcare Research and Quality.

Kahn, J. (2002). Preventing hepatitis A and hepatitis B virus infections among men who have sex with men. *Clinical Infectious Diseases, 35*(11), 1382–1387. doi:10.1086/343044

King, B. A., Dube, S. R., & Tynan, M. A. (2012). Current tobacco use among adults in the United States: Findings from the National Adult Tobacco Survey. *American Journal of Public Health, 102*(11), e93–e100. doi:10.2105/AJPH.2012.301002

King, M., Semlyen, J., Tai, S. S., et al. (2008). A systematic review of mental disorder, suicide, and deliberate self harm in lesbian, gay and bisexual people. *BMC Psychiatry, 8*(1), 1–17. doi:10.1186/1471-244x-8-70

Knight, D. A., & Jarrett, D. (2015). Preventive health care for men who have sex with men. *American Family Physician, 91*(12), 844–851.

Kroger, A. T., Atkinson, W. L., Marcuse, E. K., et al. (2006). General recommendations on immunization: Recommendations of the Advisory Committee on Immunization Practices (ACIP). *Morbidity and Mortality Weekly Report: Recommendations and Reports, 55*(RR-15), 1–47.

Lakkis, J., Ricciardelli, L. A., & Williams, R. J. (1999). Role of sexual orientation and gender-related traits in disordered eating. *Sex Roles, 41*(1–2), 1–16. doi:10.1023/A:1018829506907

Lampinen, T. M., Chan, K., Anema, A., et al. (2008). Incidence of and risk factors for sexual orientation-related physical assault among young men who have sex with men. *American Journal of Public Health, 98*(6), 1028–1035. doi:10.2105/AJPH.2007.122705

Landovitz, R. J., & Currier, J. S. (2009). Postexposure prophylaxis for HIV infection. *New England Journal of Medicine, 361*(18), 1768–1775. doi:10.1056/NEJMcp0904189

Laska, M. N., Vankim, N. A., Erickson, D. J., et al. (2015). Disparities in weight and weight behaviors by sexual orientation in college students. *American Journal of Public Health, 105*(1), 111–121. doi:10.2105/AJPH.2014.302094

Lee, J. G., Griffin, G. K., & Melvin, C. L. (2009). Tobacco use among sexual minorities in the USA, 1987 to May 2007: A systematic review. *Tobacco Control, 18*(4), 275–282. doi:10.1136/tc.2008.028241

Lefevre, M. L. (2014). Behavioral counseling to promote a healthful diet and physical activity for cardiovascular disease prevention in adults with cardiovascular risk factors: U.S. Preventive Services Task Force recommendation statement. *Annals of Internal Medicine, 161*(8), 587–593. doi:10.7326/m14-1796

Leitzmann, M. F., Platz, E. A., Stampfer, M. J., et al. (2004). Ejaculation frequency and subsequent risk of prostate cancer. *JAMA, 291*(13), 1578–1586. doi:10.1001/jama.291.13.1578

Lim, F. A., Brown, D. V., Jr., & Jones, H. (2013). Lesbian, gay, bisexual, and transgender health: Fundamentals for nursing education. *Journal of Nursing Education, 52*(4), 198–203. doi:10.3928/01484834-20130311-02

Lin, K., & Sharangpani, R. (2010). Screening for testicular cancer: An evidence review for the U.S. Preventive Services Task Force. *Annals of Internal Medicine, 153*(6), 396–399. doi:10.7326/0003-4819-153-6-201009210-00007

Lipton, B. (2004). Gay men living with non-HIV chronic illnesses. *Journal of Gay & Lesbian Social Services, 17*(2), 1–23. doi:10.1300/J041v17n02_01

Markwald, R. R., Melanson, E. L., Smith, M. R., et al. (2013). Impact of insufficient sleep on total daily energy expenditure, food intake, and weight gain. *Proceedings of the National Academy of Sciences, 110*(14), 5695–5700. doi:10.1073/pnas.1216951110

Mast, E. E., Weinbaum, C. M., Fiore, A. E., et al. (2006). A comprehensive immunization strategy to eliminate transmission of hepatitis B virus infection in the United States: Recommendations of the Advisory Committee on Immunization Practices (ACIP) Part II: Immunization of adults. *Morbidity and Mortality Weekly Report: Recommendations and Reports, 55*(RR-16), 1–33.

Mays, V. M., & Cochran, S. D. (2001). Mental health correlates of perceived discrimination among lesbian, gay, and bisexual adults in the United States. *American Journal of Public Health, 91*(11), 1869–1876. doi:10.2105 /Ajph.91.11.1869

McCall, H., Adams, N., Mason, D., et al. (2015). What is chemsex and why does it matter? *BMJ, 351*, 1–2. doi:10.1136/bmj.h5790

Meyer, I. H. (2003). Prejudice, social stress, and mental health in lesbian, gay, and bisexual populations: Conceptual issues and research evidence. *Psychology Bulletin, 129*(5), 674–697. doi:10.1037/0033-2909.129.5.674

Millett, G. A., Peterson, J. L., Wolitski, R. J., et al. (2006). Greater risk for HIV infection of black men who have sex with men: A critical literature review. *American Journal of Public Health, 96*(6), 1007–1019. doi:10.2105/ajph.2005 .066720

Molina, J.-M., Capitant, C., Spire, B., et al. (2015). On-demand preexposure prophylaxis in men at high risk for HIV-1 infection. *New England Journal of Medicine, 373*(23), 2237–2246. doi:10.1056/NEJMoa1506273

Mosca, L., Barrett-Connor, E., & Wenger, N. K. (2011). Sex/gender differences in cardiovascular disease prevention: What a difference a decade makes. *Circulation, 124*(19), 2145–2154. doi:10.1161/CIRCULATIONAHA.110.968792

Moyer, V. A. (2013). Screening for hepatitis C virus infection in adults: U.S. Preventive Services Task Force recommendation statement. *Annals of Internal Medicine, 159*(5), 349–357. doi:10.7326/0003-4819-159-5-201309030 -00672

National Institute on Alcohol Abuse and Alcoholism. (1998). Alcohol and sleep. Retrieved from https://pubs.niaaa.nih.gov/publications/aa41.htm

National Institute on Alcohol Abuse and Alcoholism. (2016a). Alcohol facts and statistics. Retrieved on April 24 from http://www.niaaa.nih.gov/alcohol -health/overview-alcohol-consumption/moderate-binge-drinking

National Institute on Alcohol Abuse and Alcoholism. (2016b). Drinking levels defined. Retrieved from http://www.niaaa.nih.gov/alcohol-health/overview -alcohol-consumption/moderate-binge-drinking

Obedin-Maliver, J., Goldsmith, E. S., Stewart, L., et al. (2011). Lesbian, gay, bisexual, and transgender–related content in undergraduate medical education. *JAMA, 306*(9), 971–977. doi:10.1001/jama.2011.1255

Obergefell v. Hodges. *United States Reports*, volume 576 (United States Supreme Court, 2015).

Office of Disease Prevention and Health Promotion. (2014). Healthy people 2020. Department of Health and Human Services. Retrieved on April 24 from https://www.healthypeople.gov/

Ott, J. J., Stevens, G. A., Groeger, J., et al. (2012). Global epidemiology of hepatitis B virus infection: New estimates of age-specific HBsAg seroprevalence

and endemicity. *Vaccine, 30*(12), 2212–2219. doi:10.1016/j.vaccine.2011
.12.116

Palefsky, J. M., Giuliano, A. R., Goldstone, S., et al. (2011). HPV vaccine against
anal HPV infection and anal intraepithelial neoplasia. *New England Journal of Medicine, 365*(17), 1576–1585. doi:10.1056/NEJMoa1010971

Petrosky, E., Bocchini, J. A., Jr., Hariri, S., et al. (2015). Use of 9-valent human papillomavirus (HPV) vaccine: Updated HPV vaccination recommendations
of the Advisory Committee on Immunization Practices. *Morbidity & Mortality Weekly Report, 64*(11), 300–304.

Reisner, S. L., Van Wagenen, A., Gordon, A., et al. (2014). Disparities in safety
belt use by sexual orientation identity among US high school students.
American Journal of Public Health, 104(2), 311–318. doi:10.2105/
AJPH.2013.301745

Rothman, E. F., Exner, D., & Baughman, A. L. (2011). The prevalence of sexual
assault against people who identify as gay, lesbian, or bisexual in the United
States: A systematic review. *Trauma Violence Abuse, 12*(2), 55–66.
doi:10.1177/1524838010390707

Russell, S. T., & Joyner, K. (2001). Adolescent sexual orientation and suicide risk:
Evidence from a national study. *American Journal of Public Health, 91*(8),
1276–1281.

Saini, R., Saini, S., & Sharma, S. (2010). Oral sex, oral health, and orogenital
infections. *Journal of Global Infectious Diseases, 2*(1), 57–62. doi:10.4103
/0974-777X.59252

Seaborne, L .A., Prince, R. J., & Kushner, D. M. (2015). Sexual health education in
U.S. physician assistant programs. *Journal of Sexual Medicine, 12*(5),
1158–1164. doi:10.1111/jsm.12879

Silenzio, V. M. B. (2002). Ten things gay men should discuss with their healthcare provider. Retrieved from http://glma.org/index.cfm?fuseaction=Page
.viewPage&pageID=690.

Simon, M. S., Weiss, D., & Gulick, R. M. (2013). Invasive meningococcal disease in
men who have sex with men. *Annals of Internal Medicine, 159*(4), 300–301.
doi:10.7326/0003-4819-159-4-201308200-00674

Simon Rosser, B. R., Merengwa, E., Capistrant, B. D., et al. (2016). Prostate cancer
in gay, bisexual, and other men who have sex with men: A review. *LGBT
Health, 3*(1), 32–41. doi:10.1089/lgbt.2015.0092

Siu, A. L. (2015). Screening for abnormal blood glucose and type 2 diabetes mellitus: U.S. Preventive Services Task Force recommendation statement.
Annals of Internal Medicine, 163(11), 861–868. doi:10.7326/M15-2345

Smith, B. D., Morgan, R. L., Beckett, G. A., et al. (2012). Recommendations for the
identification of chronic hepatitis C virus infection among persons born
during 1945–1965. *MMWR Recommendations and Reports, 61*(RR-4),
1–32.

Smith, D. K., Herbst, J. H., Zhang, X., et al. (2015). Condom effectiveness for HIV
prevention by consistency of use among men who have sex with men in the
United States. *Journal of Acquired Immune Deficiency Syndromes, 68*(3),
337–344. doi:10.1097/QAI.0000000000000461

UCLA Sleep Disorders Center. (2015). Sleep and men. Retrieved from http://sleepcenter.ucla.edu/body.cfm?id=62

U.S. Department of Health and Human Services & U.S. Department of Agriculture. (2015). 2015–2020 Dietary Guidelines for Americans. Retrieved from http://health.gov/dietaryguidelines/2015/guidelines/

Volk, J. E., Marcus, J. L., Phengrasamy, T., et al. (2015). No new HIV infections with increasing use of HIV preexposure prophylaxis in a clinical practice setting. *Clinical Infectious Diseases, 61*(10), 1601–1603. doi:10.1093/cid/civ778

Wheaton, A. G., Chapman, D. P., Presley-Cantrell, L. R., et al. (2013). Notes from the field: Serogroup C invasive meningococcal disease among men who have sex with men—New York City, 2010–2012. *Morbidity and Mortality Weekly Report, 61*(51–52), 1048.

Wilkin, T. (2015). Clinical practice: Primary care for men who have sex with men. *New England Journal of Medicine, 373*(9), 854–862. doi:10.1056/NEJMcp1401303

Woody, G. E., Vanetten-Lee, M. L., McKirnan, D., et al. (2001). Substance use among men who have sex with men: Comparison with a national household survey. *Journal of Acquired Immune Deficiency Syndromes, 27*(1), 86–90.

World Health Organization. (2010). Violence and injuries: The facts. Geneva, Switzerland: World Health Organization.

Yaphe, S., Bozinoff, N., Kyle, R., et al. (2012). Incidence of acute hepatitis C virus infection among men who have sex with men with and without HIV infection: A systematic review. *Sexually Transmitted Infections, 88*(7), 558–564. doi:10.1136/sextrans-2012-050566

Yelland, C., & Tiggemann, M. (2003). Muscularity and the gay ideal: Body dissatisfaction and disordered eating in homosexual men. *Eating Behaviors, 4*(2), 107–116. doi:10.1016/S1471-0153(03)00014-X

9

Sexual Health for Women

Tonia Poteat, Dawn Harbatkin, and Alexis D. Light

Wanting sex and having sex are important parts of the human experience. Historically, many cultures have viewed female sexuality as subordinate to male sexuality and something to be controlled through restrictions on female behavior (e.g., enforced modesty, chastity belts) (Baumeister & Twenge, 2002). The feminist movement and increasing social status of women in modern society have led to women's sexuality being reassessed as a subject in its own right.

Traditionally, lesbians have been subjected to studies that confirm our gendered understanding of sex between straight couples—that women don't really like sex as much as men do and therefore, two women together must be far less interested in and having much less sex than anyone else. But more recent studies show that this is not true. A recent "Lesbian Sex Survey" of 8,566 women who have sex with women reported that lesbians do have less sex than heterosexuals, but not that much less (Riese, 2015a). The more sex women had, the more likely they were to report "ecstasy" or "happiness" in their relationships. Women who were having sex every day or multiple times a day described their sex lives the most positively, but having sex this often did not usually last past the first year or so of the relationship. Still, this does not seem to affect the degree of happiness experienced within relationships. Lesbians have less sex than heterosexuals, though the sexual encounters usually last longer (Riese, 2015).

Lesbian and bisexual women have a broad range of ways that they experience attraction, engage in sexual behavior, enter into relationships, and self-identify—any or all of which can play a role in fulfilling this basic human need. Because sexuality is such an important part of overall health, in this chapter we explore how women meet and have sex with other women, as well as some of the main health issues that may arise as part of sexual experiences and relationships.

This chapter will address a broad range of lesbian and bisexual women's identities and experiences: queer, pansexual, polyamorous, monogamous, and others. While the experiences of trans women are included in some parts of this chapter, it is not meant to be a comprehensive place to address all of the issues around the sexuality of this group.

ATTRACTION

There are a number of factors that go into who we are attracted to and whom we choose to be with, including personality traits, interests, values, and physical appearance. Often, we cannot pinpoint exactly why we are drawn to someone.

Researchers believe that sexual attraction first begins around the age of 10 for most people and is related to activity in the anterior hypothalamus— the portion of the brain thought to process sexual cues. Some studies show that pheromones—a type of scent-bearing chemical secreted in sweat and other bodily fluids that are known to be involved in sexual attraction in animals—may also play a role for people (Gregolre, 2015).

Previously, it was thought that women needed emotional connection and established intimacy to be turned on, while men were more responsive to visual stimuli. A study by Chivers, Reiger, Latty, and Bailey published in 2004 showed that this was in fact untrue. Women in the study were attached to a plethysmograph (which measures volume changes of an organ, in this case by detecting vaginal blood flow) and shown a variety of pornography clips, such as sex between men and women, women and women, men and men, and a pair of bonobos. The women, both straight and lesbian, were aroused by all of the clips, including the copulating apes. When Chivers tried a similar experiment on men, they responded in predictable patterns: straight men's arousal soared when women were on screen and not very much at all when men were on screen. Gay men had the opposite response. And neither male group responded at all to the apes. These findings suggest that in contrast to previously held beliefs, women (both straight and lesbian) responded to a much wider array of stimuli than men.

What women find attractive and to whom they are attracted has differed dramatically over time, and multiple subcultures have formed within the lesbian and bisexual community. During the 1950s and 1960s, women often engaged in more traditional masculine/feminine roles of "butch" and "femme," with "kiki" being someone who was neither. These roles were challenged by the feminists of the 1970s. Today there are sport dykes, diesel dykes, power dykes, lipstick lesbians, chapstick lesbians, studs, bois, and many other labels with which women identify. Additional labels include pillow queen (someone who likes to be on the receiving end of sex), stone butch (someone who gets pleasure from pleasing her partner but does not like to be touched sexually), gold-star lesbian (a woman who has never slept with a man and has no intention of ever doing so), and bicurious (a person who has been involved with only one sex in the past but is curious about the other). For some, these roles remain consistent throughout their life, and for others, they are fluid depending on their partner or the particular moment in time. There is no need to feel pressure to identify with any one group. Some people's identification may change frequently, while other people are very committed to these roles and attracted to women within a particular group. Regardless, it is important to note that ultimately, attraction is subjective and each person has unique sexual and romantic tastes.

SEXUAL ANATOMY AND PHYSIOLOGY

Female sexual anatomy is often thought of as limited to the genitals. However, in addition to the clitoris, vagina, and anus, there are many other parts of the body that are part of female sexuality.

The Brain

Our brains interpret the signals we receive from the outside world and from our body parts, translating them into coherent messages for us. Our brains determine whether we are interested in sex and whom we are attracted to. When we see something or are touched in a certain way, our brain takes in the information about that visual or physical cue and tells us whether we should view it as pleasurable. During sexual activity, the brain releases dopamine and oxytocin. Dopamine stimulates the pleasure sensations, and oxytocin initiates the uterine contractions that often accompany orgasm.

For some women, this cascade can be controlled by the brain alone. In 1953, Alfred C. Kinsey of Indiana University and his colleagues found that 2 percent of the 2,727 women studied could reach an orgasm by fantasy alone (Broad, 2013). Another study in 2003 by Barry R. Komisaruk looked into brain scans of 10 women thinking erotic thoughts and then masturbating. The pleasure centers lit up more or less identically whether the women reached sexual highs by hand stimulation or fantasy alone (Altman, 2010; Broad, 2013).

The brain is truly the most sexual organ in the body.

Breasts

As pictures of topless women in *National Geographic* will confirm, breasts are not sexualized in all societies. However, breasts are considered by many women to be an erogenous zone—an area with an abundance of nerve endings that increase sensitivity to touch and whose stimulation results in sexual response.

The breasts play a key role in female sexual arousal, and scientists are beginning to understand why. Nipple stimulation is processed in the same region of the brain as touch to the clitoris, vagina, and cervix (Komisaruk et al., 2011) This means that touch to the nipples can be experienced in the same way as touch to the genitalia. In fact, some women have orgasms while breastfeeding. Women report sensitivity not just in their nipples but in the skin just above the areola (the darker area surrounding the nipples). During sexual arousal, breast volume increases, causing changes in the areola and erection of the nipples (Masters & Johnson, 1966).

In our culture, breasts are viewed as a basic part of beauty and femininity. If a breast has been removed, a woman may worry about whether her partner will still find her attractive. She may also be worried about not being able to enjoy sexual stimulation in the affected breast. Breast reconstruction restores the shape of the breast, but it cannot restore normal breast sensation. The nerve that supplies feeling to the nipple runs through the deep breast tissue and is often disconnected during surgery. In a reconstructed breast, the feeling of pleasure from having the nipple touched is lost. A rebuilt nipple has much less feeling. In time, the skin on the reconstructed breast will regain some sensitivity but probably will not give the same kind of pleasure as before mastectomy (American Cancer Society, 2017).

Even after having a breast removed, some women still enjoy being stroked around the area of the healed scar. Others dislike being touched there and may no longer even enjoy being touched on the remaining breast and nipple. Breast surgery or radiation to the breasts does not physically decrease a woman's sexual desire; nor does it decrease her ability to have vaginal lubrication or normal genital feelings or to reach orgasm. Some women who have had a mastectomy may feel self-conscious in certain sexual positions where the area of the missing breast is more visible. The good news is, studies show that after two years, many breast cancer survivors recover not only physically but also note improvement in libido, erotic responsiveness, orgasms, and sexual satisfaction (Castleman, 2014; Meyerowitz, Desmond, Rowland, Wyatt, & Ganz, 1999).

Erogenous Zones

In addition to the breasts, women have many other erogenous zones, including the lips, neck, inner thighs, ears, lower back, and scalp (Turnbull, Lovett, Chaldecott, & Lucas, 2014). Erogenous zones differ from woman to woman, and stimulation of the erogenous areas that some women find pleasant and exciting may be impossible to bear for others. Stimulating the right ones in the right way increases the release of hormones like serotonin and oxytocin. The aim of exploring the female erogenous areas is to increase a woman's level of arousal in order to enjoy the act and potentially reach an orgasm.

The Clitoris

Every female mammal has a clitoris. However, humans are one of the few species that has evolved to actually use the clitoris for sexual pleasure. In fact, the clitoris is the only organ that has come to exist for the sole purpose of providing pleasure. Far from being the tiny organ many consider it, the clitoris actually extends under the skin in a *Y* shape rivaling the size of the penis.

The *glans* is the scientific name for the external portion that most people associate with the clitoris. It has a foreskin that partially covers it, which is known as the clitoral *hood*. The glans contains approximately 8,000 sensory nerve fibers—more than anywhere else in the human body and twice the number found on the glans of the penis.

The glans is connected to the body or *shaft* of the internal clitoris, which is made up of two *corpora cavernosa*. The corpora cavernosa contain erectile tissue that fill with blood during arousal and wrap around the vagina on either side. The corpora cavernosa extend farther, bifurcating again to form the two *crura*. These extend up to nine centimeters, pointing toward the thighs when at rest and stretching back toward the spine when erect. Near each of the crura on either side of the vaginal opening are the *clitoral vestibules*—internally under the labia majora. These are also made of erectile tissue, and when engorged with blood, they cuff the vaginal opening, causing the vulva to expand outward.

The clitoris actually grows during a woman's lifetime as a result of hormonal changes in the body. By the time puberty ends, the clitoris will be about 1.8 times larger than at the onset of puberty. By the time a woman is 32 years old, it will be almost four times as big. After menopause, the clitoris will be about seven times larger than it was at birth (Laurie & Kinkly, 2013). Once it matures, it maintains its sexual peak for the rest of a woman's life.

Many women wonder about their clitoris size and shape and whether it is "normal." The reality is that there is a great deal of variation in size, how much the clitoris protrudes or hides under the hood, how it responds to touch, and what happens when it is aroused. Each clitoris is as unique as the woman it is a part of.

Some women do undergo surgery to alter their clitoris, including clitoral unhooding or enlargement/reduction of clitoral size. While generally not recommended due to the risk of scarring or infection as well as potential damage to the nerves, as with other plastic surgeries, women should make an individual and informed choice.

Female genital mutilation (FGM), also known as female circumcision or female genital cutting, on the other hand, has been performed on 125 million girls still alive today—and against their will (World Health Organization [WHO], 2018). FGM refers to procedures that intentionally cause injury to the female genital organs for nonmedical reasons. FGM is prevalent in Africa, the Middle East, and Asia for cultural, religious, and social reasons. It is often motivated by the belief that it is beneficial for the girl and will reduce her libido and discourage sexual activity before marriage.

FGM is usually done by a woman with no medical training and without the use of anesthesia or antiseptics, using knives, scissors, scalpels, pieces of glass, or razor blades while the girl is forcibly restrained. For most, it is an incredibly traumatic experience. It is usually carried out on girls between infancy and the age of 15, commonly before puberty starts, and includes

- Type 1: clitoridectomy—removing part or all of the clitoris
- Type 2: excision—removing part or all of the clitoris and the inner labia (the lips that surround the vagina) with or without removal of the labia majora (larger outer lips)
- Type 3: infibulation—narrowing of the vaginal opening by creating a seal formed by cutting and repositioning the labia
- Type 4: other harmful procedures to the female genitals that include pricking, piercing, cutting, scraping, and burning the area (WHO, 2018).

There are no health benefits to FGM, and it can result in immediate consequences (e.g., pain, wound infections, bleeding, inability to urinate, damage to the nearby urethra or bowel, acquisition of HIV or hepatitis), long-term physical consequences (e.g., chronic infections, abnormal periods, infertility, complications during pregnancy, and newborn deaths), and psychological and mental health issues.

Deinfibulation refers to the practice of cutting open the sealed vaginal opening in a woman who has been infibulated, and this is often necessary for health and well-being as well as to allow intercourse or facilitate childbirth. This, however, cannot restore sensitive tissue that has been removed.

FGM is a violation of the human rights of girls and women. In the United States, there is a federal law that makes it illegal to perform FGM domestically or to knowingly transport a girl out of the United States for the purpose of inflicting FGM (18 U.S.C. § 116). Additional information and support is available through U.S. Citizenship and Immigration Services by telephone (1-800-994-9662) or the Web site.

The Vagina

The vagina is an elastic, muscular canal with a soft, flexible lining that provides lubrication and sensation. It is inside the body and connects the uterus to the outside world. The vulva and labia form the entrance, and the cervix of the uterus protrudes into the vagina, forming the interior end. The hymen is a thin membrane of tissue that surrounds and narrows the vaginal opening. It may be torn or ruptured by sexual activity or by exercise. Once broken, it does not grow back. The vagina is a self-cleaning organ and can actually be harmed by cleansing products like douches.

There are varying reports of whether or not women experience sexual pleasure from stimulation of the vagina, specifically the *G-spot*. The G-spot was named in honor of the late Dr. Ernst Gräfenberg, who in 1950 described a particularly sensitive one- to two-centimeter-wide area a few centimeters in from the vaginal opening, on the vaginal wall toward the front of a woman's body. The G-spot's existence, and existence as a distinct structure, is still under dispute, as its reported location can vary from woman to woman and appears to be nonexistent in some women. It is hypothesized to be an extension of the clitoris and therefore the reason for orgasms experienced vaginally (Balon & Seagraves, 2009, p. 258; Burri, Cherkas, & Spector, 2010; Cox, 2012; Greenberg, Bruess, & Oswalt, 2014, pp. 102–104; Kilchevsky, Vardi, Lowenstein, & Gruenwald, 2012).

Similarly, there is controversy over female ejaculation. While it is not a myth, it is an elusive phenomenon for most women. When it does happen, women may feel embarrassed, thinking that they just urinated. Research suggests that female ejaculate is the release of very scant, thick and whitish fluid from the Skene's glands (i.e., the female prostate); however, some women do report release of larger amounts (Moalem & Reidenberg, 2009; Rubio-Casillas & Jannini, 2011). The physiologic function of female ejaculation is unknown.

The Anus

The anus can be a source of great pleasure, depending on a person's interest in engaging in anal sex or anal play as well as the type of sexual activity being performed. The anus is made up of two layers of muscle called the internal and external sphincters. The external sphincter can be voluntarily controlled, but not the internal sphincter. The anus as well as the first part of the rectum is especially sensitive, though the area becomes less sensitive the further it is penetrated. The perineal area, which runs from the anus to the bottom of the vagina, is also a sensitive area.

Sexual Response

Masters and Johnson described the process of arousal and orgasm by dividing it into four stages: arousal (or excitement), plateau, orgasm, and resolution (Masters & Johnson, 1981). The four stages are preceded by desire. The first stage, arousal, can take place through any number of senses—vision, hearing, smell, or touch. This can cause the heart rate, breathing, and blood pressure to increase. Genitals receive increased blood flow, which can make the clitoris engorge both externally and internally. In the next stage, called the plateau phase, heart rate increases more and muscles tighten. Next, with orgasm, there are rhythmic muscle contractions and a sense of euphoria. After orgasm, with the resolution phase, blood pressure drops and muscles relax.

This model of the sexual response style is linear and has been suggested by some to not be as applicable to women, especially those in long-term relationships. In 2000, Rosemary Basson suggested the circular model of sexual response, which was adjusted by Katie Giles and Marita McCabe in 2009. In this model, women start from a place of "sexual neutrality." They enter into sexual situations not from a spontaneous physical/sexual desire but from a nonsexual need arising from either a need for intimacy or a need for physical well-being: emotional closeness, bonding, commitment, love, affection, acceptance, toleration, or physical closeness. This can lead to sexual arousal, which then results in a "responsive" sexual desire—a desire to continue the experience for sexual/physical reasons in response to this initial arousal. This arousal might or might not result in orgasm. Regardless, it would result in positive rewards toward intimacy, which would fuel further sexual encounters either in that moment or in the future.

Orgasm

A study published by Indiana University in 2014 showed that lesbians had more orgasms than straight or bisexual women over the 12-month study period (Indiana University Bloomington Newsroom, 2014). Some women describe having multiple orgasms—several orgasms with no break in between that occur under continued sexual stimulation—but this a relatively uncommon occurrence. However, sequential orgasms—repeated orgasms that are separated by small breaks—are common. According to Dr. Mary Jane Sherfey, a psychiatrist who specializes in female sexuality, each orgasm is followed promptly by refilling of the venous erectile chambers. This distension creates engorgement and edema, which creates more tissue tension, and the cycle continues. The supply of blood and edema fluid to the pelvis is inexhaustible. For all intents and purposes, the human female is sexually insatiable: given the right stimulation, women can have repeated orgasms indefinitely (Sherfey, 1973, p. 112). Unfortunately, the whole concept of being able to have more than one orgasm has taken on a competitive ring. And for some women, orgasm can lead to increased sensitivity that may make further stimulation uncomfortable. Although many people think of the purpose of sexual encounters as producing an orgasm, stimulation that feels good but does not lead to orgasm can be just as exciting.

Sigmund Freud promoted the theory of two kinds of female orgasms, one being a vaginal orgasm and the other being a clitoral orgasm. However, research, such as that done by Masters and Johnson (1966) and Helen O'Connell (2005), rejects this distinction (Archer & Lloyd, 2002, pp. 85–88; Marshall Cavendish Corporation, 2009, p. 590; O'Connell, Sanjeevan, & Huston, 2005; Zastrow, 2007, p. 228). Seventy to eighty percent of women require direct clitoral stimulation to achieve orgasm, though indirect clitoral stimulation may also be sufficient (Federation of Feminist Women's Health Centers, 1991, p. 46; Flaherty, Davis, & Janicak, 1993; Kammerer-Doak & Rogers, 2008; Lloyd, 2005, p. 311; Mah & Binik, 2001; Weston, 2011). Women commonly find it difficult to experience orgasms during vaginal intercourse, although the G-spot area may produce an orgasm if properly stimulated (Kilchevsky et al., 2012; Rosenthal, 2012, p. 150; Weiner, Stricker, & Widiger, 2012, pp. 172–175).

It is now believed by many authorities that all female orgasms are physiologically identical. They are triggered by stimulation of the clitoris and expressed by vaginal contractions. Accordingly, regardless of how friction is applied to the clitoris (i.e., the tongue, the woman's finger or her partner's, a vibrator, coitus) female orgasm is almost always evoked by clitoral stimulation. However, it is always expressed by circumvaginal muscle contractions (Kaplan, 1974, p. 29).

Body Image

People from every group, including those of every sexual orientation, can have negative perceptions about their bodies. Lesbian subcultures have been thought to downplay the importance of physical attractiveness and to challenge culturally prescribed norms of female beauty. In one study, lesbians were less invested in their appearance and less involved in maintaining it compared to heterosexual women or gay men (Wagenback, 2008). And yet, according to a study done in 1996, one in three lesbian women reports having a negative body image, and one in four reports engaging in disordered eating behaviors (French, Story, Remafedi, Resnick, & Blum, 1996). It remains unclear what the real norms on body image are in the community.

FINDING PARTNERS

Where do women meet other women to date and have sex? Increasingly, the answer is on the Internet. There are a multitude of sites and smartphone apps that cater to all sexual orientations. Some of them require a monthly fee in order to contact another user. Others are free of charge. A few apps allow a person to immediately connect with potential matches who are in close proximity to her current location. Although the Internet and apps are popular, they have not replaced physical venues for meeting partners. Many women meet partners at bars, LGBT events or venues, meet-up groups or sports teams, or through friends.

When deciding to enter any sexual encounter or relationship, it is important to clearly define expectations. Many couples find fulfillment in monogamous relationships while others explore sexual relationships with other partners, either together or individually. Communication about expectations and boundaries is key. For example, some women choose to have multiple committed sexual relationships while others choose to have only casual sexual encounters outside of their primary partnership. Other women are not looking for relationships at all and prefer sex without commitment.

INTIMATE PARTNER VIOLENCE

Intimate partner violence is a pattern of violence and coercive behavior where one partner seeks to control the thoughts, beliefs, and/or conduct of the other partner. It is clear that intimate partner violence within lesbian relationships is a serious social concern: 3.9 million women are physically abused by their female partners, and 20.7 million are verbally or emotionally abused (Little & Terrance, 2010). The Centers for Disease Control and Prevention (2011, p. 8) reports the lifetime prevalence of rape, physical violence, or stalking by an intimate partner is 43.8 percent for lesbians and 61.1 percent for bisexual women.

Still, intimate partner violence within lesbian relationships remains largely unnoticed and misunderstood. One myth that supports this continued invisibility is that it can often appear that abuse between two women is "mutual." However, on closer examination of the power dynamics of the relationship, this is rarely, if ever, true. There is also a myth that the more masculine partner is always the perpetrator and the more feminine partner the victim, simulating a common scenario in heterosexual couples. While not every relationship has a more feminine or masculine partner, even in those that do, this does not necessarily define the nature of the power dynamics in the relationship. A unique aspect of abuse within lesbian relationships is the use of "homophobic control" as a method of psychological abuse, with one partner threatening to disclose the other's sexual orientation without consent (West, 2008). This must be understood when helping or supporting lesbians in abusive relationships.

If someone is in an unhealthy or dangerous relationship, the most important thing is to develop a safety plan—a personalized, practical plan that includes ways to remain safe while in a relationship, while planning to leave, or after leaving. As a friend or family member of someone in an abusive relationship, acknowledge that the person is in a difficult and scary situation, be supportive, and listen in a nonjudgmental way—even if the person continues to stay in the relationship. Encourage the person to participate in activities with friends and family outside of their relationship. For those who are concerned that their behaviors may be unhealthy or harmful to their partner, there is help for them too. The first step to change is making the commitment to begin to do so. For more information and support on domestic violence, contact the National Domestic Violence Hotline: www.thehotline.org, 1-800-799-7233, or 1-800-787-3224 (TTY).

SEXUAL PRACTICES

Women have sex with each other in wide variety of ways. Within this wide variety, some sexual practices are more common than others. In 2015, Autostraddle (www.autostraddle.com) conducted a survey of their readership, and over 8,000 (mostly 35 years old and younger) queer cis and trans women responded (Riese, 2015b). Based on open-ended questions, the three most common sex acts listed by respondents included external clitoral stimulation (99 percent), oral sex (95 percent), and frottage (body rubbing) (80 percent). Women also described engaging in nipple play; strap-on, dildo, vibrator, and other sex toy play; scissoring; vaginal fisting; and external and penetrative anal play. About half of the respondents commonly incorporate spanking into their sexual practices, and more than one in five engage in bondage, domination, and sadomasochism (BDSM).

Another survey conducted by researchers at Indiana University in 2010–2011 included over 3,000 women in the United States, United Kingdom, Canada, and Australia (Schick, Resnberger, Herbenick, & Reece, 2012). This group of women was older than the Autostraddle group and was asked to pick frequent sex acts from a predetermined list. Most women in that study reported genital rubbing (99 percent), vaginal fingering (99 percent), oral sex (99 percent), scissoring (91 percent), and vaginal fisting (57 percent). Sex toy use was common, with 74 percent reporting using a vibrator, 56 percent a strap-on, and 56 percent a dildo. Anal play was also reported, with 14 percent reporting anal insertion of dildos, 11 percent use of butt plugs, and 7 percent use of anal beads.

Even though these studies did not discuss it, queer women also practice rimming (mouth-to-anus sex), anal fisting, water sports, and additional practices. Most women do not limit their sexual practices to one sex act or even one sex act at a time. For example, some women may enjoy both penetration and external stimulation simultaneously or one after the other. Regardless of what kind of sex women have, the most important aspect is communication. Understanding one's own body and what gives pleasure makes it easier to let partners know how to provide pleasure. Checking in about what partner(s) desire, enjoy, or do not enjoy helps ensure that everyone is having the kind of sex they want to have.

External Genital Stimulation

The outer vaginal lips, inner vaginal lips, clitoral hood and glans, the opening of the vagina, and the anus can be stimulated with just about anything (see section on sex toys below). Manual stimulation with the hand or fingers can bring pleasure as well as rubbing against any other part of the body (frottage or tribadism), including vulva-to-vulva contact (scissoring). Pleasure from external stimulation may be intensified by lubrication, both self-generated and with lubricant from a bottle. In addition to greater intensity, added wetness may make stimulation more comfortable and allow for longer periods of rubbing without discomfort.

Oral Sex

Oral sex includes licking, biting, sucking, kissing, and/or penetrating the vulva, anus, or perineum (space between the vagina and anus) with the mouth or tongue. Mouth-to-vulva sex is called cunnilingus, while mouth-to-anus sex is called analingus or rimming. "Sixty-nine" is a term that is used to describe a sexual position in which both partners are giving and receiving oral sex simultaneously. Oral sex can also be performed on a dildo (see section on sex toys below). Historically, women have been taught that our genitals are "dirty," and oral-anal sex has been considered especially taboo. Some women are concerned about how they smell or taste and worry about the presence of fecal matter or blood. Taking a shower or bath before sex can help, and using a latex barrier can prevent exposure to fecal matter and vaginal fluids, if so desired. Despite these concerns, many women derive their greatest sexual pleasure from giving or receiving oral sex.

Penetration

Penetration of the vagina or anus can be deeply pleasurable. Vaginal penetration stimulates the clitoris internally as well as the sensitive areas found in the outer third of the vagina, and anal penetration stimulates the multitude of sensitive nerve endings surrounding the anal sphincter and may indirectly stimulate the clitoris, depending on the angle and amount of pressure. Penetration can be done with one or more fingers (including a fist), dildos, or other sex toys. It can be deep, shallow, or anywhere in between. Penetration can feel good for the insertive partner as well, as she may enjoy the feel of her partner surrounding her fingers, hand, or dildo. As with manual stimulation, lubrication intensifies sensations of pleasure during penetration and prevents discomfort caused by dryness. Added lubricant may be necessary for fisting to take place comfortably.

The anus does not produce its own lubrication. Applied lubrication is essential for pleasurable anal penetration. Anything that enters the anus should be nonbreakable and have a flared bottom so that it can be easily retrieved. Also, in order to prevent spread of bacteria and possible infection, anything that has been inside the anus should not be used in or around the vagina until it is well cleaned.

Sex Toys

Sex toys come in a variety of forms, including vibrators, dildos (with or without a harness, together creating a "strap-on"), anal plugs, anal beads, Ben Wa balls, and more. Almost any sex toy can be used for external stimulation, and some are clearly designed for internal use. Everything described above for external genital stimulation and for penetration also applies to the use of sex toys.

BDSM/Kink/Water Sports

Water sports, playing with and/or drinking of a partner's urine, is another less often performed but much eroticized possible activity. It is often performed in the shower or bathroom to simplify cleanup. Urine as a fluid is mostly (but not always) sterile, does not frequently pass on disease, and does not carry HIV. If ingested, there are metabolites (or waste products) of medications taken by the person urinating contained in the urine that when ingested can cause allergies or reactions in the person drinking the urine.

According to *Merriam-Webster*, a kink is defined as "an unconventional sexual taste or behavior." Kink is quite common and may be broad or specific. While more conventional or conservative people may find the idea of some kinks distasteful, most experts agree that as long as kinks are undertaken with a consenting partner (or partners), they can be part of a healthy sexual life. Kink can include some of the things already discussed, such as water sports or rimming.

Role playing a particular scenario or "scene" is common in kinky sex. For example, wearing leather or other specific outfits and acting out a "master" and "slave" scene is one form of kinky role play. Bondage and discipline (BD), dominance and submission (DS), and sadism and masochism (SM) are common forms of kink and are often abbreviated as BDSM. Bondage is the tying up or restraining of a partner for sexual pleasure. Discipline is when one partner chastises, spanks, or punishes another. Dominance involves taking power and control, while submission involves relinquishing it for sexual pleasure. Sadism is when one enjoys the act of causing pain to her partner, and masochism is the erotic enjoyment of your own pain.

As previously mentioned, kinks are best explored by consenting partners with discussion in advance about expectations and limits. Partners generally agree in advance on particular limits and use of a "safe" word that will be unrelated to the "scene," so when it is used, both partners will know that the "scene" must stop or be suspended so that a discussion of physical or emotional distress can be alleviated.

There is little medical literature about specific kinks. It therefore can be a challenge to providers asked to counsel their patients. When discussing kink with clients, consider a few things: first, ask the basic question of whether the activity will cease functions that can be necessary for life, like breathing, circulation (particularly to extremities for long periods), or eating. Second, anything that alters the sensorium, like alcohol or drugs, can make risky sexual play more risky. Finally, consider a particular activity's potential for leading to infection, such as the transmission of HIV or STIs through blood in fluids during fisting or cutting activities. There is a significant amount of information related to kink on the Internet, including many groups that have come up with recommendations to minimize harm to participants in a particular kink. While these recommendations may not be evidence based, they are frequently thought out through lenses of common sense and experience.

PREVENTION OF SEXUALLY TRANSMITTED INFECTION (STI) TRANSMISSION

There is a myth perpetuated in many lesbian communities that women cannot get or give each other sexually transmitted infections (STIs). However, women can and do transmit STIs to their female partners. The most comprehensive review of STIs among women was published in 2011. According to this summary of the evidence, human papillomavirus (HPV) and herpes simplex virus (HSV) are common among women who have sex with women, while gonorrhea and chlamydia are rarer. Studies also suggest that bacterial vaginosis can be transmitted between women, as well as trichomonas, syphilis, and hepatitis A (Gorgos & Marrazzo, 2011). There have been two confirmed cases of HIV transmission between women—one reported in 2003 and the other in 2014. It is important to understand methods to protect oneself and partners. The most important step to prevent STIs is for each woman to take a realistic risk assessment of her sexual practices.

"Risk" varies depending on which sexually transmitted infection (STI) someone is trying to prevent. For example, both oral and genital herpes are very common and can be transmitted by skin-to-skin contact. Because the herpes virus can shed even when there are no sores, the best ways to reduce the chances of herpes transmission include using latex barriers (condoms, gloves, or dental dams) and/or having the partner with herpes take antiviral medications such as acyclovir, famiciclovir, or valacyclovir when she is not having any symptoms in order to reduce the frequency of viral shedding. Human papillomavirus (HPV) is another virus that can be transmitted by skin-to-skin contact. HPV comes in many types, some of which may cause genital warts and others that cause cervical cancer. Like HSV, someone may have HPV and show no signs or symptoms. The best way to prevent HPV is to get vaccinated before the age of 27. Even if a woman has had the vaccine, it is important for her to continue to get regular Pap smears to screen for HPV and/or the cervical changes that could lead to cancer. How often and whether or not to have HPV-specific testing will vary depending on age and medical history and should be discussed with a medical provider.

STIs that are transmitted by blood or vaginal secretions (such as HIV) can be prevented by keeping the fluid from one person from entering another person's body. Using latex barriers for oral sex, cleaning sex toys or changing condoms when sex toys are shared, not sharing sex toys, and wearing gloves for fingering are all ways to reduce the risk of transmitting or acquiring HIV and other bacterial STIs.

The best way to clean a sex toy depends on the material it is made from. If the type of material is not clear, it is a good idea to check the package insert or ask the salesperson or manufacturer. Good Vibrations (http://www.goodvibes.com/s/content/c/Sex-Toy-Material-Cleaning) offers the following advice for cleaning sex toys: If a toy is made of silicone, glass, stainless steel, or wood, mild soap and water can be used to clean it. Most toys made of silicone, Pyrex, glass, stainless steel, or stone can be cleaned by putting them through the dishwasher without soap or by boiling them for five minutes, as long as they are not battery or electrically operated. Washing gently with warm water and soap cleans skin-like toys (e.g., Cyberskin, Softskin, Neoskin); however, too much soap can damage the material. Toys made of soft plastic, elastomers, silicone blends, or jelly/rubber are porous and may trap bacteria even after washing with soap and water. Using a condom is the best way to keep them clean.

In addition to cleaning toys and using barriers, there is now a prescription medication that can be taken by people who do not have HIV to prevent HIV acquisition. This is called pre-exposure prophylaxis or PrEP. Daily oral Truvada, a combination of two drugs used in the treatment of HIV, has been shown to greatly reduce the risk of HIV transmission between men and in heterosexual couples in which one partner has HIV. PrEP has not been evaluated in women who have sex with women, but it is believed to be effective in any person at risk for HIV as long as they take it as prescribed. Another way to prevent HIV infection is to take medication within 48 to 72 hours after having been exposed. This is called post-exposure prophylaxis or PEP.

Syphilis is an STI that is typically transmitted through vaginal fluids, but it can also be transmitted by blood or by skin-to-skin contact with a sore or syphilitic rash. Gonorrhea and chlamydia are transmitted through vaginal and cervical fluids as well. Use of protective barriers described above should reduce the risk of transmission between women. Viral hepatitis is not typically thought of as a sexually transmitted disease. However, we know that hepatitis A can be transmitted through fecal-oral routes like rimming or getting feces from an object used in anal play into your mouth; hepatitis B can be transmitted equally via blood and sex, and hepatitis C can be transmitted through blood and less commonly through sex. Using latex barriers and being careful to avoid touching the mouth or hands after anal contact can prevent transmission of hepatitis A. The same precautions used to prevent HIV can be used to prevent hepatitis B and C.

Research shows that women use a variety of strategies to prevent transmitting or acquiring infections during sex. One study found the following: cleaning sex toys before or after use was most common (70 to 80 percent), using a condom was less common (12 to 21 percent), and using a dental dam (latex barrier for oral sex) was quite rare at less than 5 percent (Schick et al., 2012). While this study provided important information on sexual behavior between women, it did not include the entire repertoire of potential sex acts or safer-sex strategies that could be used between women. For example, researchers did not ask if participants used finger cots or gloves.

PREGNANCY

There are many ways for same-sex couples to become parents. While not always an option for a varying degree of reasons, some women will choose to undergo pregnancy. Whole books exist on conception and pregnancy for lesbians, as well as other great resources (Brill, 2006; Clunis & Green, 2003; Toevs & Brill, 2002). This is not intended to be a comprehensive description of pregnancy in lesbian relationships but rather a brief overview.

Pathways to Pregnancy

Conception occurs at the meeting of an egg (ovum) and sperm, which can be a challenge in relationships where both partners have eggs and neither have sperm. One of the first decisions to be made is determining where the sperm should come from. The two main options are using a known sperm donor or using an anonymous sperm donor (Kranz & Daniluk, 2006). Some decide to use a friend, while others choose to go through a sperm bank. Both paths come with multiple subsequent decisions. If the donor is a friend, what will their role be? Are there local regulations regarding who can be a sperm donor? Some laws specifically prohibit gay men from being donors, and other laws do not allow for medical insemination of semen that has not been washed and quarantined. If using a sperm bank, it is important to know their policies. Do they limit the number of children produced from one donor's sperm? Is there potential to contact other children conceived from the same donor? Can the child find their donor after they turn 18? It is important to be familiar with local laws and come to a decision that is best for the family.

If in a relationship where each partner has a uterus, there needs to be a decision about which one to use for the pregnancy. For some couples, this is an easy decision, and for others, this can take much discussion. Some of the many factors to consider are age (it is statistically easier and less risky to get pregnant prior to 35 years old), genetics, medical conditions, employment, and feelings on fertility and pregnancy. This is still only the beginning of the decision making (Chabot & Ames, 2004).

There are many options for how to introduce the sperm to the egg. The least medically invasive option is vaginal insemination. This can be done at home or in a medical provider's office (Haimes & Weiner, 2000). Vaginal insemination or intracervical insemination (ICI) occurs by inserting raw semen or washed sperm (done by a fertility lab) into the back of the vaginal vault, close to the cervical os (opening). The next option is intrauterine insemination (IUI), in which washed sperm is inserted through the cervical os directly into the uterine cavity. This is done by a medical provider; those qualified include nurse midwives, gynecologists, and reproductive endocrinologists (a subspecialty of gynecology). It used to be believed that IUI was more effective than ICI, but newer research is suggesting that the methods have comparable success with conception (Carroll & Palmer, 2001; Kop et al., 2015).

In vitro fertilization (IVF) is another option—and the only option for couples who want to have a reciprocal pregnancy (using one partner's eggs and the other's uterus) (Marina et al., 2010; Woodward & Norton, 2006; Zeiler & Malmquist, 2014; Pelka, 2009). IVF is performed by reproductive endocrinologists. Oocytes are stimulated using exogenous hormones and then retrieved with a needle prior to ovulation. The oocyte or oocytes retrieved from the procedure are then combined with sperm in a petri dish, some of which will successfully combine and develop into embryos. Embryos are frozen and later thawed for transfer or are transferred fresh into an awaiting uterus. IVF allows for unique possibilities besides reciprocal pregnancies, such as preimplantation genetic diagnostic testing (PGD), where embryos are screened for significant abnormalities prior to implantation (Tafas, Ichetovkin, Kilpatrick, & Tsipouras, 2008). Not all IVF clinics are created equal when it comes to their interactions with same-sex couples (Ross, Steele, & Epstein, 2006a). While clinics and providers are being encouraged to create more supportive environments (Ross, Steele, & Epstein, 2006b), doing advance research on a clinic or provider's policies and the experiences of other same-sex couples before pursuing their services may allow for a better experience.

It is important to remember that infertility issues in same-sex partnerships may go beyond not having sperm. Infertility is defined as one year of trying without conception and can stem from multiple causes, including genetic issues in the oocytes or problems with ovulation, the fallopian tubes, or the uterine cavity (Smith, Pfeifer, & Collins, 2003). Any fertility issues faced by heterosexual women are also faced by lesbians (Donovan, 2008). Struggling with infertility can place a large emotional weight on an individual and on relationships. While some infertility issues can be overcome with the help of medical professionals, not all are surmountable. One study suggests that women in same-sex relationships may have an easier time accepting infertility and adapting to alternate forms of creating a family due to already fitting into a nontraditional family model (Goldberg, Downing, & Richardson, 2009).

Sex during Pregnancy

Many wonder if they can continue to be sexually intimate while pregnant. The simple answer is yes. It is important to remember that sexual desires will shift and evolve throughout the course of the pregnancy. For some, pregnancy hormones increase their libido. For others, pregnancy symptoms such as nausea and vomiting as well as a changing body can decrease sexual desire. Overall, sex during pregnancy is common, especially early on. Later, as the belly swells, engaging in sex may take ingenuity and creativity (Jones, Chan, & Farine, 2011). There does tend to be a decline in sexual activity in late pregnancy (von Sydow, 1999). It is important to mention that there are a few medical exceptions, which include those at high risk for preterm labor and those with placenta previa (a placenta overlying the cervical opening). For those that are pregnant and concerned, it is always safest to directly ask a pregnancy health care provider.

Breastfeeding

Breastfeeding is widely encouraged and supported by many, including the American College of Obstetricians and Gynecologists (ACOG) and the American Academy of Pediatrics (AAP) (R. A. Lawrence & R. M. Lawrence, 2010). Current recommendations from the AAP advocate "exclusive breastfeeding for about 6 months, followed by continued breastfeeding as complementary foods are introduced, with continuation of breastfeeding for 1 year or longer as mutually desired by mother and infant" (Eidelman & Schanler, 2012). Benefits of breastfeeding are many and include passage of antibodies to the infant, increased metabolic need for lactation with quicker return to prepregnancy weight, and reduced cost compared to formula (Gartner et al., 2005). It is important to remember that breastfeeding is not always easy and not always possible, for various physiological and societal reasons. There are many excellent resources for breastfeeding, including Breastfeeding Resource Center (http://breastfeedingresourcecenter .org/), La Leche League (http://www.llli.org/), Milk on Tap (https://milkontap .com/), and Milk Junkies (http://www.milkjunkies.net/)—which is specifically focused on chest feeding from a transgender perspective.

An area of growing interest and research for nongestating women is lactation induction (Wahlert & Fiester, 2013; Farrow, 2014). This is relevant for those in female same-sex families and for adoptive mothers. Lactation induction is often performed through a combination of medications and mechanical stimulation with the use of a breast pump. It can be difficult to initiate and often does not produce adequate supply, but when successful, it can be a rewarding bonding experience for the parent and infant (Wittig & Spatz, 2008). Co-nursing (where more than one caregiver nurses) can help bonding among members of families where not all are biologically related (Zizzo, 2009). More research needs to be performed in order to better understand the most effective way to achieve lactation in a nongestating parent.

MENOPAUSE

Menopause is the time in life when menstruation ceases and is defined as starting 12 months after the last menstrual cycle. It is a natural life cycle transition that occurs because the ovaries stop producing estrogen. The median age that women in the United States enter menopause is 51 years old (Gold et al., 2001). The time preceding menopause, known as the perimenopausal years, is often accompanied by irregular menstrual cycles caused by fluctuations in estrogen levels produced by the ovaries. Research has shown that perimenopausal and menopausal experiences are similar between heterosexual women and lesbian and bisexual women (Danielson et al., 2000)

Symptoms

In over 50 percent of American women, menopause is accompanied by significant physical and emotional symptoms (American College of Obstetricians and Gynecologists, 2014). These symptoms include vasomotor symptoms, sleep disruption, vaginal symptoms, urinary issues, mood swings, depression, and weight gain. Vasomotor symptoms include hot flashes and night sweats. Hot flashes are intense short episodes (commonly one to five minutes) of flushing to the face, neck, and chest. Ninety percent of women experience hot flashes for a few months to a few years; a small minority will continue to experience them for many years after menopause (Grady, 2006). Vaginal symptoms include dryness and atrophy, which can negatively impact sexual activity. Additionally, mood swings and feelings around changing body image can affect a person's sexual responsiveness and sexual desires during menopause (Bachmann & Leiblum, 2004).

Symptom Management

Since menopausal symptoms are caused by a decrease in hormones produced by the ovaries, the most effective treatment for these symptoms is to replace these hormones. However, hormone replacement therapy (HRT) received quite a bit of public scrutiny in the early 2000s after findings from the Women's Health Initiative study were released (Aubuchon & Santoro, 2004; Notman & Nadelson, 2002). Over the years since the release of that research, there has been significantly more research, thought, and discussion over how to best respond to menopausal symptoms. Expert opinion supports estrogen replacement as the most effective way to provide symptomatic relief. Current practice is to use low doses of estrogen for as long as symptoms require treatment. Most women undergo less than five years of HRT with estrogen before symptoms fade to a tolerable level and treatment is no longer necessary (American College of Obstetricians and Gynecologists, 2014).

HRT can be administered in many different ways. Some of these include via pills or patches, topically, and with vaginal creams. HRT is not the right option for every woman. Women who have had or are at high risk for breast cancer and blood clots, or have acute liver disease, should not use HRT (Grady, 2006).

There is a cornucopia of other nonhormonal methods to treat menopausal symptoms. Other prescription medications, including antidepressants and gabapentin, have been shown to be helpful in relieving bothersome vasomotor symptoms (North American Menopause Society, 2004). While complementary and alternative methods have generally not been researched in large trials, for some women, they provide symptomatic relief. Some of these options include exercise, acupuncture, black cohosh, Chinese herbs, and vaginal lubricants (Kronenberg & Fugh-Berman, 2002). A complete medical history, as well as an inventory of symptoms, goals, and risks, should be reviewed before trying any medical intervention.

Libido

Changes in sexual desire during menopause are common. A decrease in sexual desire can cause a decrease in sexual satisfaction as well as partner satisfaction and can even have a negative impact on other areas of a person's health (Leiblum et al., 2006; Dennerstein et al., 2006). There is no specific research on changes in sexual desire for women who have sex with women during menopause (Kelly, 2007). These authors hypothesize that having two women adjusting to changing body image, changes in libido, and fluctuating menopausal symptoms may further extenuate decreases in sexual desire beyond that of women in heterosexual relations. As the entire U.S. population continues to age and more research is done on same-sex relationships, this is hopefully an area that will be further researched (Fredriksen-Goldsen et al., 2013).

SUBSTANCE USE AND SEX

Regardless of whether they are prescription or nonprescription medications, or legal or illegal drugs, many medications and drugs have the potential to be abused. Some of the substances that are commonly abused have effects on sexual function. Substance abuse is often divided into two major categories—abuse and dependence. Abuse is typically thought of as substance use that causes one to make bad decisions affecting personal life, work, or school. Dependence can involve tolerance (needing more of the substance to achieve the same effect), an inability to cut down, and withdrawal symptoms when a person tries to stop using.

Alcohol

The most commonly abused substance in the United States is alcohol, likely because it is legal to use. Alcohol is potentially one of the most harmful drugs to abuse, as it lowers inhibitions and decreases coordination, leading to thousands of motor vehicle accidents each year. It is commonly used as a social lubricant for people who have anxiety finding partners or making conversation. There are socially acceptable limits on alcohol use—beyond which one is more likely to engage in risky behaviors and make bad decisions.

In the long term, alcohol has many negative physiologic effects, including liver damage, high blood pressure, stroke, and certain types of cancer (including breast cancer). In fact, women are at higher risk for developing alcohol-associated liver disease, brain damage, and heart disease even if the woman has been drinking less alcohol or for a shorter length of time than a man. With sustained use, alcohol in large quantities can ultimately lead to liver failure, requiring a liver transplant (National Institute on Alcohol Abuse and Alcoholism, 2017). In the short term, alcohol can have a number of effects on the body. It can also increase a woman's risk of becoming a victim of violence and sexual assault.

National guidelines recommend lower levels of drinking for women than men. As alcohol passes through the digestive tract, it is dispersed in the water of the body. Women have less water in their bodies than men, and so a woman's brain and other organs are exposed to more alcohol and more toxic byproducts from alcohol breakdown. Therefore, national guidelines indicate that women should be consuming no more than one drink per day. High-risk drinking for women is more than 3 drinks in a sitting or 7 drinks in a week.

Club Drugs

"Club drugs," named because of their association with dance clubs, include drugs like cocaine, MDMA (ecstasy), methamphetamine, ketamine,

LSD, and GHB (gamma-hydroxybutyrate). In one study of 1,104 female club attendees in New York City, lesbian and bisexual women used club drugs significantly more than their heterosexual peers. Of lesbian respondents, 76 percent had ever used an illegal drug and 20.5 percent had used within the past three months. The most commonly used drugs were MDMA and cocaine (Parsons, Kelly, & Wells, 2006).

MDMA, also known as "ecstasy," is a drug that causes euphoria, decreased anxiety, and increased feelings of social connectedness. Though it can increase erotic sensations, it can also cause difficulties with sexual arousal. In the study mentioned above, MDMA was the most commonly used club drug, with 49.2 percent of lesbian/bisexual respondents having ever used MDMA. Several studies have failed to find gender differences in rates of MDMA use (Boyd, McCabe, & d'Arcy, 2003). Yet, young adult females are at greater risk of experiencing harm (Topp et al., 1999) and report more negative consequences given that they generally take the same amount but have smaller bodies and different physiology compared to men (Liechti, Gamma, & Vollenweider, 2001).

In the short term, taking ecstasy can lead to hyperthermia, sweating, and dehydration. Many people know this and drink water to try to compensate. And yet, some people drink too much water, reducing the levels of salt in their bodies to dangerously low levels, resulting in seizures and death. In the long term, the way that the brain processes serotonin is affected, but there is debate about the significance of this effect. Evidence suggests that MDMA can permanently and negatively affect memory and result in depression (Rogers et al., 2009).

Taking selective serotonin reuptake inhibitor (SSRI) antidepressants with MDMA can decrease the effects of the MDMA, making it less likely the user will get high (Liechti, Bauman, Gamma, & Vollenweider, 2000; Tancer & Johanson, 2007; Farre et al., 2007). But, more important, there have been reports of this combination causing serotonin syndrome, a syndrome of hyperthermia and muscle twitches that can lead to death (Dobry, Rice, & Sher, 2013). Anyone taking this medication should avoid MDMA.

Cocaine is a commonly used drug of abuse. In one study in the United Kingdom, lesbian and bisexual women were three times as likely to have used cocaine compared to their heterosexual peers (Doward, 2010). Cocaine induces pleasurable feelings and increases sex drive. However, women are less sensitive to the drug's effects. This is thought to be due to a tendency to absorb it less well when taken intranasally and to metabolize it more quickly (Bowersox, 1996). Cocaine can have numerous immediate dangers as well as more long-term consequences, including effects on heart rhythm, heart attacks, strokes, seizures, and even sudden death. Binge use can lead to panic attacks, paranoia, and full-blown psychosis. Use of cocaine also increases the risk of contracting HIV, hepatitis B, and hepatitis C.

Prescription Medications

Alcohol and drugs can affect sexual function, but we often forget about the many medications we receive from health care providers. Many medications are suspected of interfering with sexual function, although it is unusual for them to be the sole cause. Notorious for causing sexual side effects are medications like antidepressants and blood pressure medications.

Antidepressants

While recent studies do not show increased rates of depression among lesbians, especially lesbians who are out, bisexual women have been shown to have significantly poorer mental health than lesbians or heterosexual women (DeAngelis, 2002). Antidepressants are some of the most commonly prescribed medications. Many antidepressants, especially selective serotonin reuptake inhibitors (SSRIs) such as fluoxetine (Prozac) and citalopram (Celexa), can cause sexual side effects, including decreased interest in sex (decreased libido) and inability to orgasm. At times, these side effects may be confused with the effects of depression itself. Depression can lead to decreased interest in sex but should not cause orgasmic difficulties if aroused. Many providers forget to ask about these side effects, and they can be potentially embarrassing to bring up, but it is important to talk about them because they can often be treated by switching to another antidepressant.

Blood Pressure Medications

Sexual dysfunction is more common in women with hypertension compared to women who are normotensive (Doumas, et al, 2006). The effect of high blood pressure medication on women's sexual functioning is less well understood. Diuretics can decrease forceful blood flow to the genitals, making it difficult to get aroused or achieve orgasm. Beta blockers, in particular, such as metoprolol and propranolol, have the potential to cause decreased interest in sex and problems with orgasm. These medications may be able to be switched, although they may be the best category of blood pressure medication for people with a particular health history. Other blood pressure medications, such as angiotensin II receptor blockers, may actually help with sexual functioning in the setting of high blood pressure (Bloom, 1998). If a provider says it is acceptable, it may be possible to stop taking blood pressure medications temporarily to see if one's sex life improves; however, close monitoring of blood pressure will be needed to make sure it stays in a safe range.

Contraceptives

Oral contraceptives decrease circulating free testosterone and therefore may decrease desire in women, though there is little evidence to support this. Depot medroxyprogesterone, a birth control shot, can cause vaginal atrophy, pain with sex, and decreased libido. If these symptoms occur, considering changing to another form of contraception.

There are a number of other types of medications used less commonly that can affect sexual function, so the best thing to do when there are noticeable changes in sexual interest or function is to speak with a health care provider.

A SYMPTOM-BASED APPROACH TO SEXUAL HEALTH CONCERNS

It can be difficult to know when to see a health care provider about symptoms. Some people are reluctant to see a provider, so they minimize problems, while others do not make the connection that symptoms may be sexually related. Health care providers may forget to ask about sexual activity. Furthermore, when people try to educate themselves about symptoms from sexually transmitted diseases, information is often presented in the form of more extreme cases or technical information about specific bacteria and viruses. What follows is an extensive (but by no means comprehensive) description of some common infections and conditions that can result from sexual activity and should be discussed with a health care provider.

Mouth and Throat

Sore Throat: A sore throat is very common and does not usually indicate that someone has a sexually transmitted infection. Often it is the result of a virus similar to the ones that cause the common cold. On occasion, if the symptom is isolated in the throat and does not have cough or body aches associated with it, it can be the result of a bacterial infection. This might lead to a red, painful throat, pain with swallowing, and even pus in the back of the throat. A commonly seen infection of this sort is strep throat, caused by group A streptococcus or *Streptococcus pyogenes.* In rare cases, however, one could get this type of sore throat from gonorrhea or chlamydia contracted during oral sex. In some cases, these infections may have no symptoms or may feel like a cold or allergy. If a woman has gonorrhea or chlamydia in her throat, even if she does not have symptoms, it may be possible to pass this infection on to her sexual partner. There are several different tests for gonorrhea and chlamydia in the throat, but a "routine" throat culture will likely not pick up this infection, so it is important to discuss any risks with a health care provider.

Ulcers: "Sores" outside the mouth around the lips are more noticeable than sores inside the mouth or in the throat. Painful sores around the mouth (sometimes called "fever blisters") are likely caused by the herpes virus. Herpes is a very common infection, with more than two-thirds of all adults carrying it in their bodies (although not all have symptoms). In contrast, a painless sore around or inside the mouth might come from an early infection with syphilis. Syphilis can be easily treated and cured in the early stages, but can be very dangerous as it progresses, so it is important to see a health care provider upon noticing a painless sore. In fact, a sore inside the mouth or in the back of the throat that is painless can easily go unnoticed. Other common noninfectious causes of painful ulcers in the mouth include aphthous ulcers or "canker" sores, which are not sexually transmitted but can be brought on by local trauma or stress.

Lumps and Bumps: HPV, the virus that causes warts and leads to some cancer, can infect the mouth and throat. In those who smoke or use tobacco products, quitting can help to prevent HPV-associated cancers. Vaccination against HPV may help protect one against cancers in the mouth and throat as well as in the genital area. It is important to address any new or growing lumps and bumps with a dentist or other health care provider.

Bladder and Urinary Tract

Infections of the bladder and urinary tract infections (UTIs) are common among women. UTIs are not sexually transmitted infections; however, some women notice that they get them after having sex, both oral and penetrative. UTIs can cause burning with urination; pain in the lower abdomen or back; cloudy, dark, or bloody urine; and the need to urinate frequently and urgently but with very little urine output. If these symptoms are present, seeing a health care provider is important because untreated bladder infections may travel up the urinary tract to the kidneys and cause serious illness. Certain vaginal infections may also cause burning with urination, so it is important to be tested for STIs as well as a UTI. A few things can help lower the chances of getting a UTI: drinking plenty of water, wiping from front to back after urinating, and emptying one's bladder after sex. A few research studies have found that unsweetened cranberry juice reduces the chances of getting a UTI. For frequent urinary tract infections, consider switching out the types of lubricants, toys, or other products used during sex, as they may be irritating the urethra (the tube that transports urine from the bladder to outside the body).

Vulva, Vagina, Cervix

Itching, pain, discharge: Pain, itching, or discharge in the genitals can raise concerns about sexually transmitted infections (STIs). It is important to remember that some STIs can occur without any symptoms or with symptoms that go unnoticed. It is also important to know that not all symptoms are caused by a sexually transmitted infection. Some amount of vaginal discharge is normal. Normal discharge changes in consistency as hormone levels change during the menstrual cycle and as a part of aging. It can be clear to white, pasty to creamy, and is typically thick and tacky during the most fertile time of the cycle. Brown discharge for a day or so after menstruation is also normal. Discharge that has a foul odor, is unusually heavy, or associated with itching, pain, or burning is abnormal and should prompt a visit to a health care provider. Vigorous penetrative sex can lead to irritation, pain, and/or discharge that can take hours and sometimes even a day or so to resolve. However, pain or discharge that goes on for more than a day should be evaluated by a health care professional.

There are many possible reasons for itching on the vulva or vagina. One of the most common reasons is candidiasis, commonly known as a yeast infection. Typical symptoms include itching that can be quite intense, swelling, redness or irritation, and a thick white discharge that may resemble cottage cheese. It is theoretically possible to transmit a yeast infection from one vulva to another during genital rubbing; however, yeast infections are generally not sexually transmitted. Instead, they are usually caused by an imbalance in the normal microorganisms that live in the vagina. Yeast infections are easy to treat with over-the-counter medications. However, if symptoms do not improve after a week of over-the-counter treatment, consult a health care provider. Trichomonas is a sexually transmitted infection that sometimes causes itching, burning with urination, and a discharge with a fishy odor. Bacterial vaginosis (BV) may also cause a fishy-smelling discharge or itching. BV is not classified as a sexually transmitted infection; however, there is some evidence that it may be more common in lesbians and transmitted between female partners, so female partners should be treated together (Evans et al., 2007). Chlamydia and gonorrhea are sexually transmitted infections that may cause discharge, and if they travel from the vagina and cervix to the upper reproductive tract, they can cause a serious illness called pelvic inflammatory disease (PID) that can lead to infertility. Chlamydia and gonorrhea may be present without a discharge or any symptoms at all. That is one of the reasons the Centers for Disease Control and Prevention recommends annual screening for these infections in all sexually active women younger than 25 years as well as older women with new or multiple sex partners, or a sex partner who has a sexually transmitted infection.

Lumps and Bumps: The most common sexually transmitted cause of lumps and bumps on the vulva is genital warts, usually caused by the human papilloma virus (HPV). HPV-related warts often have a rough, cauliflower-like texture and may show up as a single bump or a cluster. If there are multiple bumps, they may be near each other or scattered around. There are also nontransmissible causes of bumps on the vulva. Occasionally, a hair follicle can become blocked and an infection can develop, called folliculitis, which looks similar to a pimple. These are more common in women who trim and shave their genital area, as trimming or shaving flattens the head of the hair and can cause the hair to irritate the skin or even grow under the skin.

There are also noninfectious causes of bumps on the vulva. For example, on the labia, some women can develop blocked sebaceous glands that lead to smooth white or yellow dots called Fordyce spots, which are also harmless and not contagious. These do not require treatment.

Ulcers: Ulcers on the vulva or in the vagina are almost always from sexual transmission. Painful ulcers are generally caused by herpes. They can come once and disappear forever, or remain and come out during times of stress. Herpes can be passed by skin-to-skin contact, even when there is no outbreak. Most people with herpes feel a tingling or burning sensation that precedes the sore or ulcer by one to three days. It is at this point that medication is most successful at shortening the course of the outbreak. Another rare infection that can lead to a single painful ulcer on the vulva is an infection called chancroid, which is caused by the bacteria *Haemophilus ducreyi*. This infection requires antibiotics to heal.

Painless ulcers on the vulva or inside the vagina may develop from primary infection with syphilis. These sores will go away on their own without treatment and may go unnoticed, especially if they are inside the vagina or covered by hair on the labia. However, even though the sore from syphilis goes away on its own, the infection remains in the body unless treated. These sores are very infectious by skin-to-skin contact and should not be overlooked. Untreated syphilis advances to affect other organs in the body, including the skin, heart, lungs, and bone. Syphilis should be tested for if there is suspected exposure, and is easily treated in early stages with antibiotics.

Other noninfectious causes of genital ulcers and sores include abrasions, chafing, and trauma from aggressive sex or even trauma from a zipper in women who do not wear underwear.

Anus and Rectum

Pain: Anal pain can be a cause for concern and anxiety. Often, these symptoms may come from issues as benign as hemorrhoids. Hemorrhoids are frequently associated with some itching and bright red blood tracking along the outside of a formed stool. In some cases, a few drops of blood can turn the water in the toilet bowl bright red. In more severe cases, people with hemorrhoids can end up with fissures (cracks or tears in the skin around the anus) or sinus tracts (tunnels or holes) that run from the intestine to the anus. These can be more difficult to heal and involve seeing a specialist. Pain from these conditions tends to worsen after a bowel movement (BM) or straining to have a BM and may involve some blood or mucus in the toilet.

Herpes of the anus or rectum follows a similar pattern to other herpes infections, beginning with an itch or a tingle around the anus and leading to a sharp or burning pain. Vesicles, or clear blisters, may form and quickly result in ulcers. If pain is more internal in the rectal area, sometimes felt as a pelvic or lower abdominal pain, it could be gonorrhea or chlamydia. Rectal gonorrhea and chlamydia sometimes also cause tenesmus (an urgency to make stool), even when little comes out. These infections may produce pus or blood on or in stool.

Lumps and Bumps: There are several different causes for lumps or bumps around the anus. Hemorrhoids are benign and common causes of such symptoms. Skin tags, extra pieces of skin formed either by chafing or from prior hemorrhoids, may lead to lumps or bumps. These can be surgically removed but are not dangerous, and if they are not causing symptoms are likely best left alone. Another possible cause of bumps around the anus is genital warts caused by the HPV virus. The types of HPV that cause warts are different than the types known to predispose to anal cancer. However, anal warts imply that the HPV virus is present and may be transmitted to sex partners who come in contact with it.

Breasts

Pain: Following aggressive nipple play (with or without piercings or clamps), it is not uncommon to have bruising or pain for several days. Additionally, nipple piercings can make breasts more sensitive, or they can cause someone to lose nipple sensation as a result of scarring. New piercings may take several weeks to months to heal and can be quite raw and vulnerable to infection early on. If there is redness, irritation, increasing pain, swelling, or discharge from the site of a piercing, it is probably best to be checked by a health care provider to see if it has become infected.

Lumps and Bumps: Lumps and bumps in the breasts may be caused by benign conditions such as fibrocystic breast changes. Tenderness and the presence or absence of lumps within the breast may change over the course of the menstrual cycle as hormone levels change. These breast changes may become more or less intense during menopause. If a breast lump persists or has any suspicious signs (cannot be easily moved around under the skin, feels firm or hard rather than rubbery, grows in size, or causes changes in the skin), it should be brought to the attention of a health care provider, particularly if there is a family history of breast, colon, or ovarian cancer,

Discharge: Discharge is a normal part of breast function during pregnancy or breastfeeding. It can also happen during menstrual hormone changes or in response to vigorous breast stimulation, especially if a person has been pregnant in the past. However, bloody nipple discharge is never normal. Other signs of abnormality include nipple discharge from only one breast and discharge that occurs spontaneously without anything stimulating or irritating the breast.

Total Body Symptoms

There are some symptoms that affect more than just the genitals that can be transmitted through sex. Rashes over the chest or whole body should be evaluated for secondary syphilis or HIV. Persistent gastrointestinal symptoms such as diarrhea, bloating, or loose stools, may come from a parasite contracted during oral-anal contact. Abdominal pain, diarrhea, and jaundice (or yellowing of the skin) may indicate infection with hepatitis. Vaccination against hepatitis B is recommended for all adults and vaccines against hepatitis A are recommended for people at risk.

CONCLUSION

Sexuality is an important part of the human experience, yet it can be difficult for women to find practical and accurate information about sex between women. In this chapter, we have attempted to address this by providing information on various aspects of sexual health for lesbian, bisexual, and queer women—from attraction and meeting partners to sexual practices and potential signs of infection. Knowledge is power, and we hope that the information in this chapter empowers women to have healthier and more fulfilling sexual lives.

REFERENCES

18 U.S. Code § 116 - Female genital mutilation, Pub. L. 104-208, 110 Stat. 3009-709, codified as amended at 18 U.S.C. § 116.

Altman, M. (2010). Rutgers lab studies female orgasm through brain imaging. *Inside Jersey Magazine*. Retrieved from http://www.nj.com/insidejersey /index.ssf/2010/04/science_consciousness_and_the.html

American Cancer Society. (2017, August 23). Body image and sexuality after breast cancer. Retrieved from https://www.cancer.org/cancer/breast-cancer /living-as-a-breast-cancer-survivor/body-image-and-sexuality-after -breast-cancer.html#references

American College of Obstetricians and Gynecologists. (2014). Management of menopausal symptoms. Practice Bulletin No. 141. *Obstetric Gynecology, 123*, 202–216.

Archer, J., & Lloyd, B. (2002). *Sex and gender.* Cambridge, UK: Cambridge University Press.

Aubuchon, M., & Santoro, N. (2004). Lessons learned from the WHI: HRT requires a cautious and individualized approach. *Geriatrics, 59*(11), 22–26.

Bachmann, G. A., & Leiblum, S. R. (2004). The impact of hormones on menopausal sexuality: A literature review. *Menopause, 11*(1), 120–130.

Balon, R., & Seagraves, R. T. (2009). *Clinical manual of sexual disorders.* Washington, DC: American Psychiatric.

Basson, R. (2000). The female sexual response: A different model. *Journal of Sex and Marital Therapy, 26*(1), 51–65.

Baumeister, R. F., & Twenge, J. M. (2002). Cultural suppression of female sexuality. *Review of General Psychology, 6*(2), 166–203.

Black, M. C., Basile, K. C., Brieding, M. J., Smith, S. G., Walters, M. L., . . . Stevens, M. R. (2011). *National intimate partner and sexual violence survey (NISVS): 2010 summary report.* Atlanta, GA: Centers for Disease Control and Prevention.

Bloom, B. S. (1998). Continuation of initial antihypertensive medication after 1 year of therapy. *Clinical Therapy, 20*(4), 671–681.

Bowersox, J. A. (1996). Cocaine Affects Men and Women Differently, NIDA Study Shows. Retrieved from https://archives.drugabuse.gov/NIDA_Notes/NN Vol11N1/CocaineGender.html

Boyd, C. J., McCabe, S. E., & d'Arcy, H. (2003). Ecstasy use among college undergraduates: Gender, race and sexual identity. *Journal of Substance Abuse Treatment, 24*(3), 209–215.

Brill, S. A. (2006). *The new essential guide to lesbian conception, pregnancy, and birth.* New York: Alyson.

Broad, W. J. (2013). I'll have what she's thinking. *New York Times Sunday Review.* Retrieved from http://www.nytimes.com/2013/09/29/sunday-review/ill -have-what-shes-thinking.html?pagewanted=all&_r=2&

Burri, A. V., Cherkas, L., & Spector, T. D. (2010). Genetic and environmental influences on self-reported G-spots in women: A twin study. *Journal of Sexual Medicine, 7*(5), 1842–1852.

Carroll, N., & Palmer, J. R. (2001). A comparison of intrauterine versus intracervical insemination in fertile single women. *Fertility and sterility, 75*(4), 656–660.

Castleman, M. (2014, February). *Sex after breast cancer* [Blog post]. Retrieved from https://www.psychologytoday.com/blog/all-about-sex/201402/sex-after -breast-cancer

Chabot, J. M., & Ames, B. D. (2004). It wasn't "let's get pregnant and go do it": Decision making in lesbian couples planning motherhood via donor insemination. *Family Relations, 53*(4), 348–356.

Chivers, M. L., Reiger, G., Latty, E., & Bailey, J. M. (2004). A sex difference in the specificity of sexual arousal. *Psychological Science, 15*(11), 736–744.

Clunis, D. M., & Green, G. D. (2003). *The lesbian parenting book: A guide to creating families and raising children.* Berkeley, CA: Seal Press.

Cox, L. (2012, January 19). G-spot does not exist, 'without a doubt,' say research-
     ers. *Huffington Post*. Retrieved from https://www.huffingtonpost.com
     /2012/01/19/g-spot-does-not-exist_n_1215822.html

Danielson, M, E., Aaron, D. J., Markovic, N., Schmidt, N. J., & Janosky, J. E.
     (2000). Wednesday, November 15, 2000-3: 12 PM Abstract# 13218 Meno-
     pausal characteristics of lesbian and bisexual women: The ESTHER pro-
     ject. The 128th Annual Meeting of American Public Health Association.
     Boston, MA.

DeAngelis, T. (2002). New data on lesbian, gay and bisexual mental health. *Mon-
     itor on Psychology*, 33(2), 46. Retrieved from http://www.apa.org/monitor
     /feb02/newdata.aspx

Dennerstein, L., Koochaki, P., Barton, I., & Graziottin, A. (2006). Hypoactive sex-
     ual desire disorder in menopausal women: A survey of Western European
     women. *The Journal of Sexual Medicine*, 3(2), 212–222.

Dobry, Y., Rice, T., & Sher, L. (2013). Ecstasy use and serotonin syndrome: A
     neglected danger to adolescents and young adults prescribed selective
     serotonin reuptake inhibitors. *International Journal of Adolescent Medi-
     cine & Health*, 25(3), 193–199. doi:10.1515/ijamh-2013-0052

Donovan, C. (2008). It's not really seen as an issue, you know, lesbian infertility it's
     kind of 'what's that?': Lesbians' unsuccessful experiences of medicalised
     donor insemination. *Medical Sociology Online*, 3(1), 15–24.

Doumas, M., Tsakiris, A., Douma, S., Grigorakis, A., Papadopoulos, A., Hounta,
     A., . . . Giamarellou, H. (2006). Beneficial effects of switching from beta-
     blockers to nebivolol on the erectile function of hypertensive patients.
     Asian Journal of Andrology, 8, 177–182.

Doward, J. (n.d.). Gay men and lesbians are putting their health at risk by abusing
     drugs. Retrieved from http://www.theguardian.com/society/2010/jul/25
     /gay-lesbians-drug-use-report

Eidelman, A. I., & Schanler, R. J. (2012). Breastfeeding and the use of human milk.
     Pediatrics, 129(3), e827–e841.

Evans, A. L., Scally, A. J., Wellard, S. J., & Wilson, J. D. (2007). Prevalence of bacte-
     rial vaginosis in lesbians and heterosexual women in a community setting.
     Sexually Transmitted Infections, 83(6), 470–475.

Farre, M., Abanades, S., Roset, P. N., Peiro, A. M., Torrens, M., O'Mathúna,
     B., . . . de la Torre, R. (2007). Pharmacological interaction between
     3,4-methylenedioxymethamphetamine (ecstasy) and paroxetine: Pharma-
     cological effects and pharmacokinetics. *Journal of Pharmacology and
     Experimental Therapeutics*, 323, 954–962.

Farrow, A. (2014). Lactation support and the LGBTQI community. *Journal of
     Human Lactation*, 31(1), 26–28. doi:10.1177/0890334414554928.

Federation of Feminist Women's Health Centers. (1991). *A new view of a woman's
     body*. San Diego: Feminist Health Press.

Flaherty, J. A., Davis, J. M., & Janicak, P. G. (1993). *Psychiatry: Diagnosis & ther-
     apy. A Lange clinical manual*. New York: Appleton & Lange.

Fredriksen-Goldsen, K. I., Hyun-Jun, K., Barkan, S. E., Muraco, A, & Hoy-Ellis,
     C. P. (2013). Health disparities among lesbian, gay, and bisexual older

adults: Results from a population-based study. *American Journal of Public Health, 103*(10), 1802–1809.

French, S. A., Story, M., Remafedi, G., Resnick, M. D., & Blum, R. W. (1996). Sexual orientation and prevalence of body dissatisfaction and eating disordered behaviors: A population-based study of adolescents. *International Journal of Eating Disorders, 19*(2), 119–126.

Gartner, L. M., Morton, J., Lawrence, R. A., Naylor, A. J., O'Hare, D., Schanler, R. J., . . . American Academy of Pediatrics Section on Breastfeeding. (2005). Breastfeeding and the use of human milk. *Pediatrics, 115*(2), 496–506.

Giles, K. R., & McCabe, M. P. (2009). Conceptualizing women's sexual function: Linear vs. circular models of sexual response. *Journal of Sexual Medicine, 6*(10), 2781–2771.

Gold, E. B., Bromberger, J., Crawford, S., Samuels, S., Greendale, G. A., Harlow, S. D., & Skurnick, J. (2001). Factors associated with age at natural menopause in a multiethnic sample of midlife women. *American Journal of Epidemiology, 153*(9), 865–874.

Goldberg, A. E., Downing, J. B., & Richardson, H. B. (2009). The transition from infertility to adoption: Perceptions of lesbian and heterosexual couples. *Journal of Social and Personal Relationships, 26*(6–7), 938–963.

Gorgos, L. M., & Marrazzo, J. M. (2011). Sexually transmitted infections among women who have sex with women. *Clinical Infectious Disease, 53*, S84–S91.

Grady, D. (2006). Management of menopausal symptoms. *New England Journal of Medicine, 355*(22), 2338–2347.

Greenberg, J. S., Bruess, C. E., & Oswalt, S. B. (2014). *Exploring the dimensions of human sexuality.* Burlington, MA: Jones and Bartlett.

Gregolre, C. (2015, February 20). The strange science of sexual attraction. *Huffington Post.* Retrieved from http://www.huffingtonpost.com/2015/02/14/science-of-attraction-_n_6661522.html

Haimes, E., & Weiner, K. (2000). "Everybody's got a dad . . .": Issues for lesbian families in the management of donor insemination. *Sociology of Health & Illness, 22*(4), 477–499.

Indiana University Bloomington Newsroom. (2014, August 21). Study: Orgasm rates for single women less predictable than men's, vary by sexual orientation. *IU Bloomington Newsroom.* Retrieved from: http://archive.news.indiana.edu/releases/iu/2014/08/sexual-orientation-orgasm-rates.shtml

Jones, C., Chan, C., & Farine, D. (2011). Sex in pregnancy. *Canadian Medical Association Journal, 183*(7), 815–818.

Kammerer-Doak, D., & Rogers, R. G. (2008). Female sexual function and dysfunction. *Obstetrics and Gynecology Clinics of North America, 35*(2), 169–183.

Kaplan, H. S. (1974). *The new sex therapy.* New York: Brunner/Mazel.

Kelly, L. (2007, November). Sexual intimacy and relationship negotiation between lesbians during the menopausal transition. In *Women's health and social issues.* Session conducted at the 39th Biennial Convention of Sigma Theta Tau International, Baltimore, MD.

Kilchevsky, A., Vardi, Y., Lowenstein, L., & Gruenwald, I. (2012). Is the female G-spot truly a distinct anatomic entity? *Journal of Sexual Medicine, 9*(3), 719–726.

Komisaruk, B. R., Wise, N., Frangos, E., Liu, W. C., Allen, K., & Brody, S. (2011). Women's clitoris, vagina, and cervix mapped on the sensory cortex: fMRI evidence. *Journal of Sexual Medicine, 8*(10), 2822–2830.

Kop, P. A., van Wely, M., Mol, B. W., de Melker, A. A., Janssens, P. M., Arends, B., . . . Mochtar, M. H. (2015). Intrauterine insemination or intracervical insemination with cryopreserved donor sperm in the natural cycle: A cohort study. *Human Reproduction, 30*(3), 603–607.

Kranz, K. C., & Daniluk, J. C. (2006). Living outside of the box: Lesbian couples with children conceived through the use of anonymous donor insemination. *Journal of Feminist Family Therapy, 18*(1–2), 1–33.

Kronenberg, F., & Fugh-Berman, A. (2002). Complementary and alternative medicine for menopausal symptoms: A review of randomized, controlled trials. *Annals of Internal Medicine, 137*(10), 805–813.

Laurie, C., & Kinkly. (2013). 9 interesting things you may not know about the clitoris [Blog post]. Retrieved from https://www.alternet.org/9-interesting -things-you-may-not-know-about-clitoris

Lawrence, R. A., & Lawrence, R. M. (2010). *Breastfeeding: A guide for the medical professional.* New York: Elsevier Health Sciences.

Leiblum, S. R., Koochaki, P. E., Rodenberg, C. A., Barton, I. P., & Rosen, R. C. (2006). Hypoactive sexual desire disorder in postmenopausal women: US results from the Women's International Study of Health and Sexuality (WISHeS). *Menopause, 13*(1), 46–56.

Liechti, M. E., Baumann, C., Gamma, A., & Vollenweider, F. X. (2000). Acute psychological effects of 3,4-methylenedioxymethamphetamine (MDMA, "ecstasy") are attenuated by the serotonin uptake inhibitor citalopram. *Neuropsychopharmacology, 22*, 513–521.

Liechti, M. E., Gamma, A., & Vollenweider, F. X. (2001). Gender differences in the subjective effects of MDMA. *Psychopharmacology, 154*(2), 161–168.

Little, B., & Terrance, C. (2010). Perceptions of domestic violence in lesbian relationships: Stereotypes and gender role expectations. *Journal of Homosexuality, 57*(3), 429–440.

Lloyd, E. A. (2005). *The case of the female orgasm: Bias in the science of evolution.* Cambridge, MA: Harvard University Press.

Mah, K., & Binik, Y. M. (2001). The nature of human orgasm: A critical review of major trends. *Clinical Psychology Review, 21*(6), 823–856.

Marina, S., Marina, D., Marina, F., Fosas, N., Galiana, N., & Jové, I. (2010). Sharing motherhood: Biological lesbian co-mothers, a new IVF indication. *Human Reproduction, 25*(4), 938–941.

Marshall Cavendish Corporation. (2009). *Sex and Society* (Vol. 2). Singapore: Marshall Cavendish.

Masters, W. H., & Johnson, V. E. (1966). *Human sexual response.* Boston: Little Brown.

Masters, W. H., & Johnson, V. E. (1981). *Human sexual response* (2nd ed.). New York: Bantam.

Meyerowitz, B. E., Desmond, K. A., Rowland, J. H., Wyatt, G. E., & Ganz, P. A. (1999). Sexuality following breast cancer. *Journal of Sex and Marital Therapy, 25*(3), 237–250.

Moalem, S., & Reidenberg, J. S. (2009). Does female ejaculation serve an antimicrobial purpose? *Medical Hypotheses, 73*(6), 1069–1071.

National Institute on Alcohol Abuse and Alcoholism. (2017). Alcohol: A Women's Health History. Retrieved from https://pubs.niaaa.nih.gov/publications/womensfact/womensfact.htm

North American Menopause Society. (2004). Treatment of menopause-associated vasomotor symptoms: Position statement of the North American Menopause Society. *Menopause (New York, NY), 11*(1), 11.

Notman, M. T., & Nadelson, C. (2002). The hormone replacement therapy controversy. *Archives of Women's Mental Health, 5*(1), 33–35.

O'Connell, H. E., Sanjeevan, K. V., & Huston, J. M. (2005). Anatomy of the clitoris. *Journal of Urology, 174*(4 Pt 1), 1189–1195.

Parsons, J. T., Kelly, B. C., & Wells, B. E. (2006). Differences in club drug use between heterosexual and lesbian/bisexual females. *Addictive behaviors, 31*(12), 2344–2349.

Pelka, Suzanne. (2009). Sharing motherhood: Maternal jealousy among lesbian co-mothers. *Journal of Homosexuality, 56*(2), 195–217.

Riese. (2015a, March 30). How often do queer women have sex? [Blog post]. Retrieved from http://www.autostraddle.com/how-often-do-lesbians-have-sex-283731/

Riese. (2015b, August 25). Lesbian sex: Your 15 favorite ways to have it [Blog post]. Retrieved from https://www.autostraddle.com/how-do-lesbians-have-sex-288982/

Rogers, G., Elston, J., Garside, R., Roome, C., Taylor, R., Younger, P., Zawada, A., & Somerville, M. (2009). The harmful health effects of recreational ecstasy: A systematic review of observational evidence. *Health Technology Assessment, 13*(6), iii–iv, ix–xii, 1–315. doi:10.3310/hta13050

Rosenthal, M. (2012). *Human sexuality: From cells to society*. Boston: Cengage Learning.

Ross, L. E., Steele, L. S., & Epstein, R. (2006a). Lesbian and bisexual women's recommendations for improving the provision of assisted reproductive technology services. *Fertility and Sterility, 86*(3), 735–738.

Ross, L. E., Steele, L. S., & Epstein, R. (2006b). Service use and gaps in services for lesbian and bisexual women during donor insemination, pregnancy, and the postpartum period. *Journal of Obstetrics and Gynaecology Canada/ Journal d'obstetrique et gynecologie du Canada, 28*(6), 505–511.

Rubio-Casillas, A., & Jannini, E. A. (2011). New insights from one case of female ejaculation. *Journal of Sexual Medicine, 8*(12), 3500–3504.

Schick, V., Resnberger, J. G., Herbenick, D., & Reece, M. (2012). Sexual behavior and risk reduction strategies among a multinational sample of women who have sex with women. *Sexually Transmitted Infections, 88*(6), 407–412.

Sherfey, M. J. (1973). *The nature and evolution of female sexuality*. New York: Vintage Books.

Smith, S., Pfeifer, S. M., & Collins, J. A. (2003). Diagnosis and management of female infertility. *JAMA, 290*(13), 1767–1770.

Tafas, T., Ichetovkin, I., Kilpatrick, M., & Tsipouras, P. (2008). Pre-Implantation Genetic Diagnosis Test. U.S. Patent Application No. 11/833,678.

Tancer, M., & Johanson, C. E. (2007). The effects of fluoxetine on the subjective and physiological effects of 3,4-methylenedioxymethamphetamine (MDMA) in humans. *Psychopharmacology, 189*, 565–573.

Toevs, K., & Brill, S. A. (2002). *The essential guide to lesbian conception, pregnancy, and birth*. New York: Alyson.

Topp, L., Hando, J., Dillon, P., Roche, A., & Solowij, N. (1999). Ecstasy use in Australia: Patterns of use and associated harm. *Drug and Alcohol Dependence, 55*(1–2), 105–115.

Turnbull, O. H., Lovett, V. E., Chaldecott, J., & Lucas, M. D. (2014). Reports of intimate touch: Erogenous zones and somatosensory cortical organization. *Cortex, 53*, 146–154.

von Sydow, K. (1999). Sexuality during pregnancy and after childbirth: A metacontent analysis of 59 studies. *Journal of Psychosomatic Research, 47*(1), 27–49.

Wagenback, P. (2008). Lesbian body image and eating issues. *Journal of Psychology & Human Sexuality, 4*, 205–227.

Wahlert, L., & Fiester, A. (2013). Induced lactation for the nongestating mother in a lesbian couple. *The Virtual Mentor, 15*(9), 753.

Weiner, I. B., Stricker, G., & Widiger, T. A. (2012). *Handbook of psychology, clinical psychology*. Hoboken, NJ: John Wiley & Sons.

West, C. M. (2008). Lesbian intimate partner violence. *Journal of Lesbian Studies, 6*(1), 121–127.

Weston, L. C. (2011, February 22). Can't orgasm? Here's help for women. *WebMD*. Retrieved from https://www.webmd.com/sexual-conditions/features/cant-orgasm-heres-help-for-women#1

Wewomen. (n.d.). The lesbian kama sutra: 100 sex positions for women. *WeWomen.com*. Retrieved from http://www.wewomen.com/relationships/album962601/lesbian-kama-sutra-100-sex-positions-for-women-0.html#p13

Wittig, S. L., & Spatz, D. L. (2008). Induced lactation: Gaining a better understanding. *MCN: The American Journal of Maternal/Child Nursing, 33*(2), 76–81.

Woodward, B. J., & Norton, W. J. (2006). Lesbian intra-partner oocyte donation: A possible shake-upin the Garden of Eden? *Human Fertility, 9*(4), 217–222.

World Health Organization. (2018). *Female genital mutilation*. Retrieved from http://www.who.int/mediacentre/factsheets/fs241/en/

Zastrow, C. (2007). *Introduction to social work and social welfare: Empowering people*. Boston: Cengage Learning.

Zeiler, K., & Malmquist, A. (2014). Lesbian shared biological motherhood: The ethics of IVF with reception of oocytes from partner. *Medicine, Health Care and Philosophy, 17*(3), 347–355.

Zizzo, G. (2009). Lesbian families and the negotiation of maternal identity through the unconventional use of breast milk. *Gay and Lesbian Issues and Psychology Review, 5*(2), 96.

10

Sexual Health for Men

Laura Erickson-Schroth, Richard E. Greene, and David Hankins

Sexual desire and sexual activity are important parts of the human experience. This chapter will focus on cisgender men who have sex with other men. Sex between men may occur in many contexts, from long-term relationships to casual encounters—any or all of which can play a role in fulfilling this basic human need. Because sexuality is such an important part of overall health, in this chapter we explore how men meet and have sex with other men and some of the main health issues that may arise as part of sexual experiences.

COMMUNITY, ATTRACTION, AND SEXUAL ROLES

Romantic and erotic attraction are complicated processes formed over a lifetime. It is important to note that attraction is subjective, and each individual has sexual and romantic tastes that differ minimally to dramatically from his neighbor. Within the gay and bisexual community, many men identify themselves by their preferred sexual position during anal sex—either "top" or "bottom" (i.e., insertive or receptive partner during anal intercourse), or "vers" for versatile. For some, this identification is strictly a matter of physical position during sex, and for others, it is accompanied by generalized (and often inconsistent) role-defining characteristics, including dominance or submissiveness, or aggressiveness or passiveness. For some, these roles remain consistent throughout their lives, and for others, they are fluid depending on their partner or the particular moment in time, or they may even change during the course of a single sexual encounter.

The gay community has also famously subidentified into smaller groups or communities depending on personal identifications with others of a group. An older or more aggressive man may be considered a "daddy," or a younger, slimmer-built man may be a "twink." "Bears" are generally larger men with more overall body hair. There is no need for one to feel pressure to identify with any one group, and one person's identification may change frequently, but some are very committed to these roles and attracted to men within a particular group. The "bear" culture is thought to have formed either as a reaction to a perception of a narrowly accepted body ideal by men who felt more comfortable carrying more weight or by men who felt it was a more "masculine" look.

SEXUAL ANATOMY AND PHYSIOLOGY

Male sexual anatomy is often thought of as limited to the genitals. However, in addition to the penis, testicles, and anus, there are many other parts of the body that are part of male sexuality.

The Brain

Perhaps the most sexual organ in the body is the brain. Our brains interpret the signals we receive from the outside world and from our body parts, translating them into coherent messages for us. Our brains determine whether we are interested in sex and whom we are attracted to. When we see something or are touched in a certain way, our brain takes in the information about that visual or physical cue and tells us whether we should view it as pleasurable. This means that context is very important to whether we will feel aroused or will orgasm. Some people, including some whose spinal cords are not functioning, can orgasm without any stimulation of their bodies, which tells us that the final pathway for an orgasm is through the brain.

Erogenous Zones

Aside from our brains and our genitals, we each have different parts of our bodies that are particularly sensitive. These areas may have large numbers of nerve endings and are sometimes called erogenous zones. For example, for many people, the chest is a sensitive area that can produce pleasurable feelings when stimulated. Nipples contain numerous nerve endings, as do other parts of our chests. Earlobes can be very sensitive areas that respond sexually to licking and sucking.

The Penis

Penises come in all shapes and sizes. Many men have specific areas that are most sensitive and certain ways they enjoy being touched. However, there are some basics that can be applied to many people.

The shaft of the penis is made up of two kinds of cylindrical tissue. The corpus spongiosum is located on the underside of the penis and surrounds the urethra, the tube through which urine and semen leave the body. In addition to the corpus spongiosum, there are two corpora cavernosa on the top of the penis that are made of erectile tissue which fills with blood with arousal. (See Figure 10.1.)

The most sensitive areas of the penis are often the glans (tip) of the penis, the coronal ridge (the back edge of the glans), the frenulum (the elastic tissue on the underside of the penis near the glans), and the raphe (the line on the underside of the penis).

Many men wonder about their penis size and shape, whether they are "normal," and what the average size is. Gay male culture places a strong emphasis on penis size. In a study of over 1,500 men in the United States, self-measurement produced an average reported erect penis length of 5.6 inches (Wessells, Lue, & McAninch, 1996). The same authors identified another research group that measured the penis length of 80 men in a medical office and found an average length of 5.1 inches. These numbers

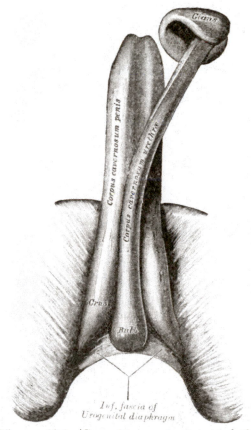

Figure 10.1 (Gray, Henry. *Anatomy of the Human Body*. Philadelphia: Lea & Febiger, 1918, p. 1248, figure 1154.)

are in contrast to the overwhelming number of personal ads in which men report much longer lengths. Men who have sex with men and feel their penises are below average size often struggle with self-doubt (Grov, Parsons, & Bimbi, 2010). Penis size, like any other feature, varies considerably.

Circumcision is a tradition in many cultures. It involves cutting away the foreskin to expose the glans. Worldwide, about a third of men are circumcised. The highest rates are in Africa and the Middle East, with low rates in Europe, Asia, and South America. The rate of circumcision in the United States is high and is estimated to be between 76 and 92 percent (World Health Organization, 2008). There are some men who find other men more attractive if they are either circumcised or uncircumcised, but many are interested in partners either way.

On an individual basis, circumcision can potentially affect the sensitivity of the penis, making it less sensitive. However, most circumcised men are content with their level of sensitivity (Morris & Krieger, 2013). Circumcised penises are easier to clean, but uncircumcised penises are easily kept clean with good hygiene. There is evidence that circumcision decreases rates of urinary tract infections (UTIs) in infants, penile cancer in adults, and possibly HIV transmission in adults.

There is some debate over whether circumcision should be recommended in order to help prevent the spread of sexually transmitted infections (STIs). Studies of adult men who have sex with women in Africa have shown that circumcision decreases the rate of HIV transmission (Hayashi & Kohri, 2013; Van Howe, 2013). The American Academy of Pediatrics recommends that circumcision be presented as an option and made accessible to parents of newborn males but does not believe that the benefits outweigh the risks enough to recommend routine circumcision (Blank et al., 2012).

The Testicles

The testicles (or testes) hang below the penis in a sack known as the scrotum. Functionally, the testes produce sperm, the genetic material used in reproduction. They are coated in a sensitive sheath, and each testis is connected to a spermatic cord (the epididymis) and blood vessels that feed it. The spermatic cord is similar in texture to a coiled piece of pasta attached to the back of the testis. Semen, the fluid that makes up ejaculate in which sperm swims, is produced in the prostate and travels into the spermatic cords during ejaculation.

In terms of sexual pleasure, each person experiences different levels of pleasure from the testicles. Some find the experience of having their testicles touched or handled to be wholly unpleasant. Others find it to be a very erotic experience. Most men fall somewhere in the middle, enjoying gentle stroking or licking of the scrotum as an adjunct to other forms of sexual activity.

The Anus and Prostate

The anus can be a source of great pleasure, depending on the type of sexual activity and whether men are interested in engaging in anal sex or anal play. The anus is made up of two layers of muscle called the internal and external sphincters. We can control the external sphincter but not the internal sphincter, both important mechanisms of continence. The anus is especially sensitive, as well as the first part of the rectum, and the area becomes less sensitive the further it is penetrated. The anus does not produce its own lubrication. Lube is often necessary for pleasurable anal play. The perineal area, which runs from the anus up to the bottom of the penis, is also a sensitive area.

Internally, our rectum is close to a number of other organs that, when pressure is applied, can produce a pleasurable sensation. An example is the prostate. The prostate is about the size of a walnut and surrounds the urethra just below the bladder. It produces fluid that combines with sperm and seminal fluid to produce semen. The prostate pushes up against the front of the rectum and can be felt with a finger placed inside the rectum and pointed toward the front of the body.

Sexual Response

The process of arousal and orgasm has been divided into four stages. In the first stage, one becomes aroused, which can take place through any number of senses—vision, hearing, smell, or touch. Heart rate, breathing, and blood pressure increase. Genitals receive increased blood flow, which can make the penis begin to become erect. In the next stage, called the plateau phase, heart rate increases more, and muscles can tighten. Next, as orgasm begins, one experiences rhythmic muscle contractions and a sense of euphoria. Semen is expelled from the body. After orgasm, one enters the resolution phase, where blood pressure drops and muscles relax. Most men have a refractory period where they cannot orgasm again for a period of time. Although many people think of the purpose of sexual encounters as producing an orgasm, stimulation that feels good but does not lead to orgasm can be just as exciting.

FINDING PARTNERS

Where do men meet other men to date and have sex with? The answer is a complicated one, as in-person venues for meeting sexual partners such as bars, clubs, and parties are increasingly complemented or replaced by online "venues" such as Web sites and smartphone apps that track users' location using global positioning satellites (GPS). According to multiple studies, a significant percentage of men who have sex with men (MSM) have said they use electronic means to meet sexual partners, and they use it for both casual partner-seeking and romantic partner-seeking (Liau, Millett, & Marks, 2006). Recent studies have confirmed that younger MSM are now meeting their first sexual partners more often on the Internet than anywhere else, leading to a corresponding decrease in the number of MSM meeting their first sexual partner by all other methods including gay venues, school, telephone chat lines, or public sex environments (Bolding, Davis, Hart, Sherr, & Elford, 2007). In one study, 60 percent of men said that online partner-seeking had reduced the amount of time they spent trying to meet other men in person (Bauermeister, Leslie-Santana, Johns, Pingel, & Eisenberg, 2011).

Dozens of GPS-based smartphone apps have burst onto the gay scene in the last decade, allowing for real-time conversation with potential sexual partners sorted by distance from one's current location. Men use these apps to engage in different kinds of sex: a majority in one study reported using apps or the Internet for condomless anal intercourse, but 44 percent also used the apps exclusively for manual or oral sex (Grosskopf, LeVasseur, & Glaser, 2014).

Many of these smartphone apps cater to specific subsets of the MSM community. For example, men using *Grindr*, the most popular of these apps, appear to be younger than the MSM population as a whole (Burrell et al., 2012). Other apps are aimed at bears (Bear Social Network), older men (MR X.), or those looking for condomless sex (BarebackRT.com).

Although the Internet and apps are hugely popular, they have not replaced physical venues for meeting partners. While a majority of MSM report using online means to meet sex partners, a majority also report using venues such as bars, clubs, bathhouses, or sex parties to meet partners (Grov, Parsons, & Bimbi, 2007), suggesting that for many MSM, Internet use is an additional tool for meeting partners and not their only tool.

Monogamy and Nonmonogamy

When deciding to enter a relationship, it is important to define expectations around monogamy or nonmonogamy. Many gay couples find fulfillment in monogamous relationships, while other gay couples freely explore sexual relationships with other partners. Columnist Dan Savage has coined the term "monogamish" to describe couples who have sex with others together or individually, according to boundaries established in advance (Savage, 2012). Communication about expectations is key at all points of a relationship, with each partner sharing how he feels about monogamy/nonmonogamy and seeking to understand the beliefs and feelings of the other partner.

SEXUAL PRACTICES

Masturbation, Mutual Masturbation, and Frottage

Masturbation is the physical act of pleasuring oneself. The ways to masturbate are as unique as the individuals who are masturbating. For most men, this involves some kind of stimulation of the penis until orgasm is achieved. Some focus exclusively on the penis, and others take a more global approach, including their nipples, anus, and other areas. Two men can masturbate each other, either by stroking each other's penises with their hands or by rubbing their penises against each other's bodies. The latter technique is known as "frottage." Masturbation is a fairly common practice and often supported by the medical community, as it is a safe way to engage in sex with almost no risk of passing sexually transmitted infections.

Oral Sex

Oral sex, as the name implies, is the act of using one's mouth to give a partner pleasure. Most frequently, this involves using the mouth on a partner's penis. Sometimes colloquially referred to as a "blow job" or "giving head," the act involves sucking on a partner's penis. Many gay men refer to "deep throating" as a deep form of oral sex. Some givers of oral sex have less of an urge to gag, a normal reflex designed to protect against aspiration (or the unwanted ingestion of substances from the mouth and throat into the lungs). Others who wish to give their partners the sensation of deeper sucking can wrap their hand around the base of their partner's penis and use either saliva or lube to make the penis slick and slide in the giver's hand or fist. While the risk of transmitting HIV through oral sex is very small (Varghese, Maher, Peterman, Branson, & Steketee, 2002) and condoms are often not used for oral sex (Stone, Hatherall, Ingham, & McEachran, 2006; Crosby, et al., 2016), other sexually transmitted infections like gonorrhea, syphilis, and herpes can be passed through oral sex.

Anal Sex

Perhaps no aspect of gay sex is the target of more thought and consternation than anal sex. For the purposes of this discussion, we will use the terms "top" to refer to the insertive partner and "bottom" to refer to the receptive partner. Gay men who are versatile or "vers" enjoy being the top or the bottom. It is not necessary to choose, but some people have a natural preference for one position over another. Often, one's preference changes over time or depends on specific partners.

For some, the pleasure derived from anal sex is physical, derived either from the stroking and pressure on the prostate or the sensation of the insertive partner sliding in and out of the rectum. For others, this is a more psychological pleasure. Initially, there can be pain with insertion of the penis, as there is stretching of the anal opening and friction that can irritate the lining of the anal canal.

There is much written about how one should prepare to have anal intercourse. For a very complete reference, consider *The Ins and Outs of Gay Sex*, by Stephen E. Goldstone, MD (1999). One should always begin slowly. Beginning with a small dildo or sex toy can be helpful, with liberal use of lubricant. It can be helpful to have the receptive partner on top of the insertive partner initially, as this allows him to control the speed of insertion and allows him to gently guide the penis past the outer and inner sphincters of the rectum. While there may be some discomfort initially, pain should be avoided.

Inherent in the risks of anal sex is the possibility of contact with feces. While the sigmoid colon can store stool prior to a bowel movement, it is not constantly full of stool. Some men can sense the amount of stool present and thus can knowingly vary the amount of preparation prior to receptive anal sex. Others as a matter of course utilize various methods to remove stool from the rectum. Methods include store-bought enemas with sodium phosphate laxative properties. Enema overuse can lead to elevated phosphate in the blood and other electrolyte abnormalities. Tap water enemas can serve a similar purpose without this risk. Some men will also use antidiarrheal preparations like loperamide to slow the movement of stool in the colon to postpone the need for additional efforts at hygiene. There is no clear medical recommendation about if and how one should prepare for receptive anal sex. Whichever mechanism one chooses, caution and good judgment should be used.

Analingus, aka Rimming

Stimulation of the anus with the mouth and tongue is another way many people experience pleasure. Some enjoy this as the receptive partner, others as the insertive partner, and many as both. Analingus carries with it the risk of passing on infections that may be in the gastrointestinal tract, including parasites like giardia and entamoeba, and viral infections like hepatitis A. There is a fairly low risk of HIV transmission from rimming. One can use a barrier protection like a dental dam when rimming to reduce the risk of disease transmission.

Sex Toys

Many gay and bisexual men use sex toys, like dildos and other objects, to enhance sex play. They may be used alone for autoerotic stimulation instead of, or in conjunction with, masturbation. With partners, they can be a way to engage in anal sex when one partner is unable to get an erection or when both partners prefer to be receptive. They can also be used to supplement sex between two partners when the bottom prefers a larger phallus than his partner has naturally. Toys allow for both partners to stay engaged in sex while alleviating the pressure on one man to have or maintain an erection. There are also sex toys that slide over the penis to give it more stiffness, length, or girth. Sex toys must be cleaned between uses with soap and warm water. When sharing sex toys, clean between partners or have each partner use their own condom on the sex toy.

There has been some controversy surrounding phthalates, which have been used to make some sex toys more pliable (Centers for Disease Control and Prevention, n.d.). These are being phased out of sex toys; however, one should take care to read the label before buying one.

Fisting

Fisting, or the insertion of the hand or fist into a partner's rectum, is a rare but sometimes eroticized activity. There is very little in the medical literature about the health risks of fisting, but among them is possible intestinal perforation, which is a medical emergency. Damage to the internal anal sphincter can lead to fecal incontinence, although this occurs much less frequently than the general population may imagine. Blood from tearing of the rectal lining, if making contact with open sores on the insertive partner's skin, creates risk for transmitting HIV and hepatitis C.

Urophilia, aka "Water Sports"

Water sports, or playing with and/or drinking of a partner's urine, is another less often performed (Scorolli, Ghirlanda, Enquist, Zattoni, & Jannini, 2007), but much-eroticized possible activity in which gay men may engage. It is often performed in the shower or bathroom to simplify clean up. Urine as a fluid is mostly (but not always) sterile and does not frequently pass on disease and does not carry HIV. If ingested, there are metabolites (or waste products) of medications taken by the person urinating contained in the urine that when ingested can cause allergies or reactions in the person drinking the urine.

BDSM and Kink

According to Merriam-Webster, a kink is defined as "an unconventional sexual taste or behavior." Kinks are quite common and may be broad or specific. Kinks can include some of the things already discussed, like water sports or rimming.

One of the more common kinks involves role playing in the form of a "scene" or particular scenario. Common forms of kinks include bondage and discipline or sadism and masochism (BDSM). Bondage is the tying up or restraint of one partner by another for pleasure. Discipline is when one partner chastises, spanks, or punishes another partner. Sadism is when one enjoys the act of causing pain to his partner, and masochism is the enjoyment of one's own pain for erotic or sexual pleasure. Another kink may be the wearing of leather or particular costumes or uniforms and acting out a specific scene. The wearing of women's clothing for sexual pleasure is more common among heterosexually identified men than it is among gay and bisexual men (Docter & Prince, 1997), although gay and bisexual men are more likely to cross-dress for purposes of entertainment, such as in "drag." As previously mentioned, kinks are best explored by consenting partners with discussion in advance about expectations and limits. Partners generally agree in advance on particular limits, and use of a "safe" word that is unrelated to the "scene" so that when it is used, both partners will know that the "scene" must stop or be suspended so that any physical or emotional distress can be alleviated.

There is little medical literature about specific kinks, and therefore providers may feel challenged when asked to counsel their patients. Consider first the basic question of whether the activity will cease functions that can be necessary for life, such as breathing, circulation (particularly to extremities for long periods), or eating. Anything that alters the sensorium, like alcohol or drugs, is discouraged and potentially unsafe when engaging in risky sexual play. Finally, consider the potential for infection when engaging in a particular activity, including the transmission of HIV or STIs through blood in fluids during fisting or cutting activities. When all else fails, one can thoughtfully consult information on the Internet for ideas. There are many groups and societies that have come up with recommendations to minimize harm to participants in a particular kink. While these recommendations may not be evidence based, they are frequently thought out through lenses of common sense and experience.

PREVENTION OF SEXUALLY TRANSMITTED INFECTION (STI) TRANSMISSION

Barrier Methods

Condoms, when correctly used, will help prevent diseases spread through contact with bodily fluids, including chlamydia, gonorrhea, and HIV, but are less useful in stopping the transmission of infections spread through skin-to-skin contact—such as herpes, human papillomavirus

(HPV), and syphilis (Cohen, 2011). Condoms are made with a variety of materials, including latex, polyurethane, polyisoprene, and lambskin. Latex condoms are the most commonly used. Many latex condoms contain a spermicide such as Nonoxynol-9, which can help prevent pregnancy but has not been shown to reduce transmission of HIV or other STIs (Richardson et al., 2001). About 1 to 2 percent of people, and more among those working in health care (Sussman & Beezhold, 1995), have an allergy to latex and should choose another kind of condom. Polyurethane condoms have been shown to be just as effective as latex ones in blocking semen (Macaluso et al., 2007). Polyisoprene condoms are the newest kind on the market; they are effective against STIs and another good option for those with latex allergies. Lambskin condoms are discouraged for most MSM; they are effective in preventing pregnancy but do not protect against STIs, including HIV (Workowski & Bolan, 2015).

To use a condom effectively, the direction of roll must be determined by placing the condom on your finger and unrolling a very small amount; if it resists this movement, try the other side. Next, place the condom on the tip of the erect penis. If the condom does not have a reservoir, pinch the tip about half an inch to leave room for semen. Unroll the condom all the way to the base of the penis. It should fit snugly, but not too tightly, to make sure that the condom stays on throughout sex and does not break. If you feel the condom break at any point, pull out and put on a new condom. It is important to use a new condom for every sexual act.

Some people who do not use condoms attempt to "pull out" before they orgasm. While this technique may reduce the likelihood of STI transmission from a "top" to a "bottom" partner, it is important to know that even before orgasm, fluids are passed between partners. Pre-ejaculate or "precum" is fluid that is released in advance of an orgasm and can spread HIV and other STIs.

When using lubricant ("lube") with condoms, it is important to use a water- or silicone-based lubricant, since oil-based lubricants (petroleum jelly, lotion) can damage condoms and render them ineffective (Voeller, Coulson, Bernstein, & Nakamura, 1989).

Some MSM use the so-called "female condom" for anal sex (Kelvin et al., 2011). One advantage to this type of condom is that the receptive partner ("bottom") can self-insert the condom before sex, giving him more control over the use of protection. However, research has shown that these condoms may be more prone to slippage and may lead to more discomfort for the receptive partner than male condoms when used for anal sex. Their overall effectiveness against STIs has also not been firmly established (Renzi et al., 2003), and they are not FDA approved for anal sex.

Dental dams can be used during oral sex or analingus (licking the anus) to prevent the transmission of STIs. Dental dams are typically made of latex and are used by holding them over the genitals or anal area while a partner's mouth is in contact with it.

Improvised or homemade methods of barrier protection, such as plastic wrap or rubber gloves, have not been scientifically evaluated to the extent that condoms and dental dams have been. The FDA in 1993 found that Saran Wrap (the brand-name product was specifically tested) can prevent the transmission of virus-sized particles (Winks & Semans, 2002). So, while scientific testing of improvised barrier methods has not been as extensive as testing done on condoms and dental dams, Saran Wrap is a possible alternative to these for use during oral sex or analingus.

PEP and PrEP

Beginning in 2005, anyone with a possible exposure to HIV could request HIV post-exposure prophylaxis (PEP), typically consisting of a four-week regimen of an approved HIV medication or medications. This included those who were concerned about sexual contact with a partner of unknown HIV status (Smith et al., 2005). Despite the strong evidence in support of PEP, medical providers' knowledge of PEP's availability and how to correctly prescribe and monitor the medications is not universal, and it continues to be underutilized (Rodriguez et al., 2013).

In 2012, the Centers for Disease Control approved the use of a once-daily combination pill containing the medications tenofovir and emtricitabine, sold under the brand name of Truvada, for use as pre-exposure prophylaxis (PrEP) for HIV. PrEP has been shown to significantly reduce the risk of new HIV infection among those who take it every day. PrEP may be especially helpful in preventing HIV transmission among MSM who have condomless anal intercourse with casual partners (Grant et al., 2010), and MSM who are injection drug users (Strathdee et. al, 2012).

"What Are My Chances?"

While there may be times when it is obvious that a potential partner has a sexually transmitted infection (i.e., a syphilis chancre or urethral discharge caused by gonorrhea), in most cases, you cannot determine a partner's HIV or STI status just by looking. Disclosure of HIV status can be particularly challenging for those who are HIV positive because of concern about stigma, with recent studies suggesting that 15 to 30 percent of HIV-positive MSM may not disclose their status to new partners (Du et al., 2015; Przbyla et al., 2013).

If you are HIV negative and intend to have condomless anal intercourse with a partner, the evidence is inconclusive about whether asking your partner's HIV status will actually reduce your chances of getting HIV. This process of "serosorting" potential partners based on their stated or perceived HIV status has been shown to be much less effective in preventing the spread of HIV than consistent and correct use of condoms (van den Boom et al., 2014; Golden, Dombrowski, Kerani, & Stekler, 2012). Having condomless anal intercourse with a partner whom you assume to have the same HIV status as you may also place you at greater risk of contracting other sexually transmitted infections such as gonorrhea, chlamydia, and syphilis (Hotton, Gratzer, & Mehta, 2012).

If you do decide to have condomless anal intercourse with a partner, what are your chances of acquiring HIV? It is only possible to estimate, but not using a condom appears to be about 20 times riskier than using a condom, and receptive anal intercourse ("bottoming") is 7 to 8 times riskier than insertive anal intercourse ("topping"). In the case of oral sex, being the receptive partner (the one taking a penis into the mouth) is estimated to be twice as risky as being the insertive partner (Varghese, Maher, Peterman, Branson, & Steketee, 2002).

Gay men often guess about a partner's HIV status without actually discussing the issue together. Making the assumption that a partner has the same HIV status has been shown to lead to higher rates of condomless anal intercourse, increasing the possibility of HIV transmission (Zablotska et al., 2009). It is a good idea to discuss HIV status with a potential sexual partner early, while understanding that a potential partner's self-identification as HIV negative should be considered in the context of the time since his last HIV test.

SUBSTANCE USE AND SEX

Regardless of whether they are prescription or nonprescription medications, legal or illegal drugs, many medications and drugs have the potential to be abused. Some of the substances commonly abused have effects on sexual function.

Alcohol

Lechery, sir, it provokes, and unprovokes;
It provokes the desire, but it takes away the performance.
                                        —Shakespeare, *Macbeth*, 2.3

The most commonly abused substance in the United States is alcohol, likely because it is legal to use. Alcohol is potentially one of the most harmful drugs to abuse, as it lowers our inhibitions and decreases coordination, leading to thousands of motor vehicle accidents each year. It is commonly used as a social lubricant for people who have anxiety finding partners or making conversation. There are socially acceptable limits on alcohol use, beyond which we are more likely to engage in risky behaviors and make bad decisions.

In the long term, alcohol has many negative physiologic effects, including liver damage that can lead to increased levels of estrogen, breast growth, and testicular shrinking. With sustained use, alcohol in large quantities can ultimately lead to liver failure, requiring a liver transplant.

In the short term, alcohol can have a number of effects on our bodies. Related to our sexual functioning, alcohol tends to decrease our inhibitions, which can make us more likely to engage in sexual behaviors, but it also increases the likelihood of erectile dysfunction, sometimes making us unable to perform despite our interest.

National guidelines indicate that men should be consuming no more than two drinks per day. High-risk drinking for men is more than 4 drinks in a sitting or 14 drinks in a week (Saitz et al., 2007).

Cocaine

Cocaine is also a commonly used drug of abuse. Cocaine induces pleasurable feelings and increases sex drive. However, it can also have numerous immediate dangers as well as more long-term consequences. Men who sleep with men and use cocaine are less likely to use condoms (Dirks et al., 2012), increasing the risk of contracting HIV and other STIs. Over the long term, cocaine has been linked with decreased sexual function, such as erectile dysfunction and decreased interest in sex (Cocores, Miller, Pottash, & Gold, 1988).

Crystal Meth

Methamphetamine has become a serious concern in gay male communities, catching on as a party drug but causing addiction and social and financial problems for many users. Many men use crystal to enhance sexual experiences. However, the drug can also cause what is colloquially called "crystal dick," which is an inability to maintain an erection, interfering with sexual activity. If it is difficult to maintain an erection, some people are more likely to have receptive anal sex, often without condoms.

Using meth can make it more likely for HIV to be transmitted. Men who have sex with men and use methamphetamine have been shown to have more sex partners, use condoms less often (Molitor, Truax, Ruiz, &

Sun, 1998), and be more likely to acquire HIV (Buchacz, et al., 2005). Frequent methamphetamine users are more likely to have unprotected anal sex with someone who is HIV positive if they are negative, and vice versa (Chen, Vallabhaneni, Raymond, & McFarland, 2012). Methamphetamine use is also associated with higher viral loads (C. K. Mantri, J. V. Mantri, Pandhare, & Dash, 2014).

One method of methamphetamine use, known as "booty bumping," involves inserting either powder or liquid into the anus. Methamphetamine powder can be abrasive, causing increased friction during anal sex, making it more likely for condoms to break and for diseases to be transmitted. It is possible that this practice may also increase the risk of human papillomavirus (HPV) transition to anal cancers. If using a syringe (without a needle) to insert methamphetamine in the anus, be sure not to share syringes, as this can transmit hepatitis and other infections.

Poppers

Amyl nitrite, also known as "poppers," is a drug that is inhaled and has a very rapid onset. It works by relaxing involuntary muscles, resulting in dilation of blood vessels that leads to a pleasant "head rush" and often an erection, but also to decreased blood pressure, increased heart rate, facial flushing, and headache. Some men use amyl nitrite to relax the anal sphincter for more comfortable anal sex.

Poppers should never be used at the same time as erectile dysfunction medications such as sildenafil (Viagra), vardenafil (Levitra), or tadalafil (Cialis). The combination can lead to a significant drop in blood pressure, resulting in passing out.

There is very little research into the long-term medical complications of amyl nitrite. However, its use has been linked to riskier sexual practices. For example, HIV-positive men who have sex with men and use poppers are more likely to have unprotected anal intercourse with HIV-negative men (Hatfield, Horvath, Jacoby, & Simon Rosser, 2009).

Ecstasy

MDMA, also known as "ecstasy," is a drug that causes euphoria, decreased anxiety, and increased feelings of social connectedness. Though it can increase erotic sensations, it can also cause erectile dysfunction.

There are a number of serious short-term risks with taking ecstasy. It can lead to dehydration, sweating, and hyperthermia. Many people are aware of this and attempt to compensate by drinking water. However, there have been deaths attributed to ecstasy users drinking too much water and reducing the salt in their bodies to dangerously low levels.

There is debate about the long-term effects of MDMA, but there is evidence that it can affect the way the neurotransmitter serotonin is processed in the brain. There is evidence suggesting that ecstasy can cause permanent changes in memory, as well as depression (Rogers et al., 2009).

Those who take selective serotonin reuptake inhibitor (SSRI) antidepressants should avoid using ecstasy, as there have been reported cases of serotonin syndrome (Dobry, Rice, & Sher, 2013), which causes hyperthermia and muscle twitches and can lead to death. Not only do these antidepressants increase risk of death when used with ecstasy, but they have also been shown to decrease MDMA's effects, making it less likely that the user will get high (Farré et al., 2007; Tancer & Johanson, 2007; Liechti, Baumann, Gamma, & Vollenweider, 2000).

Prescription Medications

Alcohol and drugs can affect sexual function, but so can many prescribed medications. Some, like erectile dysfunction medications, are prescribed specifically for sex-related purposes, but others, like antidepressants and blood pressure medications, can affect our sexual function as a side effect.

Antidepressants

Antidepressants are commonly prescribed and may be even more common among gay and bisexual men, who have higher depression rates (Jorm, Korten, Rodgers, Jacomb, & Christensen, 2002) due to social stigma. Many antidepressants, especially selective serotonin reuptake inhibitors (SSRIs) such as fluoxetine (Prozac) and citalopram (Celexa), can cause sexual side effects, including decreased interest in sex (decreased libido), erectile dysfunction, delayed ejaculation, and inability to orgasm. At times, these side effects may be confused with the effects of depression itself. Depression can lead to decreased interest in sex but should not cause orgasmic difficulties if aroused. Many providers forget to ask about these side effects, and they can be potentially embarrassing to bring up, but it is important to talk about them with a provider because they can often be treated by switching to another antidepressant.

Blood Pressure Medications

Blood pressure medications are another category of frequently prescribed medications that can affect sexual function. Beta blockers in particular, such as metoprolol and propranolol, have the potential to cause decreased interest in sex and problems with orgasm. These medications may also be able to be switched, although they may be the best category of blood pressure medication for people with a particular health history. There are a number of other types of medications used less commonly that can affect sexual function, so the best thing to do when there are noticeable changes in sexual interest or function is to speak with a health care provider.

Erectile Dysfunction Medications

Erectile dysfunction medications such as sildenafil and tadalafil are prescription medications but are also used by some people who do not have erectile dysfunction to prolong erections (Lowe & Costabile, 2011). Erectile dysfunction can be defined as the inability to produce an erection that is as hard or lasts as long as desired. Erectile dysfunction can be physical or psychological—and often a combination of the two. Psychological issues that can affect the ability to produce an orgasm include temporary mood issues and changes in desire toward a partner.

Erectile dysfunction medications work by opening up blood vessels, increasing blood flow to the penis. Often, brief courses of taking these medications are all that is needed. The lowest dose that works to produce a satisfactory erection should be used to avoid side effects, which can include headaches, facial flushing, and visual changes. One question that some people have is whether erectile dysfunction medications decrease the ability to have erections without them. The evidence seems to suggest that most men who use these medications continue to respond to them over time, although some need a slightly increased dose. This may be because there is a tolerance built or because the medical condition causing erectile dysfunction is getting worse.

Although erectile dysfunction medications require a prescription, they are often used recreationally. Medication for erectile dysfunction used to combat the effects of recreational drugs like methamphetamine has been linked to increased risk of HIV (Mansergh et al., 2006). There can be a potentially life-threatening interaction between nitroglycerin (prescribed for chest pain) and other nitrates like amyl nitrate ("poppers"). These medications in combination with erectile dysfunction medications can cause a dangerous drop in blood pressure that can lead to death.

At times, erectile dysfunction medications may cause an erection to last longer than is healthy, cutting off circulation to the penis and causing risk of tissue damage, a condition called priapism. There are also other prescription medications not intended as erectile dysfunction medications that can have the rare side effect of prolonged erections. If an erection lasts longer than four hours, emergency services should be sought immediately so that penile function is not lost permanently.

A SYMPTOM-BASED APPROACH TO
SEXUAL HEALTH CONCERNS

It can be difficult to know when you should see your health care provider about symptoms you have. Some people are reluctant to see a provider, so they minimize problems, while others do not make the connection that symptoms may be sexually related. Health care providers may forget to ask about sexual activity. Furthermore, when people try to educate themselves about symptoms from sexually transmitted diseases, information is often presented in the form of more extreme cases or technical information about specific bacteria and viruses. What follows is a set of extensive (but by no means comprehensive) descriptions of some common infections and conditions that can result from sexual activity and should be discussed with your doctor in the event that you have them.

Mouth and Throat

Sore Throat: A sore throat is a very common symptom and does not usually indicate a sexually transmitted infection. Often it is the result of a virus similar to the ones that cause the common cold. On occasion, if the symptom is isolated in the throat and generally does not have cough or body aches associated with it, it can be the result of a bacterial infection. This might lead to a red, painful sore throat, pain while swallowing, and even pus in the back of the throat. A commonly seen infection of this sort is strep throat, caused by group A streptococcus or *Streptococcus pyogenes*. In rare cases, however, one might contract this type of sore throat from gonorrhea picked up from oral sex. In some cases, gonorrhea in the throat can be completely without symptoms or mimic a cold or allergy. Asymptomatic men can transmit the pathogen to their partner. For people who have multiple sexual partners, even for oral sex, the Centers for Disease Control and Prevention recommends routine screening at intervals for oral gonorrhea (Centers for Disease Control and Prevention, n.d.). There are several different tests for gonorrhea in the throat, but a "routine" throat culture will likely not pick up this infection, so it is important to discuss any risks you have with your health care provider. A sore throat can also be the first sign of a new HIV infection but usually has other associated symptoms (further discussed below).

Ulcers: Sores in the mouth come in two varieties: outside the mouth around the lips and inside the mouth and throat. Outer sores are more easily noticed and may be painful or not. Painful sores around the mouth are likely caused by the herpes virus and are very common. More than two-thirds of all people have the virus that causes herpes sores (or "fever blisters") around their mouths (Xu et al., 2002). In contrast, a painless sore around or inside the mouth might come from an early infection with syphilis. In fact, a sore inside the mouth or in the back of the throat that is painless can easily go unnoticed, which makes routine screening for syphilis very important, as it a very easy infection to spread. Other common non-infectious causes of painful ulcers in the mouth include aphthous ulcers or "canker" sores, which are not sexually transmitted but can be brought on by local trauma or stress (Akintoye & Greenberg, 2005).

Lumps and Bumps: There is increasing evidence that HPV, the virus that causes warts and leads to some cancer, can infect the mouth, leading to several cancers of the head and neck (Vokes, Agrawal, & Seiwert, 2015). Quitting smoking and use of tobacco products is an essential part of preventing these cancers, and it is theorized that the new HPV vaccines may help decrease their incidence. It is important to address any new or growing lumps and bumps with your healthcare provider, particularly dentists.

Penis

Discharge: One of the first and most obvious signs of a sexually transmitted infection can be pain or discharge from the penis. These symptoms should always be brought to the attention of your health care provider. They may indicate infection with gonorrhea or chlamydia. It is important to remember that these infections can also be without symptoms. The discharge in chlamydia can be thin and clear or may be completely unnoticed. Routine screening in men who are at risk is recommended (Centers for Disease Control and Prevention, n.d.). Men who are having insertive anal sex without condoms are also at risk for urinary tract infections, which are considered rare in men and may be missed by some health care providers, but urethral exposure to colonic bacteria can increase this risk. Prostate infections can also manifest with some discharge from the urethra.

It is conversely important to know that not all burning of the urethra is by definition gonorrhea or chlamydia. The body changes the pH balance of the urethra to protect sperm during ejaculation and urination just before or after ejaculation can lead to some pain in the urethra. Also, medications can predispose to dryness of the urethra. And, swelling of the prostate can lead to the sensation that one needs to urinate (even if there is no significant amount of urine that comes out). Even trauma from aggressive insertive sex can lead to pain or irritation of the urethra that can take hours and sometimes even a day or two to resolve.

Lumps and Bumps: The most common sexually transmitted cause of lumps and bumps under the head or on the shaft of the penis are warts (generally caused by the human papillomavirus). Warts are generally notable for their rough, cauliflower-like texture and may present as a single bump or a cluster. If there are many, they may be near each other or scattered around. Occasionally, a hair follicle can get blocked and an infection can develop, called a folliculitis, which looks similar to a pimple. These are more common in men who trim and shave their genital area, as trimming or shaving flattens the head of the hair and can cause the hair to irritate the skin or even grow under the skin.

There are also many noninfectious causes of bumps on the penis. Around adolescence, some men develop a condition called "pearly papules of the penis," clusters of smooth, shiny papules or bumps that cluster under the corona or head of the penis. These bumps can cause distress in these men or their sex partners, who worry that they may be sexually transmitted, but they are in fact benign and harmless and not contagious. Similarly, toward the base of the penis, some men can develop blocked sebaceous glands and develop smooth white or yellow dots called Fordyce spots, which are also harmless and not contagious. Neither pearly papules nor Fordyce spots require treatment. In contrast, treatment can lead to scarring, disfigurement, and decreased sensation in the sensitive skin of the penis.

Ulcers: Ulcers on the penis are almost always from sexual transmission. Painful ulcers that can appear anywhere on the penis are generally caused by herpes. They can come once and disappear forever or remain and come out during times of stress. Herpes can be passed on by skin-to-skin contact, even when there is no outbreak in some cases but is more transmissable during an outbreak. Most people with herpes feel a tingling or burning sensation that precedes the sore or ulcer by one to three days. It is at this point that medication is most successful at shortening the course of the outbreak. Another rare infection that can lead to a single painful ulcer on the penis is an infection called chancroid, which is caused by the bacteria *Haemophilus ducreyi*. This infection requires antibiotics to heal.

Painless ulcers on the penis may develop from primary infection with syphilis. These sores will resolve on their own (without treatment) and may go unnoticed by some. Others may feel relieved that they "got better" and not bring them to medical attention until much later. Even if sores go away, it is important to speak to a provider about them because untreated syphilis can lead to heart and brain damage years later. Syphilis sores are very infectious by skin-to-skin contact. In men with HIV, primary syphilis may present with multiple primary ulcers. Other noninfectious causes of penile ulcers and sores include abrasions, chafing, and trauma from aggressive sex or even trauma from a zipper in men who do not wear underwear.

Another issue that many men struggle with is erectile dysfunction, defined as the inability to achieve or sustain an erection that is suitable for penetrative sexual intercourse. It is quite common for men to have fluctuations in the firmness of their erections or their libido, but erectile dysfunction is persistent. It is also very normal to have difficulty with erections when stressed or if one is not able to relax during sex—for example, in times of stress in a relationship. Worrying about erections can lead to some decrease in erectile function. Common medical reasons for persistent erectile dysfunction include diabetes, cardiovascular disease, obesity, smoking, and drug and alcohol abuse. Low testosterone is rarely a cause of erectile dysfunction but may lead to decreased libido. If erectile dysfunction is persistent and affecting the way one has sex, there are medications that may be helpful. In more difficult cases, a urologist may be helpful.

Anus and Rectum

Anal pain can be a cause for concern and anxiety. Often, these symptoms may come from issues as benign as hemorrhoids. Hemorrhoids are frequently associated with some itching and bright red blood tracking along the outside of a formed stool. In some cases, a few drops of blood can turn the water in the toilet bowl bright red. In more severe cases, gay and bisexual men can end up with fissures (cracks or tears in the skin around the anus) or sinus tracts (tunnels or holes) that run from the intestine to the anus. These can be more difficult to heal and involve seeing a specialist. Pain from these conditions tends to worsen after a bowel movement (or straining to have a bowel movement) and may involve some blood or mucus in the toilet with a BM.

Herpes of the anus or rectum follows a similar pattern to other herpes infections, beginning with an itch or a tingle around the anus and leading to a sharp or burning pain. Vesicles, or clear blisters, may form and quickly form ulcers. If pain is more internal, in the rectal area, sometimes felt as a pelvic or lower abdominal pain, this can indicate rectal gonorrhea or Chlamydia. Rectal gonorrhea and chlamydia sometimes also cause tenesmus (an urgency to make stool), even when little comes out. These infections may also produce pus or blood on or in stool. Unfortunately, rectal gonorrhea and chlamydia are most often without any symptoms at all, and people at risk should be screened as often as once every three to six months with a rectal swab by a health care provider. There are now strains of both gonorrhea and chlamydia that are harder than ever to treat, so in some but not all cases, providers may choose to do follow up testing to confirm an infection has been cured.

Some men may also develop prostatitis: inflammation of the prostate. This inflammation can be caused by an infection but can also be caused by inflammation from the mechanical rubbing or chafing of the prostate during various types of anal-receptive sex. Patients may feel a heaviness in their pelvis or even a burning or pressure when they try to urinate. It may take longer to initiate the urinary stream, or they may have a sensation of incomplete emptying of their bladder after urinating. This can be treated with anti-inflammatory medications like ibuprofen or even tamsulosin (Flomax, given for an enlarged prostate). If an infection is present or suspected, antibiotics may be given in addition. Treatment takes about three weeks.

Lumps or bumps around the anus can be a few different things. As mentioned previously, hemorrhoids are one benign reason for patients to have a lump or bump around the anus. Skin tags, extra pieces of skin formed either by chafing or from prior hemorrhoids, may lead to lumps or bumps. These can be surgically removed but are not dangerous, and if they are not causing symptoms, patients and providers may choose to not intervene on them.

Another possible cause of bumps around the anus relates to genital warts caused by the HPV virus. The serotypes of the virus that cause warts are different from the types known to predispose to anal cancer, but both can be disconcerting, and anal warts do imply that the HPV virus is present and may be contracted by sex partners who come into contact with it.

To date, there has been much discussion over the risk of anal cancer in men who have receptive anal sex. It is clear now from the literature that there is an increased risk of anal cancer in men who have receptive anal sex, especially in those who are HIV positive (Machalek et al., 2012). The question that health care providers are struggling with to date is how to manage this increased risk. The initial screening test is clear: an anal Pap test, which uses a cotton swab to take a sample of the highest-risk cells—the cells at the transition from skin to the lining of the colon. These cells, when combined with an infection like HPV, are most likely to lead to the development of cancer. However, the next step, high-resolution anoscopy, involves looking at the tissue in this area if an abnormal result is found, and possibly taking a biopsy. Here is where medicine is not entirely sure of what to do next. Too many biopsies in this area can lead to scarring, and too few might miss a cancer that could have been treated and possibly cured in its early stages. It seems likely that soon there will be a clear recommendation for providers to follow.

Many patients who are interested in having receptive anal sex have questions about the mechanics and safely of anal sex. Some wonder how to prevent feces from being present in the rectum when having sex. There are a wide range of opinions on this and unfortunately little data. Some men choose to simply hope that they are "clean" (clear of feces) by eating a high-fiber diet and timing sexual activity to their bowel movements. In a normal colon, feces are not always present but form in waves based on time since the last bowel movement. Other men choose a more active approach, using enemas from the pharmacy to douche and clean out their rectum of feces prior to having sex. These enemas contain some laxative elements (like phosphates) to help trigger contractions in the colon to evacuate what stool is there. Some use simple tap water to evacuate the contents. Others take anti-motility/antidiarrheal agents like loperamide to prevent the reaccumulation of feces over time. While this is not considered to be very dangerous, too frequent douching can strip the colon of some of its needed bacteria and cause inflammation or colitis, and even pain and rectal discharge.

As mentioned previously, there is some fear around the risk of fecal incontinence in men who have receptive anal sex. The vast majority of people who engage in receptive anal sex never have issues with incontinence. The external anal sphincter is a voluntary muscle and returns to its normal shape after anal sex. The internal anal sphincter, if torn or damaged during anal sex, may lead to issues with continence. Although this is rare, it does require the intervention of a specialist.

Testicles

The testicles are very sensitive in some people and less sensitive in others. Pain in the testicles may be from trauma incurred during sex or from abnormal twisting of the testicle (i.e., torsion). The testicle is connected to the epididymis or spermatic cord, which can also become painful if inflamed. This is often but not always caused by an infection with gonorrhea or chlamydia.

Lumps or bumps on the testicle itself may be concerning for testicular cancer. Testicular cancer is most common in men under the age of 25 and often presents as a painless bump on the surface of the testicle. These should not be confused with lumps or bumps on the spermatic cord. These may be common and not harmful, and include varicoceles and hydroceles. A varicocele is a protruding blood vessel that follows the spermatic cord and often feels wormlike (described in medical texts as a "bag of worms") (Practice Committee of the American Society for Reproductive Medicine, 2008). If painless, this does not require intervention. However, if varicoceles are painful, surgery may be performed. Hydroceles are fluid-filled sacs around the testes from an open pouch that should close during development, but because of either incomplete closure during development or surgical intervention, they may develop later in life. These hydroceles tend to feel more like enlarged, softer testicles, as the sac of fluid exists around the testicle itself.

Nipples

For some men, the nipples are a particularly erogenous zone. Some use the term "wired" to describe nipples that, when stimulated, lead these men to develop erections or instantly feel turned on and amorous. As a phenomenon, sensitive nipples seem more common in men as they age, although there is no data to support this. Some men engage in activities that make their nipples larger (piercing, or using "nipple clamps"). While there is no clear amount of nipple play that is dangerous, it should be noted that scarring may be irreversible (particularly after piercing), and caution should be taken with any partner in whom nipple play draws blood, as there are many infections that may transmitted through blood. Following aggressive nipple play, it is not uncommon to have bruising or pain of the nipples for several days.

Lumps in the nipples may be caused by gynecomastia, a condition in which female breast tissue develops in men from an excess of testosterone, which can lead the body to convert testosterone to estrogen. Gynecomastia can be quite painful, and its treatment, aside from surgery, can be unclear. It should also be noted that breast cancers can occur in men, although they are rare. Men who encounter a lump in their breast, particularly those who have family members with breast, colon, or ovarian cancer, should bring any lumps in their breast tissue to the attention of their health care provider.

Total Body Symptoms

Finally, there are some symptoms that affect more than just the genitals that can be transmitted through sex. Rashes over the chest or whole body should be evaluated for secondary syphilis or HIV by simple blood or finger-stick tests. Persistent gastrointestinal symptoms like diarrhea, bloating, or loose stools may come from a parasite contracted during oral-anal contact. Abdominal pain, diarrhea, and jaundice (yellowing of the skin) may indicate infection with hepatitis, and the CDC recommends that all gay and bisexual men should be vaccinated against hepatitis A and B (Workowski & Bolan, 2015).

CONCLUSION

Good health is not just the absence of medical problems but also a feeling of well-being that stems from engagement in relationships and behaviors that foster growth. When it comes to sex, gay men and other LGBTQ people can struggle with how to be healthy. Internalized homophobia and transphobia can lead gay men to undervalue themselves and their health, resulting in behaviors that increase risk of physical or mental health issues. Building community can help to alleviate some of this burden as can education about their bodies—both how to experience pleasure with them and how to keep them safe.

REFERENCES

Akintoye, S. O., & Greenberg, M. S. (2005). Recurrent aphthous stomatitis. *Dental Clinics, 49*(1), 31–47.

BarebackRT.com. (n.d.). Retrieved from https://www.barebackrt.com

Bauermeister, J. A., Leslie-Santana, M., Johns, M. M., Pingel, E., & Eisenberg, A. (2011). Mr. Right and Mr. Right Now: Romantic and casual partner-seeking online among young men who have sex with men. *AIDS and Behavior, 15*(2), 261–272.

The Bear Social Network. (n.d.). Retrieved from http://www.growlrapp.com

Blank, S., Brady, M., Buerk, E., Carlo, W., Diekema, D., Freedman, A., . . . Wegner, S. (2012). Circumcision policy statement. *Pediatrics, 130*(3), 585–586.

Bolding, G., Davis, M., Hart, G., Sherr, L., & Elford, J. (2007). Where young MSM meet their first sexual partner: The role of the Internet. *AIDS and Behavior, 11*(4), 522.

Buchacz, K., McFarland, W., Kellogg, T. A., Loeb, L., Holmberg, S. D., Dilley, J., & Klausner, J. D. (2005). Amphetamine use is associated with increased HIV incidence among men who have sex with men in San Francisco. *AIDS, 19*(13), 1423–1424.

Burrell, E. R., Pines, H. A., Robbie, E., Coleman, L., Murphy, R. D., Hess, K. L., . . . Gorbach, P. M. (2012). Use of the location-based social networking application GRINDR as a recruitment tool in rectal microbicide development research. *AIDS and Behavior, 16*(7), 1816–1820.

Centers for Disease Control and Prevention. (n.d.). Screening recommendations referenced in treatment guidelines and original recommendation sources. Retrieved from http://www.cdc.gov/std/tg2015/screening-recommendations.htm

Chen, Y. H., Vallabhaneni, S., Raymond, H. F., & McFarland, W. (2012). Predictors of serosorting and intention to serosort among men who have sex with men, San Francisco. *AIDS Education and Prevention, 24*(6), 564–573.

Cocores, J. A., Miller, N. S., Pottash, A. C., & Gold, M. S. (1988). Sexual dysfunction in abusers of cocaine and alcohol. *The American Journal of Drug and Alcohol Abuse, 14*(2), 169–173.

Cohen, M. S. (2011). Approach to the patient with a sexually transmitted disease. In L. Goldman & A. I. Schafer (Eds.), *Goldman's Cecil Medicine* (24th ed.): (1796–1800). Philadelphia: Saunders.

Crosby, R. A., Graham, C. A., Yarber, W. L., Sanders, S. A., Milhausen, R. R., & Mena, L. (2016). Measures of attitudes toward and communication about condom use: Their relationships with sexual risk behavior among young black MSM. *Sexually Transmitted Diseases, 43*(2), 94.

Dirks, H., Esser, S., Borgmann, R., Wolter, M., Fischer, E., Potthoff, A., . . . Scherbaum, N. (2012). Substance use and sexual risk behaviour among HIV–positive men who have sex with men in specialized out–patient clinics. *HIV Medicine, 13*(9), 533–540.

Dobry, Y., Rice, T., & Sher, L. (2013). Ecstasy use and serotonin syndrome: A neglected danger to adolescents and young adults prescribed selective serotonin reuptake inhibitors. *International Journal of Adolescent Medicine and Health, 25*(3), 193–199.

Docter, R. F., & Prince, V. (1997). Transvestism: A survey of 1032 cross-dressers. *Archives of Sexual Behavior, 26*(6), 589–605.

Du, P., Crook, T., Whitener, C., Albright, P., Greenawalt, D., & Zurlo, J. (2015). HIV transmission risk behaviors among people living with HIV/AIDS: The need to integrate HIV prevention interventions and public health strategies into HIV care. *Journal of Public Health Management and Practice, 21*(2), E1.

Farré, M., Abanades, S., Roset, P. N., Peiro, A. M., Torrens, M., O'Mathúna, B., . . . de la Torre, R. (2007). Pharmacological interaction between 3, 4-methylenedioxymethamphetamine (ecstasy) and paroxetine: Pharmacological effects and pharmacokinetics. *Journal of Pharmacology and Experimental Therapeutics, 323*(3), 954–962.

Golden, M. R., Dombrowski, J. C., Kerani, R. P., & Stekler, J. D. (2012). Failure of serosorting to protect African American men who have sex with men from HIV infection. *Sexually Transmitted Diseases, 39*(9), 659.

Goldstone, S. E. (1999). *The ins and outs of gay sex: A medical handbook for men.* New York: Dell.

Grant, R. M., Lama, J. R., Anderson, P. L., McMahan, V., Liu, A. Y., Vargas, L., . . . Montoya-Herrera, O. (2010). Preexposure chemoprophylaxis for HIV prevention in men who have sex with men. *New England Journal of Medicine, 363*(27), 2587–2599.

Grosskopf, N. A., LeVasseur, M. T., & Glaser, D. B. (2014). Use of the internet and mobile-based "apps" for sex-seeking among men who have sex with men in New York City. *American Journal of Men's Health, 8*(6), 510–520.

Grov, C., Parsons, J. T., & Bimbi, D. S. (2007). Sexual risk behavior and venues for meeting sex partners: An intercept survey of gay and bisexual men in LA and NYC. *AIDS and Behavior, 11*(6), 915–926.

Grov, C., Parsons, J. T., & Bimbi, D. S. (2010). The association between penis size and sexual health among men who have sex with men. *Archives of Sexual Behavior, 39*(3), 788–797.

Hatfield, L. A., Horvath, K. J., Jacoby, S. M., & Simon Rosser, B. R. (2009). Comparison of substance use and risky sexual behavior among a diverse sample of urban, HIV-positive men who have sex with men. *Journal of Addictive Diseases, 28*(3), 208–218.

Hayashi, Y., & Kohri, K. (2013). Circumcision related to urinary tract infections, sexually transmitted infections, human immunodeficiency virus infections, and penile and cervical cancer. *International Journal of Urology, 20*(8), 769–775.

Herbenick, D., Reece, M., Schick, V., & Sanders, S. A. (2014). Erect penile length and circumference dimensions of 1,661 sexually active men in the United States. *The Journal of Sexual Medicine, 11*(1), 93–101.

Hotton, A. L., Gratzer, B., & Mehta, S. D. (2012). Association between serosorting and bacterial sexually transmitted infection among HIV-negative men who have sex with men at an urban lesbian, gay, bisexual, and transgender health center. *Sexually Transmitted Diseases, 39*(12), 959–964.

Jena, A. B., Goldman, D. P., Kamdar, A., Lakdawalla, D. N., & Lu, Y. (2010). Sexually transmitted diseases among users of erectile dysfunction drugs. *Annals of Internal Medicine, 153*(1), 1–7.

Jorm, A. F., Korten, A. E., Rodgers, B., Jacomb, P. A., & Christensen, H. (2002). Sexual orientation and mental health: Results from a community survey of young and middle-aged adults. *The British Journal of Psychiatry, 180*(5), 423–427.

Kelvin, E. A., Mantell, J. E., Candelario, N., Hoffman, S., Exner, T. M., Stackhouse, W., & Stein, Z. A. (2011). Off-label use of the female condom for anal intercourse among men in New York City. *American Journal of Public Health, 101*(12), 2241–2244.

Liau, A., Millett, G., & Marks, G. (2006). Meta-analytic examination of online sex-seeking and sexual risk behavior among men who have sex with men. *Sexually Transmitted Diseases, 33*(9), 576–584.

Liechti, M. E., Baumann, C., Gamma, A., & Vollenweider, F. X. (2000). Acute psychological effects of 3,4-methylenedioxymethamphetamine (MDMA, "Ecstasy") are attenuated by the serotonin uptake inhibitor citalopram. *Neuropsychopharmacology, 22*(5), 513–521.

Lowe, G., & Costabile, R. (2011). Phosphodiesterase type 5 inhibitor abuse: A critical review. *Current Drug Abuse Reviews, 4*(2), 87–94.

Macaluso, M., Blackwell, R., Jamieson, D. J., Kulczycki, A., Chen, M. P., Akers, R., . . . Duerr, A. (2007). Efficacy of the male latex condom and of the female polyurethane condom as barriers to semen during intercourse: A randomized clinical trial. *American Journal of Epidemiology, 166*(1), 88–96.

Machalek, D. A., Poynten, M., Jin, F., Fairley, C. K., Farnsworth, A., Garland, S. M., . . . Templeton, D. J. (2012). Anal human papillomavirus infection and associated neoplastic lesions in men who have sex with men: A systematic review and meta-analysis. *The Lancet Oncology, 13*(5), 487–500.

Mansergh, G., Shouse, R. L., Marks, G., Guzman, R., Rader, M., Buchbinder, S., & Colfax, G. N. (2006). Methamphetamine and sildenafil (Viagra) use are linked to unprotected receptive and insertive anal sex, respectively, in a sample of men who have sex with men. *Sexually Transmitted Infections, 82*(2), 131–134.

Mantri, C. K., Mantri, J. V., Pandhare, J., & Dash, C. (2014). Methamphetamine inhibits HIV-1 replication in CD4+ t cells by modulating anti–HIV-1 miRNA expression. *The American Journal of Pathology, 184*(1), 92–100.

Molitor, F., Truax, S. R., Ruiz, J. D., & Sun, R. K. (1998). Association of methamphetamine use during sex with risky sexual behaviors and HIV infection among non-injection drug users. *Western Journal of Medicine, 168*(2), 93.

Morris, B. J., & Krieger, J. N. (2013). Does male circumcision affect sexual function, sensitivity, or satisfaction?—a systematic review. *The Journal of Sexual Medicine, 10*(11), 2644–2657.

MR X. (n.d.). Retrieved from http://www.mrxapp.com

Practice Committee of the American Society for Reproductive Medicine. (2008). Report on varicocele and infertility. *Fertility and Sterility, 90*(5), S247–S249.

Przybyla, S. M., Golin, C. E., Widman, L., Grodensky, C. A., Earp, J. A., & Suchindran, C. (2013). Serostatus disclosure to sexual partners among people living with HIV: Examining the roles of partner characteristics and stigma. *AIDS Care, 25*(5), 566–572.

Renzi, C., Tabet, S. R., Stucky, J. A., Eaton, N., Coletti, A. S., Surawicz, C. M., . . . Celum, C. L. (2003). Safety and acceptability of the RealityTM condom for anal sex among men who have sex with men. *AIDS, 17*(5), 727–731.

Richardson, B. A., Lavreys, L., Martin Jr, H. L., Stevens, C. E., Ngugi, E., Mandaliya, K., . . . Kreiss, J. K. (2001). Evaluation of a low-dose nonoxynol-9 gel for the prevention of sexually transmitted diseases: A randomized clinical trial. *Sexually Transmitted Diseases, 28*(7), 394–400.

Rodriguez, A., Castel, A. D., Parish, C. L., Willis, S., Feaster, D. J., Kharfen, M., . . . Metsch, L. R. (2013). HIV medical providers' perceptions of the use of antiretroviral therapy as non-occupational post-exposure prophylaxis (nPEP) in two major metropolitan areas. *Journal of Acquired Immune Deficiency Syndromes, 64*(1), S68–S79.

Rogers, G., Elston, J., Garside, R., Roome, C., Taylor, R. S., Younger, P., . . . Somerville, M. (2009). The harmful health effects of recreational ecstasy: A systematic review of observational evidence. *Health Technology Assessment, 13*(6), xii–338.

Saitz, R., Palfai, T. P., Cheng, D. M., Horton, N. J., Freedner, N., Dukes, K., . . . Samet, J. H. (2007). Brief intervention for medical inpatients with unhealthy alcohol use: A randomized, controlled trial. *Annals of Internal Medicine, 146*(3), 167–176.

Savage, D. (January 4, 2012). Meet the monogamish. Retrieved from http://www.thestranger.com/seattle/SavageLove?oid=11412386

Scorolli, C., Ghirlanda, S., Enquist, M., Zattoni, S., & Jannini, E. A. (2007). Relative prevalence of different fetishes. *International Journal of Impotence Research, 19*(4), 432–437.

Smith, D. K., Grohskopf, L. A., Black, R. J., Auerbach, J. D., Veronese, F., Struble, K. A., . . . Greenberg, A. E. (2005). Antiretroviral postexposure prophylaxis after sexual, injection-drug use, or other nonoccupational exposure to HIV in the United States: Recommendations from the US Department of Health and Human Services. *Morbidity and Mortality Weekly Report: Recommendations and Reports, 54*(2), 1–20.

Stone, N., Hatherall, B., Ingham, R., & McEachran, J. (2006). Oral sex and condom use among young people in the United Kingdom. *Perspectives on Sexual and Reproductive Health, 38*(1), 6–12.

Strathdee, S. A., Shoptaw, S., Dyer, T. P., Quan, V. M., Aramrattana, A., & Substance Use Scientific Committee of the HIV Prevention Trials Network. (2012). Towards combination HIV prevention for injection drug users: Addressing addictophobia, apathy and inattention. *Current Opinion in HIV and AIDS, 7*(4), 320.

Sussman, G. L., & Beezhold, D. H. (1995). Allergy to latex rubber. *Annals of Internal Medicine, 122*(1), 43–46.

Tancer, M., & Johanson, C. E. (2007). The effects of fluoxetine on the subjective and physiological effects of 3, 4-methylenedioxymethamphetamine (MDMA) in humans. *Psychopharmacology, 189*(4), 565–573.

van den Boom, W., Konings, R., Davidovich, U., Sandfort, T., Prins, M., & Stolte, I. G. (2014). Is serosorting effective in reducing the risk of HIV-infection among men who have sex with men with casual sex partners? *Journal of Acquired Immune Deficiency Syndromes, 65*(3), 375–379.

Van Howe, R. S. (2013). Sexually transmitted infections and male circumcision: A systematic review and meta-analysis. *ISRN Urology, 2013*, 1–42.

Varghese, B., Maher, J. E., Peterman, T. A., Branson, B. M., & Steketee, R. W. (2002). Reducing the risk of sexual HIV transmission: Quantifying the per-act risk for HIV on the basis of choice of partner, sex act, and condom use. *Sexually Transmitted Diseases, 29*(1), 38–43.

Voeller, B., Coulson, A. H., Bernstein, G. S., & Nakamura, R. M. (1989). Mineral oil lubricants cause rapid deterioration of latex condoms. *Contraception, 39*(1), 95–102.

Vokes, E. E., Agrawal, N., & Seiwert, T. Y. (2015). HPV-associated head and neck cancer. *Journal of the National Cancer Institute, 107*(12), djv344.

Wessells, H., Lue, T. F., & McAninch, J. W. (1996). Penile length in the flaccid and erect states: Guidelines for penile augmentation. *The Journal of Urology, 156*(3), 995–997.

Winks, C., & Semans, A. (2002). *The good vibrations guide to sex: The most complete sex manual ever written*. San Francisco: Cleis Press.

Workowski, K. A., & Bolan, G.A. (2015). Sexually transmitted diseases treatment guidelines, 2015. *Morbidity and Mortality Weekly Report, 64*(RR-03), 1–137.

World Health Organization. (2008). *Male circumcision: Global trends and determinants of prevalence, safety, and acceptability*. Geneva: World Health Organization/UNAIDS. Retrieved from http://apps.who.int/iris/bitstream/10665/43749/1/9789241596169_eng.pdf

Xu, F., Schillinger, J. A., Sternberg, M. R., Johnson, R. E., Lee, F. K., Nahmias, A. J., & Markowitz, L. E. (2002). Seroprevalence and coinfection with herpes simplex virus type 1 and type 2 in the United States, 1988–1994. *The Journal of Infectious Diseases, 185*(8), 1019–1024.

Zablotska, I. B., Imrie, J., Prestage, G., Crawford, J., Rawstorne, P., Grulich, A., . . . Kippax, S. (2009). Gay men's current practice of HIV seroconcordant unprotected anal intercourse: Serosorting or seroguessing? *AIDS Care, 21*(4), 501–510.

About the Editors and Contributors

EDITORS

JASON S. SCHNEIDER, MD, is an associate professor of medicine in the Division of General Medicine and Geriatrics at the Emory University School of Medicine. He works as a clinician educator at Grady Memorial Hospital in Atlanta, Georgia, where he provides direct care to general adult and transgender patients. Dr. Schneider has clinical interests in sexual health and sexuality; the interaction of psychiatry and general medicine; and primary care for lesbian, gay, bisexual, and transgender patients. He served on the board of directors of GLMA: Health Professionals Advancing LGBT Equality for over 13 years, serving two years as president.

LAURA ERICKSON-SCHROTH, MD, MA, is an assistant professor of psychiatry at Columbia University Medical Center and a consulting psychiatrist at Hetrick-Martin Institute, a nonprofit dedicated to empowerment, education, and advocacy for LGBTQ youth. She is the editor of *Trans Bodies, Trans Selves*, a resource guide written by and for transgender people, and coauthor of *"You're in the Wrong Bathroom!" and 20 Other Myths and Misconceptions about Transgender and Gender Nonconforming People*.

VINCENT M. B. SILENZIO, MD, MPH, is an associate professor of psychiatry, Public Health Sciences and Family Medicine, and director of the Laboratory of Informatics and Network Computational Studies (LINCS)/ Network Science Lab at the University of Rochester. He was a founding faculty member of the Columbia University Program in LGBT Health and served as coeditor of the *Journal of the Gay and Lesbian Medical Association*. His current research focuses on applications of machine learning and network analysis in suicide prevention research with LGBT adolescents and young adults and in studies of behavioral health and HIV prevention with gender and sexual minority communities in North America and around the globe.

CONTRIBUTORS

JONATHAN S. APPELBAUM, MD, FACP, AAHIVS, is the Laurie L. Dozier Jr., MD education director and professor of internal medicine and chair, Department of Clinical Sciences at Florida State University College of Medicine. His clinical and scholarly work focuses on the care of LGBT, HIV-infected, and older patients.

KELLAN E. BAKER, MPH, MA, is the centennial scholar in the Department of Health Policy and Management at the Johns Hopkins Bloomberg School of Public Health. Previously, he was a senior fellow at the Center for American Progress in Washington, DC, where he worked on LGBT health and data collection policy at the federal and state levels.

MARCI L. BOWERS, MD, is a pelvic and gynecologic surgeon specializing in the field of genital reassignment surgery and clitoral restoration after female genital mutilation (FGM). She established the first transgender surgical education program working with Mt. Sinai-Beth Israel in New York, is a member of the World Professional Association for Transgender Health (WPATH), and serves on the board of directors for both GLAAD and the Transgender Law Center.

RUSSELL G. BUHR, MD, is clinical instructor of medicine in the Division of Pulmonary and Critical Care at the David Geffen School of Medicine and a postdoctoral fellow in health services research in the Department of Health Policy and Management at the Fielding School of Public Health, both at the University of California, Los Angeles. Dr. Buhr primarily researches health care utilization patterns in lung disease and critical illness but maintains a special interest in health disparities that affect the LGBT community.

TAMAR C. CARMEL, MD, is a community psychiatrist and director of integrated care services at Metro Community Health Center in Pittsburgh, utilizing his combined training in psychiatry and family medicine to improve the health and well-being of underserved populations, including the LGBTQ+ community. Dr. T. Carmel has over a decade of experience providing training and education to medical/nursing students, residents/trainees, physicians, and other medical and mental health care providers on LGBTQ+ mental health.

MADELINE (MADDIE) B. DEUTSCH, MD, MPH, is an associate professor of family and community medicine and the director of UCSF Transgender Care at the University of California, San Francisco. She has cared for more than 1,500 transgender patients since 2006, has had several funded research studies in areas of transgender health, and more than 25 peer-reviewed publications on the topic.

TRI D. DO, MD, MPH, has been working in LGBTQ health since 1994 and served on the GLMA board from 1996 to 2006, including a term as board president. He is a medical director for HealthRight 360 (including Lyon-Martin Health Services). He is also a professor at the University of California, San Francisco, performing LGBTQ research.

MANUEL A. ESKILDSEN, MD, MPH, CMD, is a geriatrician and an associate clinical professor at the David Geffen School of Medicine at the University of California, Los Angeles. He is a clinician-educator with a practice dedicated to the care of elders recovering post hospitalization in skilled nursing facilities.

ROBERT GAROFALO, MD, MPH, is the division head of adolescent medicine at Ann & Robert H. Lurie Children's Hospital of Chicago. He is a professor of pediatrics at Northwestern University's Feinberg School of Medicine, editor in chief of the academic journal *Transgender Health*, and a former president of GLMA.

TRAVIS A. GAYLES, MD, PhD, is the chief of public health services and health officer for Montgomery County, Maryland. He is a clinically trained pediatrician focusing on adolescent and young adult medicine.

RICHARD E. GREENE, MD, is an associate professor of medicine at NYU School of Medicine, where he serves as the director of health disparities education and is an associate program director in the Primary Care Internal Medicine Residency Program. He is also the medical director of the Center for Health, Identity, Behavior and Prevention Studies (CHIBPS) at NYU's College of Global Public Health.

DAVID HANKINS, MD, MEd, is a resident in psychiatry at New York Presbyterian-Weill Cornell Medicine.

DAWN HARBATKIN, MD, is the medical director of the San Mateo Medication Assisted Treatment Program at HealthRIGHT 360, providing care to patients with alcohol- and opiate-use disorders. She has worked in LGBT health for the past 20 years, serving as the medical director of

Lyon-Martin Health Services for 12 years and as the medical director of Callen-Lorde Community Health Center for 5 years.

ALEXIS (LEXI) D. LIGHT, MD, MPH, is currently finishing her obstetrics and gynecology residency training in the Mid-Atlantic region. She received her MD and MPH from Tulane University in New Orleans. She has spent a lot of time thinking about, researching, and teaching on issues of sexuality and LGBT health. Most recently, she has coauthored multiple peer-reviewed articles on transgender reproductive health.

MEGAN C. LYTLE, PhD, is an assistant professor of psychiatry at the University of Rochester Medical Center. Dr. Lytle's clinical and research expertise is in multiculturalism, with a particular focus on the health and suicide disparities among lesbian, gay, bisexual, transgender, queer, and questioning (LGBTQQ) individuals. Her current research integrates computational methods with traditional approaches to investigate the unique experiences among diverse trans communities.

DAVID J. MALEBRANCHE, MD, MPH, is an associate professor of medicine at Morehouse School of Medicine in Atlanta, Georgia, and serves as the medical director of the Student & Employee Health and Wellness Center. He has extensive experience in the clinical prevention and treatment of HIV and STIs, men's health, correctional health, student health, LGBT health, sexual health, and the exploration of racial health inequities through qualitative research.

LARON E. NELSON, PhD, RN, FNP, FNAP, FAAN, is assistant professor of nursing and dean's endowed fellow in health disparities at the University of Rochester. He is also a scientist and the OHTN research chair in HIV Program Science with African, Caribbean, and Black Communities in the Centre for Urban Health Solutions of the Li Ka Shing Knowledge Institute at St. Michael's Hospital. Dr. Nelson's domestic and international research investigates strategies to reduce race- and sexuality-based disparities in HIV outcomes.

TONIA POTEAT, PhD, PA-C, is an assistant professor of social medicine at University of North Carolina-Chapel Hill as well as core faculty in the UNC Center for Health Equity Research. Her research, teaching, and practice focus on LGBT Health, particularly HIV/STI prevention among key populations.

ASA RADIX, MD, MPH, is the senior director of research and education at the Callen-Lorde Community Health Center in New York City and a clinical associate professor of medicine at New York University. Current research interests involve studying the impact of stigma on access to health services as well as innovations to improve clinician education on LGBT issues.

RANDALL SELL, ScD, is a professor of public health at Drexel University's Dornsife School of Public Health, where he is the director of the Program for Lesbian, Gay, Bisexual and Transgender (LGBT) Health and director of the online certificate in LGBT Health. His 30-year research career has focused on the development and testing of research methods to study sexual and gender minorities.

MARK J. SIMONE, MD, AGSF, is an assistant professor of medicine at Harvard Medical School and geriatrician at Mount Auburn Hospital in Cambridge, Massachusetts, where he is the associate program director for the Mount Auburn Internal Medicine Residency Program and director of the Primary Care Pathway. As a clinician and educator, Dr. Simone focuses on the needs of older LGBT adults.

W. CHRISTOPHER SKIDMORE, PhD, is an assistant professor in the Department of Psychiatry at Boston University School of Medicine and a psychologist in the National Center for Posttraumatic Stress Disorder Women's Health Sciences Division at VA Boston Healthcare System. He received his PhD in clinical psychology from Northwestern University.

DAVID O. STAATS, MD, is a retired academic geriatrician. He founded the Special Interest Group on Issues of Older LGBT Persons for the American Geriatrics Society.

HECTOR VARGAS, JD, is executive director of GLMA: Health Professionals Advancing LGBT Equality, a multidisciplinary membership organization of LGBT health professionals and their allies whose mission is to ensure equality in health care for lesbian, gay, bisexual, and transgender (LGBT) individuals and health care professionals. GLMA (formerly known as the Gay and Lesbian Medical Association) is a leading voice on LGBT health and employs the expertise of its health professional members in policy, advocacy, and education to advance the health and well-being of the LGBT community.

Index

Page numbers followed by *t* indicate tables and *f* indicate figures.

Abortion, 23, 28, 45–46

Abzug, Bella, 3

Advance care planning, 174–175

Affordable Care Act, 18–25, 75, 205; access to health coverage and care, 22–25; availability of insurance coverage, 20–22; constitutionality of, 21; disparities data collection, 19–20; essential health benefits, 23; health insurance marketplaces, 20, 22–25; LGBT nondiscrimination, 23–25; Medicaid expansion, 20–21; outreach to LGBT communities, 27; qualified health plans (QHPs), 22; required coverage for sex-specific preventive health services for transgender persons, 84; resources on ACA and LGBT populations, 19

AIDS Coalition to Unleash Power (ACT UP), 5

Alcohol use: and differential epidemiology, 76; and LGBT adolescents, 141; and men's sexual health, 277–278, 285; in Native American two-spirited population, 41; and sex, 209, 242, 274; and sexual kinks, 242, 274; and sexual orientation identity, 74; and sleep quality, 220; and STI transmission risk, 209, 242; and women's sexual health, 250–251

Alcoholism and alcohol abuse: in adolescents, 134; binge drinking, 41, 212; and erectile dysfunction, 285; health disparities, 41, 52, 53, 74, 141, 143, 172; and intersectionality, 52, 53; and LGBT adolescents, 141, 142, 143, 149*t*; and mental health, 93; and MSM population, 209, 212–213; and resilience, 52; and transgender populations, 93

American Academy of Pediatrics (AAP), 140, 247, 268

American Association of Physicians for Human Rights, 4. *See also* GLMA: Health Professionals Advancing LGBT Equality

American Geriatrics Society, 175

American Nurses Association, 4

American Psychiatric Association, 2, 94, 157–158. *See also Diagnostic and Statistical Manual of Mental Disorders* (DSM)

American Psychological Association, 140, 193

American Public Health Association (APHA), 4, 69, 206

Anal cancer, 73*t*, 165–166, 216, 257, 279, 286

Antidepressants, 249, 251, 252, 280

Antiretroviral therapy (ART), 170–172

Anxiety: in LGBT adolescents, 142, 146–147; in LGBT elders, 166, 167, 171; and LGBT parents, 187, 190, 191; and preventive care of MSM, 219–220; in trans population, 86, 92, 93, 95

Armesto, Jorge C., 187–188

Austin, S. Bryn, 141

Bailey, Michael, 230

Baldwin, Tammy, 18

Basson, Rosemary, 236

Beeler, Jeff, 187

Bergman, Kim, 189

Biber, Stanley, 112, 113, 119

Binge drinking, 41, 212

Black feminism, 29n5, 45

Blood pressure medication, 101, 252, 280–281

Body dysmorphic disorder, 75

Body image: of cisgender women, 98; and lesbian subcultures, 237–238; and LGBT public health, 74; during menopause, 248, 249; of MSM, 219–220; and preventive health, 219–220; and sexual health for women, 237–238; and sexual responsiveness, 248

Bondage and discipline or sadism and masochism (BDSM), 240, 241–243, 273–274

Bos, Henny, 190

Boxer, Andrew, 140

Brain, 231–232

Braveman, Paula, 12

Breast cancer: advocacy, 7–8; and alcohol use, 250; disparities in lesbian and bisexual women, 9, 164; and hormone replacement therapy, 89, 249; mastectomies for, 76, 233; in men, 217, 288; and progestagens, 102–103; and trans women, 89

Breastfeeding, 232, 247–248

Breasts; and medical care for trans population, 89–90; and women's sexual health, 232–233, 257

Brill, Stephanie, 136–139

Bullying: anti-bullying policy, 150; and children of transgender individuals, 191; and LGBT adolescents, 134, 139, 140, 142–143, 150, 151; and transgender mental health, 91, 92

Burou, Georges, 112, 113, 119

Bush, George W., 9

Cancer: and access to health insurance, 22; and alcohol use, 250; anal cancer, 73*t*, 165–166, 216, 257, 279, 286; cervical cancer, 87, 163, 164, 243; colon cancer, 86, 166, 217, 258, 272, 288; endometrial cancer, 73*t*, 88, 97, 102, 108, 166; and health disparities, 75, 76–77, 164, 205; and hormone replacement therapy, 249; and human papillomavirus (HPV), 165, 215, 216, 243, 254, 257, 283, 286; and hyperplasia (precancerous uterine overgrowth), 88; Kaposi's sarcoma, 73*t*; and LGBT elders, 163–166, 168–169; and LGBT health research, 14, 73*t*; and hepatitis B virus, 213; and hepatitis C virus, 215; lung cancer, 73*t*, 166; ovarian cancer, 73*t*, 88, 108, 217, 258, 288; penile cancer, 216, 268; as preexisting condition, 22; and preventive health in MSM, 205, 211, 213, 215, 216–217; and preventive health in trans populations, 87–91, 102, 108, 168–169; prostate cancer, 88–89, 91, 102–103, 166, 217–218; and sexual health for men, 268, 279, 283, 286–288; and sexual health for women, 243, 249–250, 254, 257–258; skin cancer, 217; testicular cancer, 169, 216–217, 287; and tobacco use, 211, 283. *See also* Breast cancer

Cardiovascular disease: and alcohol use, 172, 212, 250; disparate rates for MSM, 205, 218; and erectile dysfunction, 285; and gender, 218; and gender-affirming hormones, 166, 168; and human aging, 7, 218; in lesbian and bisexual women, 163, 172; and LGBT elders, 163–164, 166, 168, 172; and obesity, 164, 168; prevention of, 218–219; risk reduction and screening for MSM, 218–219; risk factors for, 163, 164, 168, 172, 212; and tobacco use, 168, 172; and women's health, 250

Cass identity model, 135

Center for American Progress (CAP), 195–196

Centers for Medicare and Medicaid Services (CMS), 17. See also Medicaid; Medicare

Centers for Disease Control and Prevention (CDC): and ACT UP, 5; Advisory Council on Immunization Practices guidelines, 213–216; Behavioral Risk Factor Surveillance System questionnaires, 15; chlamydia and gonorrhea screening recommendations, 255, 282, 283; hepatitis A and B vaccination recommendations, 288; HIV in older adults statistics, 170; HIV testing recommendations, 165; intimate partner violence statistics, 238; LGBT adolescent statistics, 134–135, 142–144; Office of Women's Health, 8; PrEP recommendations, 208; screening recommendations, 165, 208, 209, 255, 282, 283; Youth Risk Behavior Survey (YRBS), 15, 140–141

Cervical cancer, 87, 163, 164, 243

Cervix, 232, 235, 255; screening, 17, 87

Children of bisexual men and bisexual women, 190–191

Children of gay men, 188–189

Children of lesbian women, 189–190

Children of transgender individuals, 191–192

Chivers, Meredith L., 230

Chlamydia, 143–144, 165, 167, 207, 209–210, 243–244, 253–255, 257, 274, 277, 283, 285, 287

Choe, Ken, 26

Cisgender, definition of, 85t

Civil rights movement, 3, 51

Clitoris, 233–235

Club drugs, 250–251

Coker, Tumaini Rucker, 141

Colon cancer, 86, 166, 217, 258, 272, 288

Coming out: and culture, 46, 48, 49, 50; and homelessness, 145; and intersectionality, 46, 48, 49, 50; and LGBT adolescents, 134, 136, 145; and LGBT elders, 156, 158–159, 160, 167; and LGBT parents, 186–187, 190, 192–193; and stigma, 187; and transgender medical care, 95

Compton's Cafeteria riot, 3

Congressional Tri-Caucus, 18, 29n6

Contraceptives, 75, 99–100, 111, 163, 253

Crenshaw, Kimberlé, 11, 29n5, 45

Cross-dressing, 3, 274

Cultural competence in health care settings, 16, 18, 26–27, 40, 43, 52–53, 147, 160, 175–176, 205–206, 218–219

Culturally and Linguistically Appropriate Services (CLAS) Standards, 27

Culture: acculturation, 10; "bear" culture, 266; and categories of sexual orientation, 63; and female sexuality, 229–238; gay male culture, 266–269; gender nonconformity and cultural norms, 85t; influence on LGBT families, 186–189, 192–193, 195–196; and intersectionality, 40–53; lesbian and bisexual subcultures, 231, 237–238; LGBT characters in pop culture, 134;

and safety of transgender persons, 112; and "transgender" as a term, 63–64. *See also* Religion and spirituality

Dahlberg, Etienne G., 70
Danish Girl, The (film), 112
Data collection about LGBT population health, 13–17; administrative data, 16–17; medical records, 17; research, 13–14; survey data, 14–16
D'Augelli, Anthony R., 142
Defense of Marriage Act, 174, 194–195
Department of Health, Education, and Welfare (DHEW), 28n2; *Healthy People: The Surgeon General's Report on Health Promotion and Disease Prevention* (1979), 6–7
Department of Health and Human Services (HHS), 2, 13, 25–27; Agency for Healthcare Research and Quality, 28–29n3; and ACT UP, 5; administrative data, 16–17; and Affordable Care Act, 19–20, 22, 23; Centers for Independent Living, 17; and disparities data collection in the ACA, 19–20; and disparities paradigm, 6–7; *Healthy People 2000* (1990), 7–8, 12; *Healthy People 2010* (2000), 12, 69; *Healthy People 2020* (2010), 12; *HHS Action Plan to Reduce Racial and Ethnic Health Disparities*, 26; *HHS Strategic Plan on Addressing Health Disparities Related to Sexual Orientation*, 9; and legislative approaches to LGBT health, 18; LGBT Coordinating Committee, 25–27; LGBT Data Progression Plan, 15, 20; National Survey of Drug Use and Health, 15; nondiscrimination regulations, 23, 25–26; under Obama administration, 25–26; Office for Civil Rights (OCR), 23–25, 27–28; Office of LGBT Health, 9, 18; Office

of Minority Health, 7, 15, 17, 18; Office of the National Coordinator for Health Information Technology (ONC), 17; Office of Women's Health, 8; under Reagan administration, 10; on standards for collection of sex data, 66–67; survey data, 14, 15, 16, 66–67; Task Force on Black and Minority Health, 7; Task Force on Minority Health report (1985), 10; Task Force on Women's Health Issues, 7; under Trump administration, 27–28
Depression, 14, 17, 41, 75, 86, 92, 101, 102, 172, 187, 219; antidepressants, 249, 251, 252, 280; in LGBT adolescents, 141, 142, 146–147; in LGBT elders, 157, 162; and men's sexual health, 280; and preventive health in MSM, 219; and women's sexual health, 248, 251, 252
Diagnostic and Statistical Manual of Mental Disorders (DSM): DSM-I, 2; DSM-II, 94; DSM-III, 94; DSM-5, 94; DSM-V, 28n1, 136; gender dysphoria diagnosis, 3, 28n1, 94; gender identity disorder diagnosis, 28n1, 94, 136; homosexuality as sociopathic personality disturbance diagnosis, 2; homosexuality diagnosis removed from, 3–4, 68, 157–158; trans-related mental health diagnoses, 3, 28n1, 94, 136; transsexualism diagnosis, 94
DiProva, Vicky, 187
Disparities paradigm in LGBT health, 6–9
Djordjevic, Miroslav, 112
Dobinson, Cheryl, 190, 191
"Don't ask, don't tell" policy, 77–78, 134
Dopamine, 231
Down-low phenomenon, 47
Downing, Jordan B., 191–192

Eads, Robert, 88
Eating disorders, 41, 73, 75, 145, 219

Elbe, Lili, 112, 119
Ending LGBT Health Disparities Act
    (ELHDA), 18
Endometrial cancer, 73t, 88, 97, 102,
    108, 166
Epstein, Steven, 6, 8
Erectile dysfunction, 165–166, 278,
    284–285; medication, 279, 280,
    281–282
Erickson, Reed, 4
Erickson Educational Foundation, 4
Erogenous zones, 125, 232, 233,
    266–267, 287

Facial hair removal, 111
Family Equality Council (FEC),
    195–196
Farmer, Paul, 10–11
Federal LGBT health policy 2009–
    2016, 13–27; Affordable Care Act,
    18–25; cultural competency and
    outlook, 27–28; data collection
    about LGBT health, 13–17;
    legislative approaches to LGBT
    health, 18; nondiscrimination
    regulations, 26; reports and
    strategies, 18, 23–25, 26; staffing
    and administration, 26
Federal LGBT health policy after 2016,
    27–28; appointments of anti-LGBT
    officials, 27–28; data collection
    about LGBT health, 27; Tax Cuts
    and Jobs Act (Public Law No.
    115–97), 28
Federal Poverty Level (FPL), 20–21,
    29n7
Female genital mutilation (FGM),
    234–235
Feminism, 229, 231; black feminism,
    29n5, 45
Feminizing hormone regimens,
    98–103; basic hormone physiology,
    96–98; effects of masculinizing and
    feminizing regimens, 99t; estrogen
    therapy, 98–101; long-term
    considerations, 107–108;

progestagens, 102–103; testosterone
    blocking (anti-androgen) therapy,
    101–102
Fertility, 28, 88, 111, 115, 245–247, 255
Food and Drug Administration: and
    ACT UP, 5; and bioidentical
    hormone therapy, 106; and
    cyproterone acetate, 102; and facial
    hair reduction methods, 111; female
    condoms not approved for anal sex,
    275; and HIV transmission
    prevention, 144–145; label route for
    estrogen and testosterone injections,
    108; off-label medication use, 96;
    and pre-exposure prophylaxis
    (PrEP), 144–145; research on Saran
    Wrap as barrier protection, 276; and
    transition-related medical care, 96,
    102, 106, 108
Franciscan Alliance, Inc. v. Burwell, 23
Freud, Sigmund, 237
Fundamental cause model of health
    disparities, 72

G-spot, 115, 120, 235, 237
Gamble, Vanessa, 6, 7
Gay, Lesbian and Straight Education
    Network (GLSEN), 142–143
Gay and Lesbian Medical Association.
    See GLMA: Health Professionals
    Advancing LGBT Equality
Gay Dads Study, 188
Gender-affirmation care. See
    Transgender medical care
    in the U.S.
Gender dysphoria diagnosis, 3,
    28n1, 94
Gender-confirmation surgery and
    care. See Transgender medical
    care in the U.S.
Gender identity, definition of, 85t
Gender identity disorder diagnosis,
    28n1, 94, 136
Gender nonconformity, definition of,
    85t
Genderqueer, definition of, 85t

Giles, Katie, 236
Giovanni, Nikki, 39, 53
Gittings, Barbara, 3
GLMA: Health Professionals
   Advancing LGBT Equality, 4, 161,
   204, 206, 214
Goldberg, Abbie E., 187
Golombok, Susan, 189–190
Gonorrhea: and LGBT adolescents,
   143–144; and LGBT elders, 165, 167;
   and men's sexual health, 271, 274,
   276–277, 282–283, 285, 287; and
   preventive health for MSM, 207,
   209–210; and women's sexual
   health, 243–244, 253–255, 257
Gräfenberg, Ernst, 235
Green, Robert-Jay, 189
Green, Ronald, 4
Greenlee, Kathy, 26
Grijalva, Raúl, 18

Hall, Peter, 5
Harkin, Tom, 20
Hate crimes, 40, 47–48, 171, 194
Hatzenbuehler, Mark, 72
Health disparities: conceptual
   approaches to, 70–74; disparities
   paradigm of LGBT health policy,
   6–9; and health differences, 7; in
   LGBT adolescents, 134–135,
   140–141, 144; in LGBT elders, 156,
   159, 161–162, 170, 175–176; and
   LGBT health policy, 13–14, 18–20,
   26, 28; and LGBT parents and
   families, 194–195; and LGBT public
   health, 62, 69, 70–76, 78; mental
   health disparities in trans
   population, 92–93; and minority
   stress, 94, 157; and MSM, 204–206;
   and politics of LGBT health, 5–20,
   26, 28; and race and culture, 40–42,
   46–48, 51, 53; suicide, 40, 41, 75, 92,
   161
Health Equity and Accountability Act
   (HEAA), 18
Health equity, 10–13, 18

Health of Lesbian, Gay, Bisexual, and
   Transgender People: Building a
   Foundation for Better
   Understanding, 13–14
Health in All Policies paradigm, 6,
   9–13
Health Resources and Services
   Administration (HRSA), 9, 16–17
Healthy People: The Surgeon General's
   Report on Health Promotion and
   Disease Prevention (1979), 6–7
Healthy People 2000 (1990), 7–8, 12
Healthy People 2010 (2000), 12, 69
Healthy People 2020 (2010), 12
Heart disease. See Cardiovascular
   disease
Heckler, Margaret, 7
Hepatitis, 68, 234; hepatitis A virus
   (HAV), 207, 213, 243, 244, 272, 288;
   hepatitis B virus (HBV), 165, 166,
   209, 213–214, 244, 251, 258, 288;
   hepatitis C virus (HCV), 166,
   214–215, 244, 251, 273; and LGBT
   elders, 165, 166, 169; and substance
   use, 279; symptoms of, 258, 288; and
   transgender population, 169
Herdt, Gilbert, 140
HHS. See Department of Health and
   Human Services
HHS Action Plan to Reduce Racial and
   Ethnic Health Disparities, 26
HHS Strategic Plan on Addressing
   Health Disparities Related to Sexual
   Orientation (2001), 9
HIV/AIDS: and the Affordable Care
   Act, 22–23; and conceptualizing
   LGBT health, 39, 40–42, 46–48,
   51–52; and culture/race, 40–42, 43,
   46–48; and human rights, 5; and
   LGBT adolescents, 143–146; and
   LGBT elders, 158, 164, 165, 169–172;
   and LGBT public health, 62, 68–69,
   74, 75–76; and Medicaid, 21;
   medicalization of, 46; and Medicare,
   17; and men's sexual health, 258,
   268, 271–279, 281–282, 284, 286,

288; and politics of LGBT health, 5, 7–11, 17, 21, 22–23, 28; and preventive health for MSM, 204–210, 213–216, 218; and transgender population, 17, 169; and women's sexual health, 234, 242, 243–244, 251, 258

Homelessness, 76; and LGBT adolescents, 144, 145–146; and outing transgender persons, 86; and suicide, 145–146; Runaway and Homeless Youth Act, 27; and trans and gender-nonconforming persons, 92

Homophobia: homophobic control as psychological abuse, 239; interactions with race and culture, 42–44, 49; internalized, 72, 140, 288; and LGBT youth, 133–135, 140, 142, 144, 146; and LGBT elderly, 218–220; and preventive health, 218–220; and sexual health, 288; structural homophobia, 204, 219, 220

Homosexuality as sociopathic personality disturbance diagnosis, 2

Homosexuality diagnosis removed from, 3–4, 68, 157–158

Hooker, Evelyn, 68

Hormone therapy: basic hormone physiology, 96–98; bioidentical hormones, 105–107; effects of masculinizing and feminizing regimens, 99t; estrogen therapy, 98–101; feminizing regimens, 98–103; genderqueer and other gender nonconforming/nonbinary persons, 107; hormone blood levels, 105; long-term considerations, 107–108; masculinizing regimens, 103–107; medication administration, 108–109; progestagens, 102–103; testosterone blocking (anti-androgen) therapy, 101–102

Human papillomavirus (HPV): and cancer, 165, 166, 215, 216, 243, 254,

257; and LGBT elders, 165; and men's sexual health, 274–275, 279, 283, 286; and preventive care for MSM, 207, 210, 215, 216; and transgender medical care, 87–88; vaccine, 88; and women's sexual health, 243, 254, 256, 257

Human Rights Campaign Fund (later Human Rights Campaign), 3, 139, 159, 186

Immigration and immigrants: and health disparities, 11; and health insurance, 20; and hepatitis B screening, 214; and intersectionality, 45, 48

In vitro fertilization (IVF), 246

Indian Health Service, 27

Intersectionality, 11, 13; as promising paradigm for LGBT health, 45–52; queer intersectionality, 44; and resiliency, 47, 51–52

Institute of Medicine (IOM), 13, 84, 134

Institutionalization, forced, 3

Institutionalized discrimination, 91, 93, 158, 173, 174

Intimate partner violence, 172, 211, 238–239

Intrauterine insemination (IUI), 246

Jakes, T. D., 49

Johns Hopkins University, 4, 113, 119

Johnson, Cathryn, 135

Johnson, Virginia E., 236

Kameny, Frank, 3

Katz, Jonathan Ned, 69

Kaufman, Joanne M., 135

Kinks, 241–243, 272–274

Kinsey, Alfred C., 231–232

Koch, Ed, 3

Koh, Howard, 25–26

Komisaruk, Barry R., 232

Krieger, Nancy, 29n4

Krug, Linda L., 70

Lactation induction, 247–248

Langbehn, Janice, 25

Latty, Elizabeth, 230

Laub, Donald, 119

Lawrence v. Texas, 2

Lease, Suzanne H., 192

Lesbian and bisexual women: breast cancer disparities, 9, 164; cardiovascular disease, 163, 172; children of lesbian women, 189–190; health care needs for older lesbian and bisexual women, 163–164; lesbian subcultures, 231, 237–238. *See also* Sexual health for women

Lesbian Health: Current Assessment and Directions for the Future (Institute of Medicine), 8

LGBT adolescents, 134–135; alcohol use and abuse, 141, 142, 143, 149*t*, anti-bullying policy for, 150; definition of adolescent, 134; demographics, 140; developmental states of gender and sexual identity minorities, 136–139*t*; eating disorders and weight management, 145; health issues and concerns, 141–147; historical perspectives, 135–141; homelessness, 145–146; and homophobia, 133–135, 140, 142, 144, 146; mental illness, 146–147; policy issues, 150–151; population of, 135; and provider relationship, 147–149; sexual health and STIs, 143–145; sample questions for adolescent patient interview, 148–149*t*; smoking, 143; and stigma, 135, 140–141; and suicide, 141–143, 145–147; transgender identity policy, 150–151; and violence and bullying, 142–143

LGBT Data Inclusion Act, 18

LGBT elders, 155–156; advance care planning, 174–175; challenges for, 158–162; concealment versus "coming out," 158–159; demographics and socioeconomic status, 156–157; future policy issues and new resources for, 175; health care needs for older gay and bisexual men, 164–167; health care needs for older lesbian and bisexual women, 163–164; health care needs for older transgender women and men, 167–168; health disparities, 161–162; HIV in older adults, 169–171; housing, home care, and long-term care, 159–160; medical decision making and visitation, 173; mental health and exposure to violence, 171–173; minority stress, sexual stigma, and prejudice, 157–158; policy issues affecting, 173–175; provider-related barriers to care, 160–161; Services and Advocacy for GLBT Elders (SAGE), 156, 175; social support and family structure, 159; specific care needs for, 162–173; and stigma, 155–158, 159, 161–164, 169, 171; unequal treatment under laws, programs, and services, 173

LGBT health activism: early history of, 2–5; health professional coalitions, 4; and HIV/AIDS epidemic, 5; homosexuality removed from DSM, 3–4; "outsider" and "insider" activism, 5; national advocacy organizations, 3; Stonewall riots, 3, 50, 157–158

LGBT older adults. *See* LGBT elders

LGBT parents: children of bisexual men and bisexual women, 190–191; children of gay men, 188–189; children of lesbian women, 189–190; children of transgender individuals, 191–192; and family relationships, 186–187; influence of culture on LGBT families, 192–193; parent-child bonds, 187–192; policies that impact LGBT families, 193–194; practical recommendations, 194–196; and stigma regarding health care decisions for children, 193, 195, 196

LGBT public health and epidemiology: conceptual approaches to health and health disparities, 70–74; definition of public health, 61; framework for LGBT health research, 72, 73*t*; and fundamental cause model of public health, 72; future challenges of, 78; and health concern differences, 76–78; and health disparities, 74–76; history of, 67–70; and pathways model of public health, 72; populations served by, 61–62; reasons for, 62; and social construction of sexual orientation and gender, 62–67; and social ecological model of health, 70–72

Link, Bruce, 72

Lorde, Audre, 8

Machismo, 48

Marriage equality, 22, 25, 40, 173–174, 193–194; *Obergefell v. Hodges*, 22, 173, 194, 205

Masculinizing hormone regimens, 103–107; bioidentical hormones, 105–107; effects of masculinizing and feminizing regimens, 99*t*; hormone blood levels, 105; long-term considerations, 107–108

Masters, William H., 236

McCabe, Marita, 236

McClintock, Karen, 190

McHugh, Paul, 113

McLeroy, Kenneth R., 70

Medicaid: and Affordable Care Act, 19, 20–21, 23, 25; creation of, 19; and disparities in provisions for LGBT families, 195; establishment of LGBT-inclusive nondiscrimination policies for, 18, 25; and HIV treatment, 21; means testing for, 21; and transgender-related care, 25, 84, 114

Medical records, 17, 68, 75, 86; electronic health records (EHRs), 17; Meaningful Use of Electronic Health Records (2009), 17

Medicare: and Affordable Care Act, 19, 23; creation of, 19; establishment of LGBT-inclusive nondiscrimination policies for, 18, 25; and transgender-related care, 17, 84, 114

Meltzer, Toby, 112

Menopause, 248–249; breasts during, 257; in cisgender women, 91, 98, 107, 109; clitoris during, 234; and hormone therapy, 99, 249; libido, 249; symptom management, 248–249; symptoms, 248

Mental health: discrimination in healthcare settings, 93–94; gender dysphoria as diagnosis, 3, 28n1, 94; and LGBT adolescents, 146–147; mental health as preventive health in trans community, 91–92; mental health disparities in trans community, 92–93; question of trans diagnoses, 94–95; and resilience, 93; society's effect on transgender mental health, 91; and stigma, 91, 93, 171, 218–219, 280; and WPATH's Standards of Care, 95–96, 112, 115–117, 127. *See also* Anxiety; Depression; *Diagnostic and Statistical Manual of Mental Disorders*

Meyer, Jon, 113

Microaggressions, 48, 91–92

Movement Advancement Project (MAP), 195–196

MSM, 40, 43, 48, 53, 144–145. *See* Preventive health for gay, bisexual, and queer men; Sexual health for men

Multiple minority statuses, 93, 195

Murray, Paul D., 190

Murray, Pauli, 3, 200

National Academy of Medicine, 1, 13–14

National Coverage Determination (NCD), 84

National Gay Health Coalition (NGHC), 4

National Gay Health Education
  Foundation (later National Lesbian
  and Gay Health Association), 4
National Gay Task Force (later
  National LGBTQ Task Force), 3
*National Healthcare Disparities
  Report, Women's Health USA, the
  Health Disparities and Inequalities
  Report* (HHS), 26
National Institute for Minority Health
  and Health Disparities (NIMHD), 14
National Institutes of Health (NIH):
  and ACT UP, 5; and disparities
  paradigm, 6–9, 14; first solicitation
  for LGBT research proposals, 9; and
  IOM report, 13–14, 141; and LGBT
  public health recognition, 62; LGBT
  Research Coordinating Committee,
  14; NIH Revitalization Act (1993),
  8, 28–29n3; Office of Minority
  Health and Research, 7; Office of
  Research on Women's Health, 8;
  percentage of funded studies
  concerning LGBT population, 13;
  sexual and gender minorities
  (SGM) used by, 2n; Sexual and
  Gender Minority Research Office,
  14; transgender-related research
  funding, 84; and 21st Century
  Cures Act (2016), 18
National Lesbian and Gay Health
  Association, 4
National March on Washington for
  Lesbian and Gay Rights, 4
National Resource Center on LGBT
  Aging, 27, 175
Nonbinary, definition of, 85t

Obama, Barack, federal LGBT health
  policy under, 18–25; data collection,
  13–17; HHS policies, 25–27; hospital
  visitation rights for LGBT families,
  174, 195; legislation, 18–25. *See also*
  Affordable Care Act
Obamacare. *See* Affordable Care Act
Obergefell v. Hodges, 22, 173, 194, 205

Osteoporosis, 88, 91, 104, 107, 108,
  164, 168, 170
Ovarian cancer, 73t, 88, 108, 217, 258,
  288
Ovaries, 87, 88, 91, 97–99, 104, 106,
  108, 217, 248, 258, 288
Oxytocin, 231, 233

Padrón, Elena, 189
Parents and parenting. *See* LGBT
  parents
Pathways model of health disparities,
  72
Patient Protection and Affordable Care
  Act of 2010. *See* Affordable Care Act
Patterson, Charlotte J., 188–189
Penile cancer, 216, 268
Pepper, Rachel, 136–139
Perovic, Sava, 112
Phelan, Jo, 72
Pilkington, Neil, 142
Pituitary gland, 88, 90, 97–99, 100,
  102–103
Politics of LGBT health: disparities
  paradigm, 6–9; early LGBT health
  activity, 2–5; federal LGBT health
  policy 2009–2016, 13–27; federal
  LGBT health policy after 2016,
  27–28; Health in All Policies
  paradigm, 6, 9–13; policy
  paradigms, 5–13
Pond, Lisa, 25
Poverty: Federal Poverty Level (FPL),
  20–21, 29n7; and hepatitis, 169; and
  HIV health disparities, 144; and
  LGBT families of color, 195; and
  transgender older adults, 167
Pregnancy, 21, 41, 75, 102, 111, 115,
  134, 234, 245–247
Preventive health for gay, bisexual, and
  queer men: alcohol and substance
  use, 212–213; bacterial meningitis,
  215; body image, 219–220; cancer,
  205, 211, 213, 215, 216–217;
  cardiovascular risk detection and
  screening, 218–219; hepatitis A

virus (HAV), 213; hepatitis B virus (HBV), 213–214; hepatitis C virus (HCV), 214–215; and homophobia, 218–220; influenza, 216; papillomavirus (HPV), 215; infection prevention and vaccination, 213–216; injury prevention and violence, 210–211; mental health, 219–220; screening and preventing STIs and HIV, 206–210; special needs and risks, 204–206; tobacco use, 211–212

Preventive health in trans populations, 86–91, 167

Pro-choice movement, 45–46

Prostate, 268, 269, 272: cancer, 88–89, 91, 102–103, 166, 217–218; enlargement, 165, 283; exams; 165–166, 169, 217; infections, 269, 283; inflammation, 285–286; and transgender population, 88–89, 91, 101, 110, 120

Race and culture: biases in LGBT health, 50–51; color" as descriptive term," 50; cultural competency, 16, 18, 27, 40, 43, 52–53, 176; health research and intervention agenda, 51l; intersectionality, 45–53; racialized stigma, 48; religion and spirituality, 42–45; resiliency approach to LGBT health, 51–52; role of in LGBT health, 40; and social identities, 45–53

Reagan, Ronald, 10, 204

Rehabilitation Act, 23

Reiger, Gerulf, 230

Religion and spirituality: and bullying (Title IX and Title IV protections), 150; Christianity, 44–45, 49, 193; definition of religion, 43; definition of spirituality, 43; and female genital mutilation, 234; Hinduism, 193; homophobia, 42–44, 49; influence of on LGBT families, 192–193; and intersectionality, 43–53; Islam, 43–44, 49, 53, 193; Judaism, 193; and LGBT health, 42–45, 47, 48–53; and objections by health care providers to specific services, 28; and race/culture, 42–53; and resiliency, 42–45; Santeria, 44; spiritual and religious identities, 43. See also culture

Reparative therapy, 3, 140

Reproductive rights, 45–46

Rivera, Sylvia, 3

Ross, Lori E., 190, 191

Roux, Diez, 72

Rubio, Ritchie J., 189

Runaway and Homeless Youth Act, 27

Rustin, Bayard, 3

Schrang, Eugene, 112

Schuster, Mark, 141

Sebelius, Kathleen, 19, 25

Self-esteem, 42, 47, 48, 134, 140, 142, 157, 189, 191, 193

Self-efficacy, 48

Sell, Randall L., 72, 73t

Services and Advocacy for GLBT Elders (SAGE), 156, 175

Severino, Roger, 27–28

Sex reassignment surgery. See Gender-confirmation surgery and care

Sexual health for men: anus and rectum symptoms, 285–287; cancer, 268, 279, 283, 286–288; community, attraction, and sexual roles, 265–266; finding partners, 269–270; monogamy and nonmonogamy, 270; mouth and throat symptoms, 282–283; nipple symptoms, 287–288; penis symptoms, 283–285; prevention of sexually transmitted infection transmission, 274–277; sexual anatomy and physiology, 266–269; sexual practices, 271–274; substance use and sex, 277–282; symptom-based approach to sexual health concerns, 281–282; testicle symptoms, 287

Sexual health for women: anus, 236, 256–257; anus and rectum symptoms, 256–257; attraction and stimuli, 229–231; BDSM/kink/water sports, 241–243; bladder and urinary tract symptoms, 254; body image, 237–238; brain, 231–232; breast symptoms, 257–258; breasts, 232; cancer, 243, 249–250, 254, 257–258; clitoris, 233–235; erogenous zones, 233; external genital stimulation, 240; finding partners, 238; intimate partner violence, 238–239; menopause, 248–249; mouth and throat symptoms, 253–254; oral sex, 240–241; orgasm, 236–237; penetration, 241; pregnancy, 245–247; prevention of sexually transmitting infection transmission, 243–245; sex toys, 241; sexual anatomy and physiology, 231–238; sexual practices, 239–243; sexual response, 236; substance use and sex, 250–253; symptom-based approach to sexual health concerns, 253–258; vagina, 235; vulva, vagina, and cervix symptoms, 255–256

Sexual identity development, 135–141; developmental stages of gender and sexual identity minorities, 136–139t

Sexually transmitted infections (STIs): chlamydia, 143–144, 165, 167, 207, 209–210, 243–244, 253–255, 257, 274, 277, 283, 285, 287; gonorrhea, 143–144, 165, 167, 207, 209–210, 243–244, 253–255, 257, 271, 274, 276–277, 282–283, 285, 287; and LGBT adolescents, 143–144; and LGBT elders, 164–167, 169, 172; and men's sexual health, 274–277, 282–288; and preventive care for MSM, 206–210; syphilis, 143–144, 165, 207, 209–210, 243–244, 254, 256, 258, 271, 275, 276–277,

283–284, 288; and women's sexual health, 243–244, 253–255, 257. See also HIV/AIDS

Sherfey, Mary Jane, 237

Shulman, Julie L., 192

Silence = Death Project, 5

Silenzio, Vincent M., 72, 73t

Sleep hygiene, 220

Smoking. See Tobacco use

Social determinants of health, 10–11

Social ecological model of health, 70f, 70–72

Social identities, 45–53. See also Race and culture

Stigma, 77–78; and children of bisexual parents, 190–191; and children of transgender parents, 192; and decision to come out, 187; and health care decisions of LGBT parents, 193, 195, 196; and HIV status, 276; language of, 94–95; and LGBT adolescents, 135, 140–141; and LGBT elders, 155–158, 159, 161–164, 169, 171; and LGBT parents, 187, 190–191, 193, 195, 196; and mental health, 91, 93, 171, 218–219, 280; and multiple minority statuses, 93, 195; and sexual or physical violence, 211; and transgender medical care, 91, 93, 94–95

Stone, Deborah, 6, 7

Stonewall riots, 3, 50, 157–158

Structural homophobia, 204, 219, 220. See also Homophobia

Structural violence, 10–11

Suicidal ideation, 40, 92, 93, 137, 142, 146

Suicide and suicide attempts: and adolescent mortality, 134; and bullying, 142; and health disparities, 40, 41, 75, 92, 161; and homeless LGBT youth, 145–146; and LGBT adolescents, 141–143, 145–147; and LGBT health research, 73f; and minority stress and prejudice, 157;

and trans community, 92, 143; and transgender youth, 143

Supreme Court cases: *Lawrence v. Texas* (unconstitutionality of anti-sodomy laws), 2; *National Federation of Independent Business v. Sebelius* (constitutionality of ACA), 21; *Obergefell v. Hodges* (legalization of same-sex marriage), 22, 173, 194, 205; *United States v. Windsor* (unconstitutionality of DOMA), 194

Surgeon General, U.S., 4; *Healthy People: The Surgeon General's Report on Health Promotion and Disease Prevention* (1979), 6–7

Syndemics, 47

Syphilis, 143–144, 165, 207, 209–210, 243–244, 254, 256, 258, 271, 275, 276–277, 283–284, 288

Tasker, Fiona, 189–190

Testicular cancer, 169, 216–217, 287

Title IV, 150

Title IX, 23, 150

Tobacco use: and breast cancer, 89; electronic cigarettes, 212; and gender-confirmation surgery, 116; and health disparities, 10, 40–41, 75; and LGBT adolescents, 141, 142, 143, 146, 148, 149; and LGBT elders, 163, 164, 166, 168, 172; and LGBT public health, 71; and men's sexual health, 283, 285; and MSM population, 211–212; and sexual identity, 74; and women's sexual health, 254

Tornello, Samantha L., 188–189

Trans-related mental health diagnoses, 3, 28n1, 94, 136

Transfeminine spectrum surgery options, 116–122; body contouring, 118; breast augmentation, 117–118; feminization surgery (FFS), 116–117; genital surgery, 118–119; liposuction, 118; labiaplasty, 122;

nongenital surgery, 116–118; orchiectomy, 119–120; scrotectomy, 119; vaginoplasty, 119–122; vocal cord surgery, 118

Transgender, definition of, 85*t*

Transgender medical care in the U.S.: and Affordable Care Act, 84; choice to undergo gender-confirmation surgery, 113–114; effects of masculinizing and feminizing regimens, 99t; facial hair removal, 111; feminizing hormonal regimens, 98–103; gender-confirmation surgery and WPATH Standards of Care, 115–116; gender-confirmation surgery for gender-nonconforming individuals, 126–127; compared with other nations, 83; history of, 83; history of transgender surgery, 112–113; hormonal care, 96–109; insurance coverage for, 84; masculinizing hormonal regimens, 103–105; mental health as preventive health, 91–96; nonsurgical transition-related treatments, 111–112; originating in universities, 83; preoperative requirements, 116; preventive care, 86–91; and safety, 85–86; sexual health, 109–111; speech modification, 111–112; and stigma, 91, 93, 94–95; surgical aftercare, 126; trans-competent and affirming health care environments, 85–86; transfeminine spectrum surgery options, 116–122; and transgender terminology, 85*t*; transition-related medical care, 96–109, 111–112; transmasculine spectrum surgery options, 122–126; WPATH Standards of Care, 95–96, 112, 115–117, 127

Transition, definition of, 85*t*

Transmasculine spectrum surgery options, 122–126; Adam's apple augmentation, 123;

chest surgery, 122–123; classical meta (CM), 124; facial masculinization surgery, 123; free flap phalloplasty, 125; genital surgeries, 123–126; glansplasty, 125; metoidioplasty, 115, 123, 124, 127; monsplasty, 125–126; nongenital surgeries, 122–123; pectoplasty, 123; phalloplasty, 113, 115, 123–125; ring meta, 124; scrotoplasty, 124, 125; simple meta, 124; simple phalloplasty, 125; vaginectomy, 115, 124, 125

Transsexual, definition of, 85*t*

Transsexualism diagnosis, 94

Trump, Donald, federal LGBT health policy under, 16–17, 27–28

Tuskegee syphilis experiments, 68

21st Century Cures Act (2016), 18

University of California at San Francisco (UCSF) Transhealth Protocols, 86

Uterus, 87–88, 97, 105, 108, 235, 245, 246

Varnum v. Brien, 193

Violence: against trans patients, 86; and alcohol, 250; and intersectionality approach, 45, 47; intimate partner violence, 75, 172, 211, 238–239; against LGBT elders, 162, 167, 169, 171–173; and LGBT youth, 134, 141–143; and mental health in trans population, 91, 92; and minority stress, 157; and preventive health for MSM, 210–211; and public health, 75, 76; and social ecological model of health, 70; and stigma, 211; structural violence, 10–11. *See also* Bullying

Virchow, Rudolf, 1

White House Conferences on Aging, 175

Whitehead, Margaret, 7

Wilchins, Riki Anne, 142

Women's rights movement, 3, 29n5

Women's sexual health. *See* Sexual health for women

Women's studies, 45

World Health Organization (WHO): accident and trauma statistics by gender, 210; and American health policy, 1; circumcision statistics, 268; definition of "Health in All Policies," 11–12; enjoyment of health as fundamental right, 4; female genital mutilation statistics, 234

World Professional Association for Transgender Health (WPATH), 95–96, 112, 115–117, 127

Yip, Andrew K. T., 49–50